Contemporary Approach to Lower Extremity Reconstruction

Editor

LEE L.Q. PU

CLINICS IN PLASTIC SURGERY

www.plasticsurgery.theclinics.com

April 2021 • Volume 48 • Number 2

ELSEVIER

1600 John F. Kennedy Boulevard • Suite 1800 • Philadelphia, Pennsylvania, 19103-2899

http://www.theclinics.com

CLINICS IN PLASTIC SURGERY Volume 48, Number 2
April 2021 ISSN 0094-1298, ISBN-13: 978-0-323-79438-1

Editor: Stacy Eastman
Developmental Editor: Nicole Congleton

Clinics in Plastic Surgery (ISSN 0094-1298) is published quarterly by Elsevier Inc., 360 Park Avenue South, New York, NY 10010-1710. Months of issue are January, April, July, and October. Business and Editorial Offices: 1600 John F. Kennedy Blvd., Suite 1800, Philadelphia, PA 19103-2899. Periodicals postage paid at New York, NY and additional mailing offices. Subscription prices are $543.00 per year for US individuals, $1210.00 per year for US institutions, $100.00 per year for US students and residents, $607.00 per year for Canadian individuals, $1252.00 per year for Canadian institutions, $675.00 per year for international individuals, $1252.00 per year for international institutions, $100.00 per year for Canadian and $305.00 per year for international students/residents. To receive student/resident rate, orders must be accompanied by name of affiliated institution, date of term, and the *signature* of program/residency coordinator on institution letterhead. Orders will be billed at individual rate until proof of status is received. Foreign air speed delivery is included in all *Clinics* subscription prices. All prices are subject to change without notice. **POSTMASTER:** Send address changes to *Clinics in Plastic Surgery*, Elsevier Health Sciences Division, Subscription Customer Service, 3251 Riverport Lane, Maryland Heights, MO 63043. **Customer Service: 1-800-654-2452 (US and Canada). From outside of the United States and Canada, call 314-447-8871. Fax: 314-447-8029. E-mail: JournalsCustomerService-usa@elsevier.com (for print support); JournalsOnline-Support-usa@elsevier.com (for online support).**

Reprints. For copies of 100 or more of articles in this publication, please contact the Commercial Reprints Department, Elsevier Inc., 360 Park Avenue South, New York, New York 10010-1710. Tel.: +1-212-633-3874; Fax: +1-212-633-3820; E-mail: reprints@elsevier.com.

Clinics in Plastic Surgery is covered in *Current Contents, EMBASE/Excerpta Medica, Science Citation Index, MEDLINE/PubMed (Index Medicus), ASCA, and ISI/BIOMED.*

Contributors

EDITOR

LEE L.Q. PU, MD, PhD, FACS, FICS
Professor of Surgery, Division of Plastic
Surgery, Department of Surgery, University of
California Davis Medical Center, Sacramento,
California, USA

AUTHORS

CHRISTOPHER E. ATTINGER, MD
Professor, Department of Plastic Surgery,
MedStar Georgetown University Hospital,
Washington, DC, USA

JENNA C. BEKENY, BA
Research Fellow, Department of Plastic
Surgery, MedStar Georgetown University
Hospital, Washington, DC, USA

JORDAN T. BLOUGH, MD
Division of Plastic Surgery, Baylor Scott &
White Health, Scott & White Memorial Hospital,
Temple, Texas, USA

KAREN K. EVANS, MD
Associate Professor, Department of Plastic
Surgery, MedStar Georgetown University
Hospital, Washington, DC, USA

KENNETH L. FAN, MD
Assistant Professor, Department of Plastic
Surgery, MedStar Georgetown University
Hospital, Washington, DC, USA

ANDREAS GOHRITZ, MD
Department of Plastic, Reconstructive,
Aesthetic and Hand Surgery, University
Hospital Basel, Basel, Switzerland

ARIN K. GREENE, MD
Department of Plastic and Oral Surgery,
Boston Children's Hospital, Harvard
Medical School, Boston, Massachusetts,
USA

ALEXANDER HAUMER, MD, PhD
Department of Plastic, Reconstructive,
Aesthetic and Hand Surgery,
University Hospital Basel, Basel,
Switzerland

JOON PIO HONG, MD, PhD, MMM
Professor, Department of Plastic Surgery, Asan
Medical Center, University of Ulsan, Songpa-
Gu, Seoul, Korea

YUN-HUAN HSIEH, MBBS, MS (PRS)
Plastic and Reconstructive Surgery
Registrar, Head and Neck Clinical Institute,
Epworth Eastern Hospital, Box Hill, Victoria,
Australia

CHUNG-CHEN HSU, MD
Associate Professor, Department of Plastic
and Reconstructive Surgery, Linkou Medical
Center, Chang Gung Memorial Hospital, Chang
Gung University, Gueishan, Taoyuan, Taiwan,
ROC

SENG-FENG JENG, MD, FACS
Department of Plastic and Reconstructive
Surgery, E-Da Hospital, Kaohsiung City,
Taiwan, ROC

Z-HYE LEE, MD
Department of Plastic Surgery, The University
of Texas MD Anderson Cancer Center,
Houston, Texas, USA

L. SCOTT LEVIN, MD, FACS
Paul B. Magnuson Professor, Chairman,
Department of Orthopedic Surgery, Professor
of Surgery (Plastic Surgery), University of
Pennsylvania, Philadelphia, Pennsylvania, USA

JAMIE P. LEVINE, MD
Associate Professor, Hansjörg Wyss
Department of Plastic Surgery, NYU Langone
Health, New York, New York, USA

CHENG-HUNG LIN, MD, FACS
Professor of Plastic and Reconstructive
Surgery, Department of Plastic and
Reconstructive Surgery, Chang Gung
Memorial Hospital, Chang Gung Medical
College and Chang Gung University, Taoyuan,
Taiwan, ROC

CHIH-HUNG LIN, MD
Professor and Deputy Superintendent,
Department of Plastic and Reconstructive,
Surgery, Linkou Chang Gung Memorial
Hospital, Taoyuan, Taiwan, ROC

**CHARLES YUEN YUNG LOH, MBBS, MS,
MSc, MRCS**
Plastic Surgery Registrar, Addenbrooke's
Hospital, Cambridge, United Kingdom

IAN MCCULLOCH, MD, MRes
The Massachusetts General Hospital and
Harvard Medical School, Boston,
Massachusetts, USA

HEATHER A. MCMAHON, MD
Resident, Department of Plastic and
Maxillofacial Surgery, UVA Health,
Charlottesville, Virginia, USA

RIK OSINGA, MD
Department of Plastic, Reconstructive,
Aesthetic and Hand Surgery, University
Hospital Basel, Centre for Musculoskeletal
Infections, University Hospital Basel, Basel,
Switzerland

CHANGSIK JOHN PAK, MD, PhD
Assistant Professor, Department of Plastic
Surgery, Asan Medical Center, University of
Ulsan, Songpagu, Seoul, Korea

MARIOS PAPADAKIS, MD, PhD, MBA
Department of Plastic and Reconstructive
Surgery, E-Da Hospital, Kaohsiung City,
Taiwan, ROC

RAJIV P. PARIKH, MD, MPHS
Fellow, Microsurgery and Oncological
Reconstruction, Plastic and Reconstructive
Surgical Service, Center for Advanced
Reconstruction, Memorial Sloan Kettering
Cancer Center, New York, New York,
USA

LEE L.Q. PU, MD, PhD, FACS, FICS
Professor of Surgery, Division of Plastic
Surgery, Department of Surgery, University of
California Davis Medical Center, Sacramento,
California, USA

JUSTIN M. SACKS, MD, MBA
Chief, Division of Plastic and
Reconstructive Surgery, Sydney M. Jr. and
Robert H. Shoenberg Chair, Department of
Surgery, Washington University School of
Medicine in St. Louis, St Louis, Missouri,
USA

MICHEL H. SAINT-CYR, MD, FRCSC
Division of Plastic Surgery, Baylor Scott &
White Health, Texas, USA

DIRK JOHANNES SCHAEFER, MD
Department of Plastic, Reconstructive,
Aesthetic and Hand Surgery, University
Hospital Basel, Centre for Musculoskeletal
Infections, University Hospital Basel, Basel,
Switzerland

HSIANG-SHUN SHIH, MD
Department of Plastic and Reconstructive
Surgery, E-Da Hospital, Kaohsiung City,
Taiwan, ROC

PING SONG, MD
Resident Surgeon, Division of Plastic
Surgery, Department of Surgery, University of
California, Davis Medical Center, University of
California, Davis, Sacramento, California,
USA

JOHN S. STEINBERG, DPM
Associate Professor, Department of Plastic
Surgery, MedStar Georgetown University
Hospital, Washington, DC, USA

ZVI STEINBERGER, MD
Staff Physician, Department of Hand and
Microsurgery, Sheba Medical Center, Tel
Hashomer, Israel

JOHN T. STRANIX, MD
Assistant Professor, Department of Plastic and
Maxillofacial Surgery, UVA Health,
Charlottesville, Virginia, USA

CHRISTOPHER L. SUDDUTH, MD
Department of Plastic and Oral Surgery,
Boston Children's Hospital, Harvard Medical
School, Boston, Massachusetts, USA

HYUNSUK PETER SUH, MD, PhD
Assistant Professor, Department of Plastic
Surgery, Asan Medical Center, University of
Ulsan, Songpagu, Seoul, Korea

AMIR H. TAGHINIA, MD
Department of Plastic and Oral Surgery,
Boston Children's Hospital, Harvard Medical
School, Boston, Massachusetts, USA

PAUL J. THERATTIL, MD
Plastic Surgeon, Department of Plastic and
Reconstructive Surgery, Hackensack

University Medical Center, Hackensack, New
Jersey, USA

IAN VALERIO, MD, MS, MBA, FACS
The Uniformed Services University of the
Health Sciences, Bethesda, Maryland,
USA; Captain, Medical Corps, US Navy
Active Reserve Component, Division of
Plastic and Reconstructive Surgery,
Massachusetts General Hospital, Harvard
Medical School, Boston, Massachusetts,
USA

FU-CHAN WEI, MD, FACS
Distinguished Chair Professor, Department of
Plastic and Reconstructive Surgery, Linkou
Medical Center, Chang Gung Memorial
Hospital, Chang Gung University, Gueishan,
Taoyuan, Taiwan, ROC

MATTHEW R. ZEIDERMAN, MD
Resident Surgeon, Division of Plastic
Surgery, Department of Surgery, University of
California, Davis Medical Center, University of
California, Davis, Sacramento, California,
USA

ELIZABETH G. ZOLPER, BS
Research Fellow, Department of Plastic
Surgery, MedStar Georgetown University
Hospital, Washington, DC, USA

Contents

> Locoregional flaps play an important role in soft tissue reconstruction of the lower extremity and should be considered an effective option in soft tissue reconstruction. The medial hemisoleus muscle flap and the distally based sural artery flap can be elevated because of unique vascular anatomy and more advanced surgical techniques in flap dissection. Each flap can replace free tissue transfer as the first choice for soft tissue reconstruction of a less extensive wound in the distal third of the leg. Patient selection and detailed knowledge of the flap and its advanced technique for flap dissection are keys to success.

> Propeller flaps represent an outstanding alternative to conventional pedicled and free flap options in lower extremity reconstruction, offering significant advantages over the latter. An understanding of the perforasome concept, hot and cold perforator locations, and basic flap design enable the surgeon to readily harvest flaps based on any clinically relevant perforator in freestyle fashion. The purpose of this article is to review fundamentals of propeller flap design and harvest in the lower extremity and discuss reconstructive strategies by level of injury.

> The perforator-plus flap is a new concept for lower extremity reconstruction. It combines a perforator flap with a traditional skin rotation flap. It can be another option for lower extremity soft tissue defects since the flap has an augmented blood supply. The ability to detect cutaneous perforators has improved with the Duplex scan imaging technique. These advances have made the perforator-plus flap a viable option for soft tissue reconstruction. It can be versatile and reduces donor site morbidity; it is technically simple to perform and faster than traditional free flaps. It achieves durable soft tissue coverage for lower extremity wounds.

> The freestyle local perforator flap is an advanced version of the conventional island pedicle flap. Intramuscular dissection can provide a longer pedicle, which allows restoration of defects that are future from the donor site. Without microsurgery, the flap can be either rotated or advanced toward the defect, making it particularly useful for reconstructing soft tissue defects in the lower third of the leg. Careful preoperative design with vessel mapping, skillful intramuscular dissection of the

pedicle, and a well-considered backup plan in case of unexpected difficulty are crucial for freestyle local perforator flaps to be successful.

Free tissue transfer to the lower extremity for limb salvage remains challenging. A comprehensive approach includes patient selection, flap selection, selection of the recipient vessels, flap dissection, flap preparation, microvascular anastomosis, flap inset, immediate postoperative care, intermediate postoperative care, and further follow-up care. Each step in this comprehensive approach has its unique considerations and should be executed equally to ensure an optimal outcome. Once acquired, some clinical experience along with adequate microsurgical skill, good surgical judgment, well instructed and step-by-step intraoperative execution, and a protocol-driven practice, successful free tissue transfer to the lower extremity can be accomplished.

Improved knowledge of vascular anatomy has enabled surgeons to preoperatively identify perforators and design free-style flaps based on that perforator. Options for choosing the optimal donor site tissues are increased with the free-style technique. This reduces donor site morbidity while providing the same reconstructive success as traditional free skin flaps. The free-style technique allows the surgeon to successfully complete reconstruction when aberrant anatomy is encountered. With the necessary skills in perforator flap dissection and supermicrosurgery, the armamentarium of the reconstructive microsurgeon has been expanded with the introduction of free-style perforator free flaps.

The superficial circumflex iliac artery perforator flap is evolved from the groin flap, which was one of the early free flaps with a good concealed donor site. By further understanding the anatomy of perforators and elevating the flap based on it, this will provide added advantage of being a thin flap, harvesting as a composite flap, and help estimate the limit of skin paddle dimension. Despite these advantages, the relatively short pedicle still remains a challenge where long pedicle flaps are needed. One should select the flaps based on the recipient defect condition along with surgeons' experience, knowledge, and preference.

The anterolateral thigh (ALT) flap is a popular flap for lower extremity reconstruction despite its varied pedicle anatomy. Beyond its use for soft tissue coverage, using the chimeric flap concept, the ALT flap is useful for tendon and ligament reconstruction and the creation of a gliding surface with the fascia lata component. The vastus lateralis muscle can be included for dead-space obliteration. The main pedicle is long and is a similar size match for major artery reconstruction. If several perforators are available, a split flap could be fashioned into a multitude of shapes all arising from the same pedicle.

Medial sural artery perforator (MSAP) flap is a thin, pliable, and versatile flap. It is a fasciocutaneous flap with chimeric design capacity. The donor site permits the synchronous harvesting of nonvascularized tendons and nerves. Free MSAP flap is suitable for foot, ankle, and distal one-third of the leg reconstructions. Pedicled MSAP flap is an alternative flap for knee and proximal two-thirds of leg defects, covering classical lower limb reconstruction territories of soleus, medial, and lateral gastrocnemius muscle flap. Computed tomography angiography, indocyanine green, and endoscopic-assist dissection enhances MSAP flap surgical planning and reduces its technical adversities and complications.

Marko Godina in his landmark paper in 1986 established the principle of early flap coverage for reconstruction of traumatic lower extremity injuries to minimize edema, fibrosis, and infection while optimizing outcomes. However, with the evolution of microsurgery and wound management, there is emerging evidence that timing of reconstruction is not as critical as once believed. Multidisciplinary care with a combined orthopedic and reconstructive approach is more critical for timely and appropriate definite treatment for severe lower extremity injuries.

Gustilo IIIC injuries of the lower extremity pose a significant challenge to the reconstructive surgeon. Key principles include early vascular repair and serial debridement followed by definitive coverage within 10 days. Primary reconstructive options following vascular repair include the anterolateral thigh flap or the latissimus dorsi muscle flap. Complications include elevated rates of microvascular thrombosis requiring return to the operating room, partial and complete flap loss, and infection. There is also an elevated rate of secondary amputation. However, in spite of higher complication rates, when approached thoughtfully and with an experienced multidisciplinary team, patients can achieve reasonable functional outcomes.

In order to address complex extremity injuries, the orthoplastic approach uses plastic, orthopedic, and microsurgical techniques and includes other disciplines to optimize limb salvage. This collaboration, if created early in treatment, allows for more expedient and individualized solutions to a variety of extremity injuries resulting in decreased hospital stay, fewer complications, and improved functional outcomes. The orthoplastic approach does not merely avoid amputation, but also improves patient function and quality of life in the short and long term.

> Daily walking stance benefits the health, whereas lower extremity reconstruction aims to accomplish balanced walking and posture control. If local flap or tendon transfer cannot provide the basic function, microsurgical reconstruction is indicated for bony, soft tissue, and sensation restoration. Wound repair can use every modality and can achieve varying wound coverage results. However, all reconstruction should have functional goals using either local flap or free flap to restore the lost function. With less recipient site secondary damage, microsurgery can provide healthy composite tissue with like-replaces-like approach to create more stable long-term results.

> Supermicrosurgery is defined as microsurgery working on vessels less than 0.8 mm, allowing applications in smaller-dimension microsurgery, such as lymphedema, minimal invasive reconstruction, small parts replantation, and application of perforator as recipient. To accommodate this technique, developments and use of finer instruments, smaller sutures, new diagnostic tools, and higher-magnification microscopes have been made. Although supermicrosurgery has evolved naturally from microsurgery, it has developed into a unique field based on different thinking and tools to solve problems that once were difficult to solve.

> Surgical resection with wide margins and perioperative radiation therapy is the standard treatment of extremity soft tissue sarcomas. This combination often results in complex wounds and functional compromise. Reconstructive surgery is integral to limb salvage after sarcoma resection. Advances in adjuvant therapy and reconstructive surgical techniques have made functional limb salvage, instead of amputation, possible for most patients. This article reviews key concepts in the multidisciplinary care of patients with extremity soft tissue sarcomas and details reconstructive surgical techniques, including locoregional and free tissue transfer, free functional muscle transfer, and vascularized bone transfer, to optimize functional limb restoration after sarcoma resection.

> Chronic lower extremity wounds are defined as wounds that fail to heal within 3 months of defect onset. Free tissue transfer offers an opportunity for limb salvage and length preservation. Preoperative optimization includes a medical and nutritional consult, complete work-up by vascular surgery, and an analysis of bony stability and gait biomechanics by podiatric surgery. In the authors' practice, the thigh has proved the workhorse donor site and offers fasciocutaneous and muscle-based flaps depending on defect characteristics. Postoperative care requires early monitoring for flap compromise and continued long-term follow-up for wound recurrence.

Video content accompanies this article at http://www.plasticsurgery.theclinics.com/.

Demand has increased for complex lower extremity reconstruction in the steadily growing elderly patient group in many highly developed countries. Microsurgery is indispensable for soft tissue reconstruction and osseous consolidation salvaging leg function and preventing amputation, with its devastating consequences. Microvascular reconstruction can be performed successfully in specialized centers with low donor-site morbidity, minimal operative time, and comparably low complication rates. However, this requires thorough multidisciplinary planning, preoperative optimization of risk factors, such as diabetes and malnutrition, and individually adapted intraoperative management. Implementing these principles can reliably restore ambulation and mobility, maintaining autonomy in this population.

Indications for lower extremity reconstruction in children are unique because most result from congenital conditions (eg, constriction ring, lymphedema, syndactyly, nevi, vascular anomalies). Like adults, pediatric patients also suffer from effects following extirpation and trauma. Principles of reconstruction are based on the condition and type of deformity. The pediatric population typically has fewer comorbidities than adults that can negatively affect outcomes (eg, diabetes, peripheral vascular disease), although children can be less compliant with postoperative care. Growth, development, appearance, and postoperative compliance are variables that especially influence operative management of children.

Evolution in extremity injury treatment often occurs during major conflicts, with lessons learned applied and translated among military and civilian settings. In recent periods of war, improvements in protective equipment, in-theater damage control resuscitation/surgery, delivery of antibiotics locally/systemically, and rapid evacuation to higher levels of medical care capabilities have greatly improved combat casualty survivability rates. Additionally, widespread application of lower extremity tourniquets also has prevented casualties from exsanguination, thus reducing hemorrhagic-related deaths. Secondary to these, a high number of combat casualties suffering lower extremity traumatic injuries have presented for functional limb reconstruction and restoration as well as residual limb care.

CLINICS IN PLASTIC SURGERY

ISSUE OF RELATED INTEREST

Facial Plastic Surgery Clinics
https://www.facialplastic.theclinics.com/
Otolaryngologic Clinics
https://www.oto.theclinics.com/

THE CLINICS ARE AVAILABLE ONLINE!
Access your subscription at:
www.theclinics.com

Preface

Contemporary Approach to Lower Extremity Reconstruction

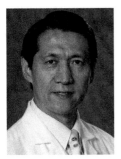

Lee L.Q. Pu, MD, PhD, FACS, FICS

Editor

Lower extremity reconstruction, as a subspecialty of plastic surgery, is an important part of the reconstructive surgery we do as plastic surgeons. For the past 20 years, many innovative techniques for lower extremity reconstruction have been discovered, for example, advanced wound management and microvascular free-tissue transfer, and development of new perforator-based flaps for lower extremity reconstruction. At many tertiary medical centers in developed countries, lower extremity reconstruction has become more than just soft tissue coverage, since functional restoration has also been emphasized through a multidisciplinary approach. It is important for reconstructive plastic surgeons to be familiar with the most recent innovations in lower extremity reconstruction so that the best possible reconstructive outcome can be provided to their patients.

As an active member of both American Society for Reconstructive Microsurgery and World Society for Reconstructive Microsurgery, I believe one of my primary responsibilities is to promote scientific exchange for reconstructive plastic surgery. For this reason, I decided to accept another invitation by Elsevier to edit a new issue of *Clinics in Plastic Surgery* on lower extremity reconstruction. I have chosen this topic because of my ongoing clinical experience on lower extremity reconstruction and expertise on editing a textbook for lower extremity reconstruction. The goal of this new issue in the *Clinics in Plastic Surgery* is to provide readers a precise but comprehensive overview on the contemporary approach to lower extremity reconstruction. For this reason, I have invited several contributors who not only are renowned experts in the field but also have published extensively in lower extremity reconstruction.

In this 19-article issue, the first 4 articles focus on refined or newly developed locoregional flaps, such as hemisoleus muscle flaps, distally based sural artery flaps, propeller flaps, perforator-plus flaps, and freestyle local perforator flaps for soft tissue reconstruction of the lower extremity. The next 5 articles focus on perforator-based microvascular free tissue transfer, including some new workhorse flaps, such as the medial sural artery perforator flap, the superficial circumflex artery perforator flap, and freestyle free perforator flaps. This is followed by another 9 articles, and each focuses on a unique issue in lower extremity reconstruction, such as the optimal timing for traumatic lower extremity reconstruction, management of Gustilo type IIIC injuries, orthoplastic reconstruction, functional restoration, super-microsurgery, lower extremity reconstruction after sarcoma resection, free tissue transfer for chronic wounds, and lower extremity reconstruction for both pediatric and elderly populations. The issue ends with a special article on the combat experience for limb salvage and functional restoration.

As guest editor, I sincerely hope that you enjoy reading this special issue of *Clinics in Plastic*

Clin Plastic Surg 48 (2021) xiii–xiv
https://doi.org/10.1016/j.cps.2021.01.010

Surgery and find it useful for your busy practice. It represents a true team effort from many world-renowned expert surgeons from United States, South Korea, Taiwan, and Switzerland. I would like to express my heartfelt gratitude to all contributors for their expertise, dedication, and responsibility to produce such a world-class issue of plastic surgery. It is certainly my privilege to work with these respected authors in this important field of plastic surgery. I would also like to express my special appreciation to the publication team of Elsevier, who has put this remarkable issue together with the highest possible standard.

Lee L.Q. Pu, MD, PhD, FACS, FICS
Division of Plastic Surgery
Department of Surgery
University of California, Davis
2335 Stockton Boulevard, Room 6008
Sacramento, CA, 95817, USA

E-mail address:
llpu@ucdavis.edu

Locoregional Flaps in Lower Extremity Reconstruction

Lee L.Q. Pu, MD, PhD

KEYWORDS

- Local flap • Regional flap • Lower extremity • Reconstruction • Soft tissue • Limb salvage

KEY POINTS

- Locoregional flaps play an important role in soft tissue reconstruction of the lower extremity.
- Either the medial hemisoleus muscle flap or the distally based sural artery flap can be a work horse for reconstruction of a soft tissue wound in the distal third of the leg.
- These flaps may be able to replace free tissue transfer as the first choice for soft tissue reconstruction of a less extensive wound in the distal third of the leg.
- Proper patient selection as well as a detailed knowledge of each flap anatomy and its advanced technique for flap dissection are the keys to the success.

INTRODUCTION

Locoregional flaps play an important role in the soft tissue reconstruction of the lower extremity and should also be considered as an effective and valid option in contemporary approach to lower extremity reconstruction. A study reviewed 290 lower extremity trauma patients over a 12-year period from a level 1 trauma center from a major tertiary hospital clearly showed that more local flaps and skin grafts were performed in general for soft tissue reconstruction of open tibia and fibula fracture wounds than free flaps.[1] In addition, local flaps for soft tissue coverage of lower extremity wounds may be more cost effective than free flaps for the same soft tissue wound in selected patients.[2]

Although free tissue transfer has become a standard choice of procedure for many soft tissue reconstructions in lower extremity reconstruction, the application of locoregional flaps for lower extremity reconstruction should be equally emphasized. Over the last 2 decades, several locoregional flaps have been refined or revisited in terms of their role in soft tissue reconstruction of the lower extremity because much more

advancement in understanding of the flap anatomy and in surgical dissection of each flap has also been made. It has become clear that local or regional flaps can also safely be chosen for soft tissue coverage in the lower extremity.[3,4] This is true because of the evolution of reconstructive flap surgery, especially a wide application of several muscle flaps, fasciocutaneous flaps, or even pedicled perforator flaps.[5–8] In addition, many locoregional flaps can be elevated because of their unique vascular anatomy and more advanced surgical technique in flap dissection. Several useful locoregional flaps are commonly designed in a reverse fashion and can, therefore, be used to reconstruct many complex wounds in the distal third of the leg wound as a good alternative to free tissue transfer.

When managing a complex soft tissue wound in the lower extremity, plastic surgeons can be divided into 2 general groups: microsurgeons and nonmicrosurgeons. Obviously, microsurgeons are capable of performing free tissue transfers and their preference for most lower extremity reconstructions are free flaps. In contrast, nonmicrosurgeons only can perform locoregional flaps for lower extremity reconstructions; for certain

Division of Plastic Surgery, University of California, Davis, 2335 Stockton Boulevard, Room 6008, Sacramento, CA 95817, USA
E-mail address: llpu@ucdavis.edu

Clin Plastic Surg 48 (2021) 157–171
https://doi.org/10.1016/j.cps.2021.01.001
0094-1298/21/© 2021 Elsevier Inc. All rights reserved.

patients, they have to transfer the care to microsurgeons in the same hospital or in a different hospital because they could not perform microsurgical procedures. It is possible that proper selection of a more suitable procedure for a lower extremity reconstruction is overshadowed by a plastic surgeon's ability and preference, but not by the actual soft tissue wound of the patient.

In this article, the author describes 2 reliable locoregional flaps, the medial hemisoleus muscle flap and the distally based sural artery fasciocutaneous flap, that have been used in his practice to manage a complex wound in the distal third of the leg. Because this author also routinely performs microvascular free tissue transfer, the selection of these 2 locoregional flaps for lower extremity reconstruction can be considered to have less bias and a free flap can be a good backup option if a locoregional flap is not successful. The indications and contraindications, preoperative evaluations, flap dissections, and management of flap-related complications are discussed as well.

INDICATIONS AND CONTRAINDICATIONS

It is critical to know the indications of a locoregional flap for reconstruction of a complex wound in the lower extremity, especially in the distal third of the leg. In general, a locoregional flap can be used to cover a relatively small (<50 cm^2) wound in the distal third of the leg (**Fig. 1**). Such a locoregional flap should not be within the zone of injury and should not have been traumatized from a previous injury or surgery.[9] The surgeons should be familiar with those flaps, including advanced techniques for flap dissection. The surgeons should also feel comfortable handling complications related to locoregional flap reconstruction.

The medial hemisoleus muscle flap and the distally based sural artery flap are 2 workhorse flaps that are used by the author to reconstruct a complex wound associated with an open fracture

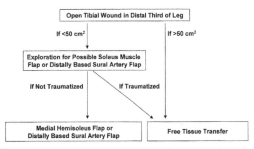

Fig. 1. A new algorithm proposed by the author for the management of a complex wound in the distal third of the leg.

or exposed bone in the distal third of the leg.[3,4] More recently, the concept of pedicled perforator flaps has been introduced in the literature. These axially based flaps can be elevated as a named perforator flap or even as a freestyle pedicled flap for various needs for soft tissue coverage in the lower extremity.[8] These flaps are described separately elsewhere in this issue.

The timing for a locoregional flap lower extremity reconstruction depends on the patient's readiness and associated medical conditions. In general, a definitive soft tissue reconstruction is commonly performed within 7 to 10 days after the initial consultation. However, because a locoregional flap is a relatively short procedure (about 2 hours) and has more straightforward postoperative care, it can be performed right after definitive bony reconstruction by orthopedic trauma service in the same operation.

Contraindications for a locoregional flap for reconstruction a complex wound in the distal third of the leg are as follows: the wound is larger (ie, >50 cm^2); more composite tissue involvement, the flap is within the "zone of injury," or significant peripheral vascular disease is present. If the patient has an occluded posterior tibial artery, a medial hemisoleus muscle flap is contraindicated. If the patient has an occluded peroneal artery, a distally based sural artery flap is contraindicated. For those conditions, free tissue transfer will be a more reliable option than a locoregional flap reconstruction. If the soft tissue injury is extensive and there is a significant trauma to the area that a locoregional flap would be based on, a free flap reconstruction may provide the only option for limb salvage in these patients.[9]

PREOPERATIVE EVALUATION AND SPECIAL CONSIDERATIONS

A complex wound in the distal third of the leg is frequently associated with an underlying tibial fracture and successful soft tissue coverage for the open fracture site provides a critical means for primary or secondary healing of the fracture as well as for limb salvage. In general, a free tissue transfer is currently the standard procedure of choice to provide meaningful soft tissue coverage in this anatomic region of the leg because there is no good local option available for such a critical soft tissue reconstruction, at least based on the classic teaching of the past 2 decades. Controversy among plastic surgeons often remains for those complex wounds in the distal third of the leg that are relatively too small for free tissue transfer, but clearly too large for primary wound closure.[10]

Although a free flap has been considered a standard procedure of choice for soft tissue coverage in the distal third of leg, certain patients may not be candidates for free tissue transfer because of their overall medical conditions after a multisystem trauma or they are not in compliance with proper postoperative care. It becomes clear to many plastic surgeons, including this author, that not every patient requires a free flap reconstruction as a standard procedure of choice, even for an open tibial wound in the distal third of the leg, and a few locoregional flaps may serve well for selected patients with a less extensive wound in the distal third of the leg.

With a better understanding of the flap anatomy and its blood supply, as well as refinements and innovations of the flap dissection, a few locoregional flaps can be used for the soft tissue coverage of a complex wound in the distal third of the leg. In the author's practice, the medial hemisoleus muscle flap has been selected more than any other local muscle flaps for soft tissue coverage of a complex wound in the distal third of the leg.[2,3,9,10] When the size of a wound is less than 50 cm^2, a medial hemisoleus muscle flap can be chosen primarily for soft tissue coverage if the soleus muscle is not traumatized. With the application of sound clinical judgment, the author has found that many orthopedic trauma patients who have an open tibial wound in the distal third of the leg with an open tibial fracture can be reconstructed successfully with a medial hemisoleus muscle flap based either proximally or distally for soft tissue coverage. When the selection of a medial hemisoleus muscle flap for a wound in the distal third of the leg, a proximally based flap can be chosen when a defect is relatively proximal, whereas a distally based flap can be selected when a defect is relatively distal.[11]

The distally based sural artery flap, a distant skin island flap,[4,5,7] has also been used frequently to provide soft tissue coverage for a complex wound in the distal third of the leg, if the flap donor site is available and the pedicle of the flap in the lesser saphenous vein territory is not traumatized. The flap itself provides a good skin coverage to a wound in both the medial and lateral aspects of the distal leg. However, the less optimal blood supply provided by a fasciocutaneous flap has been one of the main concerns for its routine use in soft tissue coverage of a complex wound in the distal third of the leg associated with an open tibial fracture.[12]

Frequently, the determination of whether a locoregional flap can be selected for lower extremity wound coverage is performed in the operating room where a complex wound is more properly explored and assessed by the surgeon. Such an intraoperative assessment can provide a critical means to the surgeon to decide whether a locoregional flap can safely be selected to reconstruct a complex wound in the lower extremity. In addition, the plastic surgeon's expertise, as well as reconstructive services provided by a hospital, can play a role in the decision-making process for the flap selection.

SURGICAL PROCEDURES
Medial Hemisoleus Muscle Flap

The soleus muscle is a bipenniform muscle located in the superficial posterior compartment of the leg. It originates from the fibula and medial aspect of the tibia and inserts into the calcaneus as a part of the Achilles tendon (**Fig. 2**). The medial hemisoleus muscle flap can provide not only adequate soft tissue coverage, but can also minimize functional loss of the foot planter flexion.[13] The bipenniform morphology of the soleus muscle and the independent neurovascular supply to either the medial or lateral belly of the muscle are important features that allow a surgeon to split the muscle longitudinally along the muscle's midline to create a muscle flap composed of only one-half the muscle (hemisoleus).[14] After splitting the muscle, the medial part of the muscle is supplied throughout its length by perforators arising from the posterior tibial vessels. This constant blood supply makes the medial part of the muscle (medial hemisoleus) reliable as a proximally or even distally based flap[13] (**Fig. 3**).

The flap dissection is done under tourniquet control. An existing wound can be extended into the incision both proximally and distally. For a proximally based medial hemisoleus muscle flap, once the medial hemisoleus muscle is identified and dissected freely from the medial gastrocnemius muscle, its insertion is divided distally at a level close to the Achilles' tendon, depending on the length of the flap rotation required. The medial half of the muscle is split longitudinally along with a midline between the bellies of the soleus muscle. To cover a wound in the distal third of the leg (**Fig. 4**), the proximally based medial hemisoleus muscle flap is elevated only to the level just below the junction between the middle and distal thirds of the leg with an emphasis on the preservation of as many major perforators to the flap as possible, even in the distal-third of the leg, while allowing an adequate arc of flap rotation (**Fig. 5**). These perforators are critical sources of blood supply to the distal portion of the medial hemisoleus muscle flap and should be preserved whenever possible. During flap dissection, only the muscular portion of the soleus muscle is used as

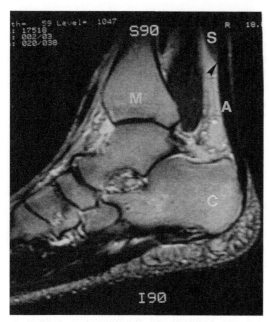

Fig. 2. An MRI shows the insertion of the soleus muscle (*arrow*) to the level of the ankle. A, Achilles; C, Calcaneous; M, Malleolus; S, Soleus.

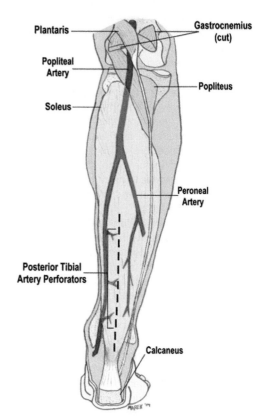

Fig. 3. A schematic diagram shows the blood supply to the medial and lateral halves of the soleus muscle as well as splitting of the muscle (*dotted line*) for the medial hemisoleus muscle flap dissection. (*From* Pu, LLQ. Successful Soft-tissue coverage of a tibial wound in the distal third of the leg with a medial hemisoleus muscle flap. Plast Reconstr Surg. 2005; 115(1):247; with permission.)

the flap; the tendinous portion of the soleus is left intact (**Fig. 6**). The spared tendon is then approximated to the remaining lateral half of the soleus muscle with nonabsorbable sutures. This technique may minimize functional loss of the leg after the flap is harvested. With these refined techniques for the flap dissection, the flap can be suitable for a more proximal defect in the distal third of the leg.

This author prefers an intraoperative dissection of the soleus muscle to confirm the level of the distal muscle insertion, although a preoperative MRI can easily identify the location of the soleus musculotendinous junction in the ankle. Once the medial hemisoleus muscle is identified and dissected freely to the level at the junction between the middle and distal thirds of the tibia, the major perforators from the posterior tibial vessels to the medial half of the soleus muscle within even distal third of the tibia should be identified (**Fig. 7**). Next, the surgeon must be attentive in the preservation of these perforators when designing the adequate arc of flap rotation to cover the target soft tissue defect or exposed hardware (**Fig. 8**). If needed, the medial hemisoleus muscle can be extended more laterally after longitudinally splitting, so that the flap can be made wide enough to cover a relatively large wound in the distal third of the leg.[15] These modifications made by the author to the surgical techniques in flap dissection emphasize the

preservation of an adequate blood supply to the distal portion of the medial hemisoleus muscle flap after flap elevation. These techniques maximize the reliability of the medial hemisoleus muscle flap and expand its role in reconstruction of distal third tibial wounds[3,10,11,15] (**Fig. 9**).

When a distally based medial hemisoleus muscle flap is planned, a preoperative angiogram can be very helpful to determine the presence of major perforators from the posterior tibial vessels to the distal portion of the medial soleus muscle (**Fig. 10**). Usually at the junction of the proximal and middle thirds of the soleus muscle, the medial half of the muscle is divided and then split longitudinally along with the midline between the medial and lateral halves of the soleus muscle to the level of the junction of the proximal and middle third of the muscle. Attention should also be taken to preserve as many major perforators from the posterior tibial vessels to the flap as possible even in the

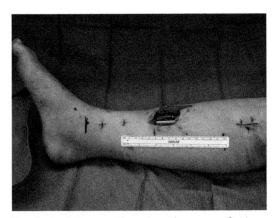

Fig. 4. An intraoperative view shows a soft tissue wound in the distal third of the leg. The wound is located in the distal third of the leg.

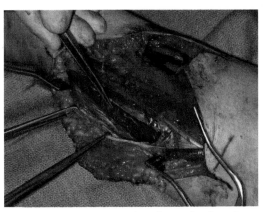

Fig. 6. An intraoperative view shows the flap dissection of a proximally based medial hemisoleus muscle flap. The tendon portion of the soleus muscle is dissected free from the muscle belly and preserved to minimize functional loss after the flap elevation.

distal and middle thirds of the tibia while allowing for adequate arc of flap turnover to cover wounds in the distal-third of the leg (**Fig. 11**). This maneuver may provide a longer arc for flap turnover because the level of these perforators serves as a pivot point for flap turnover and ultimately determines how far the flap can reach to the distal leg. With this technique, the flap can often reach the proximal border of the medial malleolus after elevation and turnover.[3,11,16]

In this author's practice, the flap can be suitable for a relatively larger and more distal tibial wound of the leg (**Fig. 12**). The flap is primarily based on the last 2 or 3 major perforators from the posterior tibial vessels. However, it also receives a blood supply from the proximal lateral half of the muscle

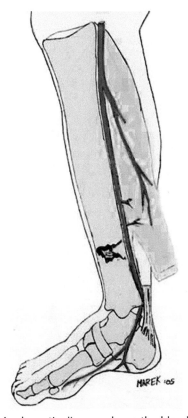

Fig. 5. A schematic diagram shows the blood supply to the proximally based medial hemisoleus muscle flap after the flap elevation. The flap can be used to cover a wound located more proximal in the distal third of the leg. (*From* Pu, LLQ. Further experience with the medial hemisoleus muscle flap for soft-tissue coverage of a tibial wound in the distal third of the leg. Plast Reconstr Surg. 2008; 121(6):2026; with permission.)

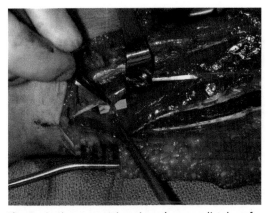

Fig. 7. An intraoperative view shows a distal perforator from the posterior tibial vessel. This perforator will be divided to allow adequate flap rotation of the proximally based medial hemisoleus muscle flap to cover an adjacent soft tissue wound.

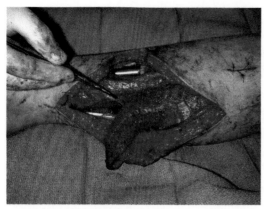

Fig. 8. An intraoperative view shows another more proximal perforator from the posterior tibial vessel. This perforator should be preserved to ensure good blood supply to the distal flap while allowing adequate flap rotation of a proximally based medial hemisoleus muscle flap to cover an adjacent soft tissue wound.

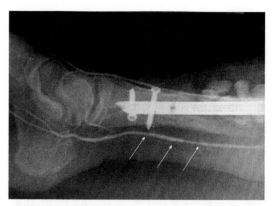

Fig. 10. An angiogram shows 3 perforators (*arrows*) from the distal posterior tibial vessel. Those perforators are the major source of blood supply for the distally based medial hemisoleus muscle flap.

in an antegrade fashion. However, the flap is still primarily based distally or reversed. More proximal perforators from the posterior tibial vessels to the medial half of the soleus muscle within the upper distal or even middle third of the tibia should be preserved while allowing adequate arc of the flap turnover to cover the target defect in the distal third of the leg. Thus, the most proximal perforator that is preserved will serve as the pivot point for the flap turnover (**Figs. 13** and **14**). Again, these techniques maximize the blood supply to the medial hemisoleus muscle flap and expand its role in the reconstruction of distal third tibial wounds[3,11,16] (**Fig. 15**).

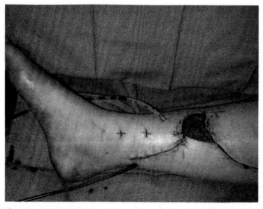

Fig. 9. An intraoperative view shows a reliable soft tissue coverage for a complex wound in the distal third of the leg with a proximally based medial hemisoleus muscle flap before placement of a skin graft to the muscle flap.

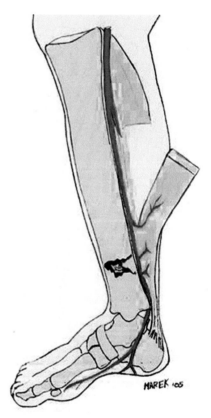

Fig. 11. A schematic diagram shows the blood supply to the distally based medial hemisoleus muscle flap after the flap elevation. The flap can be used to cover a wound located in the distal third of the leg. (*From* Pu, LLQ. Further experience with the medial hemisoleus muscle flap for soft-tissue coverage of a tibial wound in the distal third of the leg. Plast Reconstr Surg. 2008; 121(6):2026; with permission.)

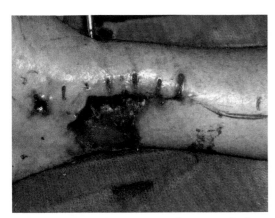

Fig. 12. An intraoperative view shows a soft tissue wound in the distal third of the leg. The wound is located more distal in the distal third of the leg.

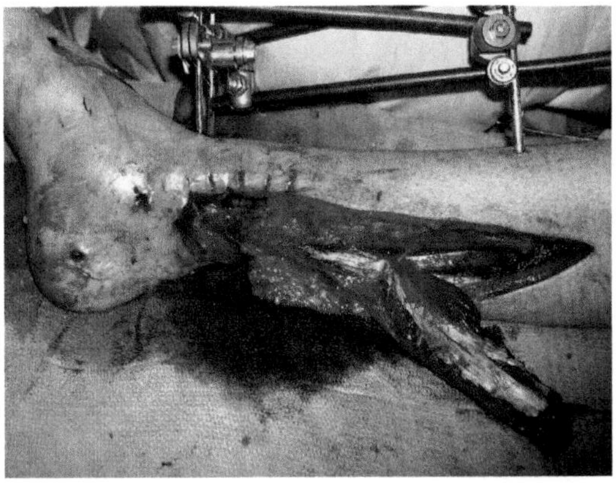

Fig. 14. An intraoperative view shows the completed flap dissection of a distally based medial hemisoleus muscle flap.

Distally Based Sural Artery Flap

The donor site of a distally based sural artery flap is centrally located in the posterior calf over the medial and lateral gastrocnemius muscles. The skin island can be harvested from the proximal two-thirds of the posterior leg. The safest size of the flap is about 12 × 8 cm, but the upper limit of the flap size remains unknown. The flap receives blood supply primarily from 3 to 6 septocutaneous perforators arising from the peroneal artery in a retrograde fashion. The most proximal end of those perforators is located 4 to 7 cm proximal to the lateral malleolus. It also receives a blood supply, again in a retrograde fashion, from the fasciocutaneous perforators from the posterior tibial

artery, venocutaneous perforators from the lesser saphenous vein, and neurocutaneous perforators from the sural nerve. Thus, the blood supplies to the flap are through the lesser saphenous vein and sural nerve systems that are included in the adipofascial pedicle once the flap is elevated. The venous outflow of the flap can either drain directly to the concomitant vein of a perforator from the peroneal artery or drain back to the less saphenous vein.[17]

The flap elevation is performed in the prone position. The pivot point of the flap turnover is marked about 5 to 6 cm above the lateral malleolus.[4,7,17] The whole course of the lesser saphenous vein is mapped with a handheld Doppler between the Achilles tendon and the lateral malleolus. The skin island flap is designed based on the size of soft tissue wound and the less saphenous vein

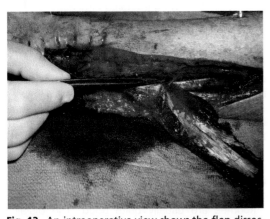

Fig. 13. An intraoperative view shows the flap dissection of a distally based medial hemisoleus muscle flap. The perforator (*pointed by a forceps*) from the posterior tibial vessels should be preserved to ensure adequate blood supply of the flap while allowing adequate turnover of the distally based hemisoleus muscle flap to cover a soft tissue wound.

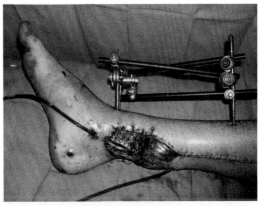

Fig. 15. An intraoperative view shows a reliable soft tissue coverage for a complex wound in the distal third of the leg with a distally based medial hemisoleus muscle flap before placement of a skin graft to the muscle flap.

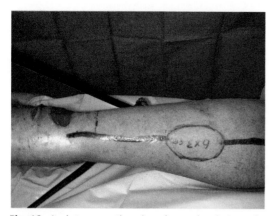

Fig. 16. An intraoperative view shows the design of a distally based sural artery flap. The pedicle of the flap is marked between the lateral malleolus and Achilles tendon and extended through the center of the flap.

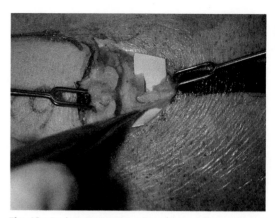

Fig. 18. An intraoperative view shows a close-up view of the isolated lesser saphenous vein and its accompanying vessels before their division.

should be included (**Fig. 16**). Under tourniquet control, the proximal incision of the flap is made first to explore the lesser saphenous vein and its accompanying vessels (**Fig. 17**). The lesser saphenous vein and its accompanying vessels are divided (**Fig. 18**). The sural nerve and its accompanied vessels are exposed next and then divided (**Fig. 19**). The skin island is elevated under the fascia and it is then completely elevated as a fasciocutaneous flap. The adipofascial pedicle of the flap, about 2 to 4 cm wide (**Fig. 20**), is dissected free and can be turned over and tunneled under the skin bridge or skin grafted over if such a tunnel is opened (**Fig. 21**). The flap can be used to cover a complex wound in the distal leg. The donor site can be closed primarily after undermining if it is less than 5 cm wide or closed with a skin graft.

POSTOPERATIVE CARE AND EXPECTED OUTCOME

The postoperative care is relatively straightforward after a locoregional flap reconstruction in the lower extremity. The postoperative care regimen in this author's practice includes bed rest with leg elevation to decrease edema and the placement of a warming unit around the leg to maintain a warm temperature for the first few days after flap reconstruction. A splint may be used to immobilize the leg. Five days of bedrest are needed when a skin graft is placed to the muscle flap. This practice allows time for the skin graft to begin revascularization. With more routine application of a vacuum-assisted closure device to immobilize skin graft over the muscle flap, a splint now is only used if there is an underlying fracture in the leg.

Elevation of the affected leg in the postoperative period is critical because early venous congestion after a distally based medial hemisoleus muscle flap or a distally based sural artery flap is relatively common. Weight-bearing status often is dictated jointly with the orthopedic trauma service. However, for simple soft tissue defects, return to weight bearing is allowed within 2 weeks, depending on follow-up clinical examinations.

The proximally based medial hemisoleus muscle flap is fairly reliable. In addition, the flap can provide just enough muscle bulk for soft tissue coverage of a tibial wound and thus reconstructive outcomes are usually quite good. The distally based medial hemisoleus muscle flap can be reliable in most healthy and compliant patients. However, the flap should not be used in patients with significant peripheral vascular disease because of the potential for poor inflow of the posterior tibial artery or with significant diabetes because of the

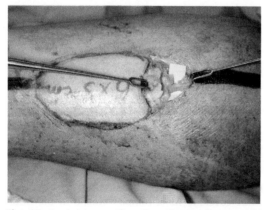

Fig. 17. An intraoperative view shows the exposed lesser saphenous vein and its accompanied vessels together after skin incision.

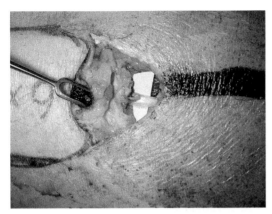

Fig. 19. An intraoperative view shows a close-up view of the exposed sural nerve and its accompanying vessels before their division. In this view, the lesser saphenous vein and its accompanied vessels have been divided.

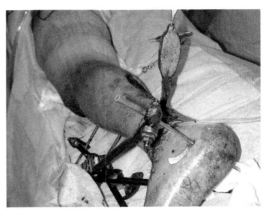

Fig. 21. An intraoperative view shows the pedicle of the flap that is completely elevated. The flap will be turned over to cover a wound in the distal third of the leg.

potential for small vessel disease. The initial venous congestion may become a problem in certain patients such as smokers or those with an inability to elevate the leg during the postoperative period. In general, distal flap necrosis occurs infrequently if the flap is based proximally, but occurs in about 20% of the patients if the flap is based distally. The flap may be bulky in the first few months after surgery, but the contour of the leg can become close to normal after 6 to 9 months.

Venous congestion after the distally based sural artery flap in the immediate postoperative period can be relatively common. However, in case of prolonged postoperative venous congestion, application of topical nitroglycerin paste or medicinal leech therapy may be used.

This author has not experienced any total flap loss for nearly 200 flaps. Both the medial hemisoleus muscle flap and the distally based sural artery flap are workhorses in managing a complex wound in the distal third of the leg. In selected patients who have a relatively less extensive soft tissue wound of their lower extremity, each flap can provide reliable soft tissue coverage and can often be performed in 2 hours.

MANAGEMENT OF COMPLICATIONS

A common complication for all locoregional flap lower extremity reconstructions is the presence of venous congestion. For a distally based sural artery flap, inspection of the flap pedicle is warranted to ensure there is no direct compression. If venous congestion persists or worsens, the flap can be inset back to the donor site or a supercharge to augment venous drainage between the proximal lesser saphenous vein and an adjacent vein in the leg can be performed with microsurgical technique.[18] Any delayed wound separation of the flap from the wound edge can be successfully treated with local wound care. However, if there is exposure of vital underlying structures or hardware, flap readvancement should be performed.

If performed properly, total flap loss of a medial hemisoleus muscle flap should not happen. However, just like any other pedicled flaps, distal flap necrosis may still occur. Fortunately, distal flap necrosis is usually insignificant and can be managed with debridement. The flap can then be readvanced adequately to cover the wound and the final outcome can still be quite good. Further advancement of the flap is possible by dividing the most proximal perforator which has served

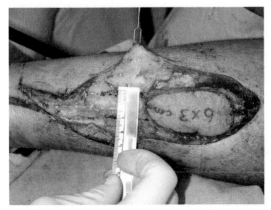

Fig. 20. An intraoperative view shows the exposed pedicle of the flap after zig-zig skin incisions. The pedicle can be as narrow as 2 cm.

as a pivot point because the flap has been delayed after initial flap elevation.[11] Occasionally, a distally based sural artery flap may have partial separation of the incision at the distal edge of the flap suture line and this can be treated successfully by reapproximation of the flap.

REVISIONS OR SUBSEQUENT PROCEDURES

The contour after a locoregional flap reconstruction in the distal third of the leg may not become an issue compared with after a free flap reconstruction in the same location. However, it can be an issue after a distally based sural artery flap because the calf tissue in some patients can be relatively thicker. Thus, the bulkiness of the flap needs to be revised so that a better contour of the leg can be achieved. It is the author's preference that a minimum of 6 months' waiting period should be expected before a debulking procedure can be considered. Unlike a skin-grafted muscle flap, the bulkiness of a fasciocutaneous flap would

not shrink any further after 6 months and a debulking procedure can be performed relatively sooner. Again, because a distally based sural artery flap is a fasciocutaneous flap, conventional liposuction can be performed first to remove any excess adipose tissue from the flap. Additional skin resection may be necessary to achieve better contour of the flap in the leg. A medial hemisoleus muscle flap, even when it is based distally, can shrink nicely. The contour in the distal third of the leg can be quite good and no debulking procedures are performed in the author's practice.

CASE EXAMPLES
Case 1

A 57-year-old female patient had an open tibial fracture of her left distal leg with a soft tissue loss secondary to a motor vehicle accident. She had a 5 × 4 cm tibial wound in the distal third of the leg with exposed fracture site (**Fig. 22**A). A rigid fixation of the distal tibial fracture was performed

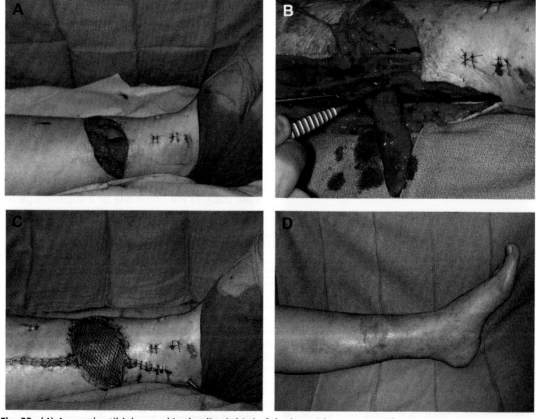

Fig. 22. (A) A complex tibial wound in the distal third of the leg with an exposed fracture site and a more extensive soft tissue wound of the leg. (B) A proximally based medial hemisoleus muscle flap is elevated and a perforator (*pointed by a forceps*) is preserved. (C) Completion of the flap inset and a skin graft to the flap and the rest of the wound. (D) Results at 2 years and 4 months of follow-up.

by the orthopedic trauma service after the initial wound debridement. She returned to the operating room 3 days late, where a laterally extended medial hemisoleus muscle flap was performed for soft tissue reconstruction (**Fig. 22**B). A split-thickness skin graft was placed over the muscle flap (**Fig. 22**C). The patient did well postoperatively, and her distal tibial wound healed primarily without complications (**Fig. 22**D). Her tibial fracture also healed afterward, and she was able to ambulate without problem.

Case 2

A 32-year-old male patient sustained infected nonunion in the distal tibia. He had a 6 × 3 cm open tibial wound in the distal third of the left leg with an exposed old tibial fracture site following multiple surgical debridements by the orthopedic trauma service (**Fig. 23**A). The definitive soft tissue reconstruction was performed successfully with a distally based medial hemisoleus muscle flap (**Fig. 23**B). A split-thickness skin graft was also performed to cover the muscle flap (**Fig. 23**C). The patient did well postoperatively, and his distal

tibial wound healed without complications (**Fig. 23**D). His fracture also healed eventually, and he was able to ambulate without problem.

Case 3

A 43-year-old male patient had a soft tissue wound in the medial aspect of his left distal leg secondary to surgical debridement of necrotic skin after open reduction and rigid fixation by the orthopedic trauma service. He had an 8 × 5 cm wound in the distal leg just above the medial malleolus with an exposed hardware and fracture site (**Fig. 24**A). The patient returned to the operating room 5 days later where a distally based sural artery flap was performed for soft tissue coverage of his distal tibial wound (**Fig. 24**B, C). The patient did well postoperatively and his distal tibial wound healed primarily without complication (**Fig. 24**D). His tibial fracture also healed a few months later. He was able to ambulate without problem.

Case 4

A 57-year-old male patient had a soft tissue wound in the lateral aspect of his left distal leg secondary

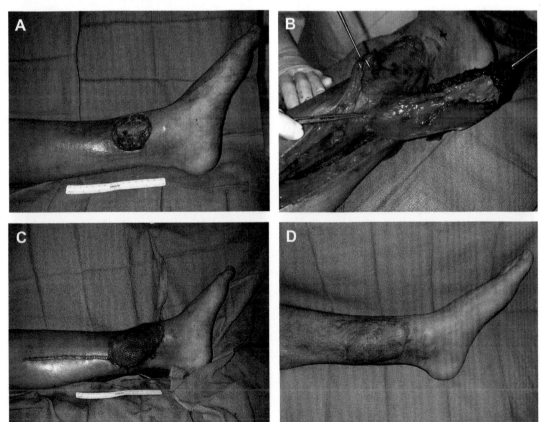

Fig. 23. (*A*) A complex wound in the distal third of the leg with an exposed tibia. (*B*) A distally based medial hemisoleus muscle flap is elevated and a perforator (*pointed by a forceps*) is preserved and served as a pivot point for flap turnover. (*C*) Completion of the flap inset and a skin graft to the flap. (*D*) Results at 5 months of follow-up.

to motor vehicle accident. He had a 6 × 3 cm wound in the distal leg just above the lateral malleolus with an exposed underlying bone (**Fig. 25**A). He also had other fractures in his left leg. A distally based sural artery flap was performed for soft tissue coverage of his distal tibial wound see (**Fig. 25**B, C). The patient did well postoperatively and his distal tibial wound healed primarily without complication (**Fig. 25**D). Other fractures in his left leg also healed a few months later. He was able to ambulate without problem.

DISCUSSION

It is important to determine whether a locoregional flap can be used safely and reliably to reconstruct a complex wound in the distal third of the leg. It is also critical to know the limitations of a selected locoregional flap and to have a back-up plan if the plan A fails. Such a back-up plan can entail further flap advancement after removing the necrotic portion of the flap, another locoregional flap, or, frequently, free tissue transfer. Based on this author's experience, the size of a wound in the lower extremity can often be a primary factor to be considered by the surgeon when selecting a locoregional flap if such an option is available. In addition, the selected locoregional flap, either the entire flap or its pedicle, should not be within the zone of injury of the lower extremity. This can frequently be a limiting factor for the selection of a locoregional flap in an orthopedic trauma patient (**Box 1**). The new treatment algorithm established by the author provides a practical guideline for soft tissue coverage of an open tibial wound in the distal third of the leg. The selected option may potentially offer a simple but more cost-effective approach to managing a complex wound in the distal third of the leg because free flap may no longer be the first choice for soft tissue reconstruction, but will only be indicated for a large open tibial wound or when a locoregional flap is contraindicated.[9]

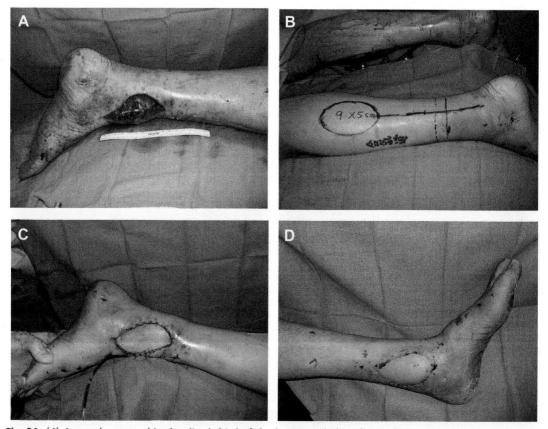

Fig. 24. (*A*) A complex wound in the distal third of the leg extended to the medial malleolus with an exposed fracture site and hardware. (*B*) The design of a distally based sural artery flap as a turnover flap. (*C*) Completion of the flap inset in the operating room. In this case, the pedicle of the flap was tunneled through the skin bridge. (*D*) Results at 2 months of follow-up.

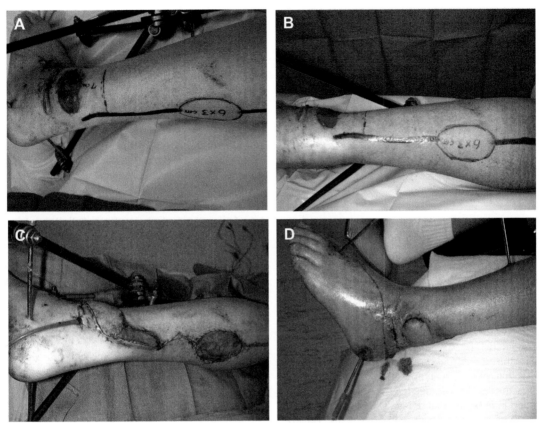

Fig. 25. (*A*) A complex wound over the lateral distal third of the leg with an exposed bone. (*B*) The design of a distally based sural artery flap as a turnover flap. (*C*) Completion of the flap inset in the operating room. In this case, the pedicle of the flap was partially tunneled through the skin bridge and partially covered with a skin graft. (*D*) Results at 6 weeks of follow-up.

When performing a proximally based hemisoleus muscle flap, any perforators from the posterior tibial vessels to the distal medial half of the soleus muscle just at or above the level of a tibial wound should be preserved while allowing for an adequate arc of flap rotation to cover a wound in the distal third of the leg. These modifications of surgical techniques emphasize the preservation of an adequate blood supply to the distal portion of the medial hemisoleus muscle flap after the flap is elevated. These techniques would maximize reliability of the medial hemisoleus muscle flap and expand its role in reconstruction of a complex wound in the distal third of the leg. Based on the author's experience, the proximally based medial hemisoleus muscle flap can be used for a relatively distal tibial wound in the junction of the middle and distal thirds or in the distal third of the leg. The flap is fairly reliable and can often be done within 2 hours. In addition, the flap can provide just enough muscle bulk for soft tissue coverage of

the tibial wound and thus reconstructive outcomes are usually quite good.[3,10,11,15]

With the aid of a preoperative angiogram, major perforators in the distal third of the leg can be identified when planning a distally based medial hemisoleus flap. The most proximal perforators from the posterior tibial vessels to the medial half of the distal soleus muscle within the distal third of the leg should be preserved while allowing adequate flap turnover to cover a tibial wound in the distal third of the leg. This perforator will serve as a pivot point for flap turnover and the level of the perforator will determine how far this flap can reach. The modified surgical techniques in flap dissection indeed emphasize the preservation of an adequate blood supply to the distal portion of the distally based flap and maximize reliability of the medial hemisoleus muscle flap even when it is based distally. The flap can be reliable in most healthy and compliant patients and can often be performed in 2 hours. However, the flap should

Box 1	
Special considerations for a locoregional flap in the distal third of the leg	
Characteristics	**Consideration**
Size of defect	Relatively small (<50 cm²)
Involvement of tissue loss	Less complicated
Adjacent or distant flap tissue	Available
Flap and/or its pedicle within "zone of injury"	Spared

not be used in smokers or in patients with significant peripheral vascular disease because of the potential poor inflow of the posterior tibial artery or in patients with significant diabetes because of the potential small vessel disease in those perforators. The initial venous congestion may become a problem in certain patients and should be managed accordingly.[3,11,16]

The distally base sural artery flap can also play a role in the reconstruction of a complex wound in the distal third of the leg. In appropriately selected patients, the flap can be used to cover a less extensive wound in either medial or lateral distal third of the leg extending to the level of the malleolus. Based on the author's experience, the flap is reliable in most healthy patients and can also be performed in 2 hours. However, the flap dissection should be done in a prone position that makes the flap inset somewhat difficulty. The pedicle of the flap, after turnover, can be skin grafted if the tunnel is too tight. In obese patients, the flap can be thicker and thus future flap debulking may be needed. Venous congestion of the flap may be encountered and a supercharge of the flap can be added to an adjacent vein in the distal leg or foot.[18] The surgical delay of the flap has also been advocated by others.[19] However, the flap, after surgical delay, can be more swollen and rigid and may be more difficult for the flap inset.

Like any other pedicled flap, distal flap necrosis may occur, but total flap loss should not occur if the flap is performed properly. Fortunately, distal flap necrosis is usually insignificant and can be managed with debridement. The flap can then be readvanced adequately to cover the wound and the final outcome can still be good. Further advancement of the flap is possible by dividing the most proximal perforator, which has served as a pivot point of the flap rotation or turnover for a medial hemesoleus muscle flap or by elevating and advancing the pedicle so that the flap can be turned over more for a distally based sural

artery flap because both flaps have been delayed after the initial flap elevation.[11,15,16]

SUMMARY

A locoregional flap can play an important role in the soft tissue reconstruction of the lower extremity, even in the distal third of the leg. It is relatively simple and straightforward, but can be reliable if the flap dissection and inset are properly done by the surgeon. Two important locoregional flaps such as the medial hemisoleus muscle flap and the distally based sural artery flap can be a work horse and can even be used to replace free tissue transfer as the first choice for soft tissue reconstruction of a less extensive wound various in the distal third of the leg. Proper patient selection as well as detail knowledge of the flap and its advanced technique for flap dissection are the keys to the success.

CLINICS CARE POINTS

- In general, vigorous post-operative care is not necessary after a locoregional flap reconstruction.
- Partial flap necrosis may occur and this complication can be managed successfully with possible flap re-advancement.
- Free tissue transfer can be a good back up option for lower extremity reconstruction if a locoregional flap fails.

DISCLOSURE

The author has no financial interests in any of the drugs, products, or devices mentioned in this article.

REFERENCES

1. Parrett BM, Matros E, Pribaz J, et al. Lower extremity trauma: trends in the management of soft-tissue reconstruction of open tibia-fibula fractures. Plast Reconstr Surg 2006;117:1315–22.
2. Thornton B, Rosenblum WJ, Pu LLQ. Reconstruction of limited soft-tissue defect with open tibial fracture in the distal third of the leg: a cost and outcome study. Ann Plast Surg 2005;54:276280.
3. Pu LLQ. Successful soft-tissue coverage of a tibial wound in the distal third of the leg with a medial hemisoleus flap. Plast Reconstr Surg 2005;115:245–51.
4. Huisinga RL, Houpt P, Dijkstra R, et al. The distally based sural artery flap. Ann Plast Surg 1998;41:58–65.

5. Gumener R, Zbrodowski A, Montandon D. The reversed fasciosubcutaneous flap in the leg. Plast Reconstr Surg 1991;88:1034–41.

6. Hughes LA, Mahoney JL. Anatomic basis of local muscle flaps in the distal third of the leg. Plast Reconstr Surg 1993;92:1144–54.

7. Hollier L, Sharma S, Babigumira E, et al. Versatility of the sural fasciocutaneous flap in the coverage of lower extremity wounds. Plast Reconstr Surg 2002; 110:1673–9.

8. Hallock GG. Lower extremity muscle perforator flaps for lower extremity reconstruction. Plast Reconstr Surg 2004;114:1123–30.

9. Pu LLQ. Soft-tissue reconstruction of an open tibial wound in the distal third of the leg: a new treatment algorithm. Ann Plast Surg 2007;58:78–83.

10. Pu LLQ. Soft-tissue coverage of an open tibial wound in the junction of the middle and distal thirds of the leg with the medial hemisoleus muscle flap. Ann Plast Surg 2006;56:639–43.

11. Pu LLQ. Further experience with the medial hemisoleus muscle flap for soft-tissue coverage of a tibial wound in the distal third of the leg. Plast Reconstr Surg 2008;121:2024–8.

12. Anthony JP, Mathes SJ, Alpert BS. The muscle flap in the treatment of chronic lower extremity osteomyelitis: results in patients over 5 years after treatment. Plast Reconstr Surg 1991;88:311–8.

13. Raveendran SS, Kumaragama KGJL. Arterial supply of the soleus muscle: anatomical study of fifty lower limbs. Clin Anat 2003;16:248–52.

14. Tobin GR. Hemisoleus and reversed hemisoleus flaps. Plast Reconstr Surg 1985;76:87–96.

15. Pu LLQ. The laterally extended medial hemisoleus flap for reconstruction of a tibial wound in the distal third of the leg. Eur J Plast Surg 2007;30:19–24.

16. Pu LLQ. The reversed medial hemisoleus muscle flap and its role in reconstruction of an open tibial wound in the lower third of the leg. Ann Plast Surg 2006;56:59–64.

17. Follmar KE, Baccarani A, Baumeiser SP, et al. The distally base sural flap. Plast Reconstr Surg 2007; 119:138e–48e.

18. MPJ Loonen, Kon MK, Schuurman AH, et al. Venous bypass drainage of the small saphenous vein in the neurovascular pedicle of the sural flap: anatomical study and clinical applications. Plast Reconstr Surg 2007;120:1898–905.

19. Kneser U, Bach AD, Polykandriotis E, et al. Delayed reverse sural flap for staged reconstruction of the foot and lower leg. Plast Reconstr Surg 2005;116: 1910–7.

Propeller Flaps in Lower Extremity Reconstruction

Jordan T. Blough, MD[a], Michel H. Saint-Cyr, MD, FRCSC[b],*

KEYWORDS

- Pedicled perforator flap • Propeller • Leg • Lower extremity • Reconstruction

KEY POINTS

- The propeller flap is a workhorse pedicled perforator flap designed as an island flap that reaches the recipient site through an axial rotation.
- Advantages to propeller flaps include minimal donor site morbidity, preserving axial blood supply to the distal extremity, excellent tissue quality match, and significantly less physiologic demands on the comorbid patient.
- Literature-reported complication rates in propeller flap reconstruction of the lower extremity compare similarly to free tissue transfer.
- An understanding of the perforasome concept, hot and cold perforator locations, and basic propeller flap design will enable the surgeon to readily harvest flaps based on any clinically relevant perforator in freestyle fashion; however, each level of injury has preferable perforator source options.

INTRODUCTION

The advent of perforator flaps has ushered in a new and exciting era for reconstructive surgery. Although not a panacea for the lower extremity, pedicled perforator flaps (PPFs), and propeller flaps in particular, have seen increased application, replacing traditional locoregional options and free tissue transfer in the appropriate settings. Most commonly, their indication includes small- to medium-sized defects of the distal third of the leg, a challenging predicament given limited local donor tissue availability; they do have utility in smaller defects of other areas of the leg also.[1–3] The propeller flap is a workhorse subset of PPFs, defined as a completely islanded flap that reaches the recipient site through an axial rotation.[4]

Propeller flaps carry significant advantages, including minimizing donor site morbidity and pain, sparing the underlying muscle, preserving axial blood supply distally, and providing excellent tissue match. Compared with free flaps, propeller flaps obviate the requirement for microsurgery and position changes; additionally, they are less morbid for unhealthy patients, and reduce operative and hospitalization time and costs.[2]

This article discusses the principles of PPFs, propeller flap design, and considerations by location along the lower extremity.

PERFORATOR FLAP ANATOMY

Understanding perforasome theory is key to propeller flap success. Areas of high perforator density are termed hot spots, while those of a relative paucity are cold spots. In the extremities, hot spots are located adjacent to articulations and at midpoints between 2 articulations; in the trunk, hot spots are parallel to the anterior and posterior midline and the midaxillary line.[1,5,6]

Perforators communicate bidirectionally with one another in series through direct (suprafascial) and indirect (subdermal plexus) linking vessels. With adequate filling pressures through 1 perforator, there is interperforator flow to the adjacent perforasome(s), thus explaining how large flaps can be based off of single perforators. Linking vessels are oriented longitudinally in the extremities

[a] Division of Plastic Surgery, Baylor Scott & White Health, Scott & White Memorial Hospital, 2401 South 31st Street, Temple, TX 76508, USA; [b] Division of Plastic Surgery, Baylor Scott & White Health, 2401 South 31st Street, Temple, TX 76508, USA
* Corresponding author.
E-mail address: Michel.Saintcyr@bswhealth.org

Clin Plastic Surg 48 (2021) 173–181
https://doi.org/10.1016/j.cps.2021.01.002

and perpendicular to midline in the trunk. Furthermore, extremity interperforator flow tends to occur away from articulations versus multidirectional for midpoint perforators. Flow also generally perfuses same-source artery perforators before other-source perforators. These principles form the basis for flap design, whereby flap length and skin paddle orientation should be based on the orientation of the linking vessels (ie, axially in the lower extremity).[7]

The angle of perfusion is another element to consider.[8] When perforators are located at the most proximal aspect of the flap (eccentric), geometric design of the proximal skin paddle (superior angle of the tissue edge proximal to the perforator) influences distal perfusion. Specifically, as the angle increases, more linking vessels are captured, thereby augmenting distal flap perfusion through enhanced interperforator flow, and vice versa. The influence of interperforator flow by the angle of perfusion is less impacted with centrally located perforators, as a more centrally based pedicle captures more linking vessels.

INDICATIONS AND CONTRAINDICATIONS

The perioperative considerations in propeller flap reconstruction of the lower extremity are nearly identical to more traditional approaches and include timing, comorbidities such as vascular disease, and nutrition, radiation, trauma mechanism, and nicotine use. Comorbidities such as diabetes and peripheral vascular disease are posited to increase flap necrosis.[9] Ultimately, although healthier patients are more ideal candidates, those with multiple comorbidities benefit from avoiding a large, complex free flap reconstruction.

In the trauma setting, the injury should be allowed to fully declare and radical debridement achieved, with early reconstruction being generally preferred.[10] The temptation to sacrifice extent of debridement to limit defect size should be avoided.

In the oncologic setting, one should consider delaying reconstruction until pathology indicates clear margins. Additionally, although propeller flaps provide durable coverage that can withstand radiotherapy, previously irradiated wounds mostly require new, well-vascularized tissue via free flap.

The principle indication for propeller flaps includes small- to medium-sized defects with exposed critical structures for which alternatives like skin grafting are inadequate. Size limitations for safe flap design are not firmly understood. Authors have suggested limitations based on clinical experience, while cadaver-based studies have sought to define perforasome areas.[11] In a 2012 systematic review, mean leg defect size reconstructed with propeller flaps was 37.4 cm^2, ranging from 4 cm^2 to 180 cm^2.[3]

PREOPERATIVE EVALUATION AND SPECIAL CONSIDERATIONS

Preoperative imaging is not routinely mandated, as flap dissection can be conducted in freestyle fashion. Nonetheless, Doppler evaluation is quick and prudent. Computed tomography (CT) angiography and other advanced modalities can be obtained as needed, such as investigating vascular integrity after trauma or backup options including free tissue transfer. Other adjuncts like smartphone-based thermography and color duplex have also been employed.[12,13]

The lower extremity represents 46% of the adult total body surface area, with a mean of 93 plus or minus 26 perforators in each extremity. Each clinically relevant perforator can theoretically be incorporated into freestyle flap design; thus flap options are virtually limitless. Here workhorse options are briefly reviewed by level including clinical examples (**Table 1**).

Table 1
Traditional flap options versus authors' preferred propeller flap options by location of defect

Location:	Traditional Flap	Propeller Flap
Groin	Sartorius, TFL, RAM	SFA
Thigh	Leg muscles, RAM, free flap	Rarely indicated; SFA, LSGA
Peripatellar/popliteal fossa	Gastrocnemius, thigh muscles	MSA, SFA/DGA, LSGA, MSFA,
Upper third leg	Gastrocnemius	MSA, PA, PTA, ATA
Middle third leg	Soleus	MSA, PA, PTA, ATA
Distal third leg/ankle	Free flap, reverse sural flap	PA, PTA, ATA

Abbreviations: ATA, anterior tibial artery; DGA, descending genicular artery; LSFA, lateral superogenicular artery; MSA, medial sural artery; PA, peroneal artery; PTA, posterior tibial artery; RAM, rectus abdominis myocutaneous; SFA, superficial femoral artery; TFL, tensor fascia lata.

Superficial Femoral Artery Perforator

The medial thigh yields numerous flaps of varying and inconsistent nomenclature based on the superficial femoral artery (SFA), medial circumflex femoral artery, and lateral circumflex femoral artery.[13,14] SFA flaps are reliably harvested from a mean of 5 perforators, roughly half musculocutaneous, for coverage ranging from the groin, distal thigh, knee, and even proximal tibia and posterior calf.[14–17] Miyamoto and colleagues[15] reconstructed groin defects with flap sizes up to 19 × 8 cm eccentrically oriented along the axis of the sartorius (approximating the SFA).

In the distal thigh, perforators from the SFA (62%) and its principle distal branches, the descending genicular (15%) and saphenous (23%) arteries, can support critical coverage of the knee and popliteal fossa (**Fig. 1**A–E, Case 1 below).[13,14,16]

Lateral Supragenicular Artery Perforator

The lateral supragenicular artery (LSGA) perforator flap represents another workhorse alternative to the gastrocnemius for locoregional coverage of the knee and popliteal fossa (**Fig. 2**A–C, Case 2)[18]. Two perforators are localized within 5 cm laterally and 7 cm proximally from the superolateral patella, and the flap is designed eccentrically from the perforator up to the mid-thigh. Compared with the distally based ALT flap, the LSGA perforator is closer in proximity to the knee and does not as easily suffer venous congestion. The senior author has designed flaps up to 270 cm^2 for knee coverage.[18]

LOWER LEG

Both musculocutaneous and septocutaneous perforators pierce the crural fascia in 4 longitudinal rows (1 row for each major source artery) along the intermuscular septa bordering the compartments of the leg (**Fig. 3**A–C).[19]

Anterior Tibial Artery

The proximal third and distal third perforators are the most reliable clusters, and there are 9.9 plus or minus 4.4 perforators on average. The proximal perforators are largest and ideal for coverage of proximal tibial defects.[20] Distal flaps can cover defects over the lateral malleolus and heel, and flaps as large as 20 × 8 cm have been reported.[20]

Posterior Tibial Artery

Most consider the posterior tibial artery (PTA) to be the most reliable and largest of the leg (4.9 ± 1.7 on average), well-equipped for coverage of the heal, medial malleolus, Achilles, and distal two-thirds tibia (**Fig. 4**A–I, Case 3).[19,21] Reliable perforators are located at each third in 80% of patients, predominantly septocutaneous in the proximal two-thirds.[19] In a 2012 systematic review, mean defect size reconstructed was 46.7 cm^2.[3] Flaps measuring 19 × 13 cm have been reported.[22] For larger flaps, the saphenous vein can be harvested for supercharging. Saphenous nerve can also be included.[22]

Peroneal Artery

There are 4.4 ± 2.3 perforators on average, of which the middle-third perforators are the most

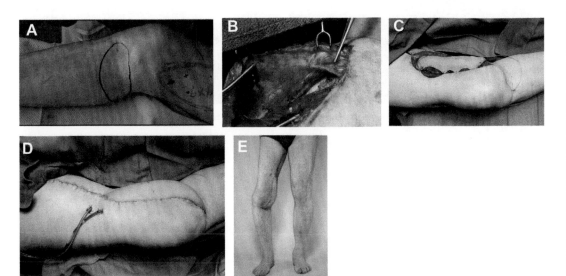

Fig. 1. (Case 1: A–E) SFA perforator emerging through vastus medialis for propeller coverage of peripatellar defect after tumor extirpation.

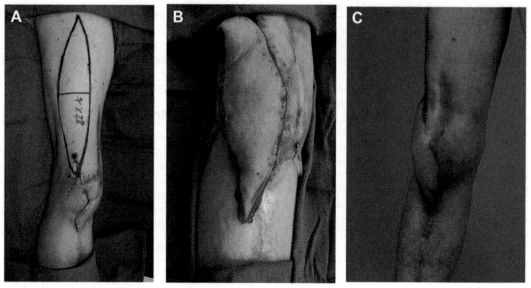

Fig. 2. (Case 2: *A–C*) LSGA perforator flap for reconstruction of a traumatic knee injury with long-term healing.

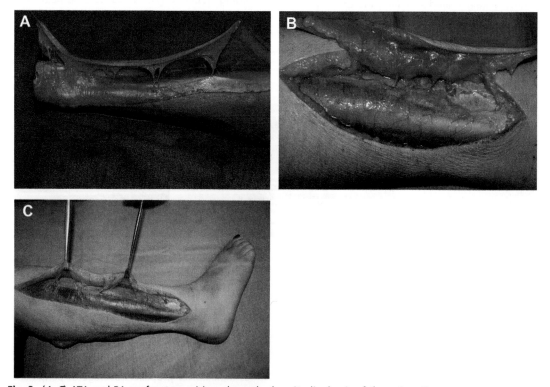

Fig. 3. (*A–C*) ATA and PA perforators arising along the longitudinal axis of the extremity.

reliable cluster (present in 93% of patients). Peroneal artery perforator dissection is the most technically challenging, and the middle-third preferential location limits the flap's clinical utility.[20] Mean defect size reconstructed on systematic review was 28.4 cm^2. However, flaps as large as 10 × 20 cm (200 cm^2) have been reported.[3,23]

Medial Sural Artery

There are 1.4 plus or minus 1.2 perforators consistently, usually paired with the medial sural cutaneous nerve and short saphenous vein.[19] Flaps have been described for coverage of the proximal tibia, knee, and even middle-third defects with a distal perforator.[24] The most proximal perforator is localized approximately 8 cm distal to the midpoint of the popliteal crease on a line drawn to the medial malleolus.[24] Inclusion of a second, more distal perforator can extend the skin paddle safely, with defects up to 15 × 8 cm covered.[25] Of note, any myocutaneous flap with a skin paddle can be converted to a propeller flap with independent rotation (eg, when the medial gastrocnemius is harvested with an overlying medial sural artery

propeller that is independently oriented to fit the defect) (**Fig. 5**A–C, Case 4 below).

SAFE HARVEST TECHNIQUE FOR PROPELLER FLAPS

Armed with knowledge regarding regional anatomy and perforator hotspots, the surgeon first localizes perforators. Strong signals are marked using Doppler, moving from the defect edge retrograde along the axial source vessel (longitudinally). The length of the skin paddle will be designed longitudinally, thereby maximizing interperforator flow from linking vessels. An initial eccentric skin paddle design is marked (see **Fig. 4**A–D).

Once the perforator is localized, dissection proceeds under loupe magnification with a tourniquet. A single, wide exploratory incision is extended from the defect according to the preliminary flap design (see **Fig. 4**E). This incision should accommodate backup flap options (eg, muscle flaps or free flap recipient site). Dissection is conducted toward deep fascia and can proceed either subfascially or suprafascially. Subfascial dissection is generally simpler and can provide a gliding surface

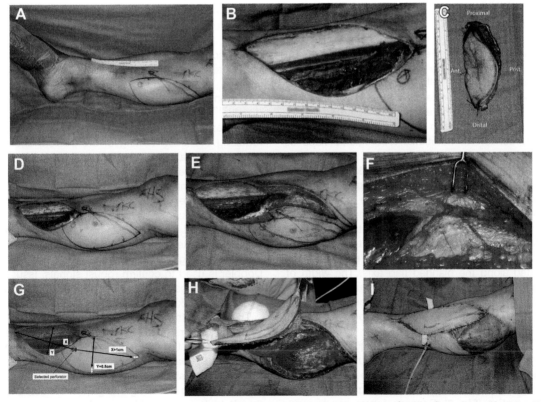

Fig. 4. (Case 3: A–I) Medial lower leg sarcoma defect reconstructed using PTA perforator flap measuring 20 × 7 cm raised on a middle third perforator emerging between the flexor digitorum longus and the soleus.

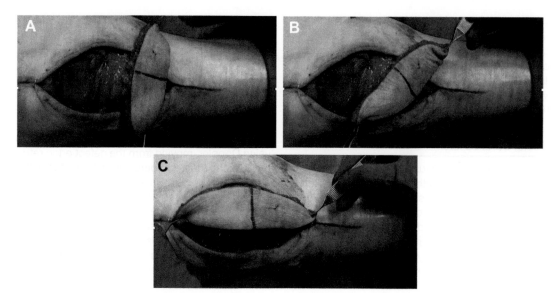

Fig. 5. (Case 4: *A–C*) Knee reconstruction using medial gastrocnemius flap with overlying skin paddle independently rotated as PPF based on an MSA perforator.

for tendons, while suprafascial dissection affords thinner flaps. All perforators near the point of rotation are preserved initially; then the tourniquet is deflated, and Doppler is used to verify arterial and venous flow. The ideal perforator is sizable, out of the zone of injury, and near the defect edge (see **Fig. 4**F). In general, the perforator closest to the defect edge is selected, thereby minimizing flap size requirement and tension on the pedicle. Multiple perforators are generally avoided in true propeller flaps because of pedicle kinking, but may be feasible in flaps rotating less than 90°. Rarely, there are no reliable perforators or flap feasibility is in question, and the surgeon may convert to traditional locoregional flaps or free flap reconstruction.

After perforator selection, flap design is reassessed. The flap is designed slightly larger in area than the defect to minimize tension. The long axis is determined by measuring the distance between the perforator and the distal edge of the defect and adding an extra centimeter. This length is then applied from the selected perforator oriented along the planned flap axis. The width of the flap is based on defect width plus a half centimeter (see **Fig. 4**G). Flaps are designed elliptically to facilitate donor site closure; however, defect templates can be employed.

After final markings, the tourniquet is inflated again, and the flap is raised. Subcutaneous veins along the distal flap edge are clipped at maximal length as potential lifeboats against venous congestion (**Fig. 6**). Sensory nerves can be preserved for neurotization. If deciding between 2

perforators, a clamp is applied to the perforator furthest from the defect to facilitate perforator selection (and vice versa if perfusion is in question). The perforator and comitantes veins are skeletonized to minimize kinking, and side branches are ligated; a small cuff of fascia can be left around the perforator to limit injury risk. Before rotating the flap, the tourniquet is deflated, and the flap is evaluated in situ. Clinical examination and adjuvant imaging as desired (eg, indocyanine green imaging or thermography) are used to monitor perfusion and excise any underperfused areas distally.[12,26]

The flap is rotated into the defect in the direction requiring the least twisting of the pedicle under direct visualization (see **Fig. 4**H). Torsion or stretching necessitate further dissection of the pedicle into muscle or septum as needed to lengthen. Longer pedicles are more robust against torsional forces; further, each flap has a preferential direction of rotation for maximal flow.[27] Most flaps are rotated 180°; however, many require less depending on orientation.[3] After rotation, Doppler is used to confirm robust signals. Issues related to vasospasm, kinking, or improper flap design are quickly apparent in the operating room.

The flap is then inset under minimal tension loosely in layers, and a penrose drain often is placed. Finally, the donor site is closed with deep fascia left unrepaired. A systematic review demonstrated donor sites 37% primary closure versus 63% requiring skin grafting.[3] The authors' threshold for skin grafting, particularly near the pedicle, is low to avoid excess pedicle

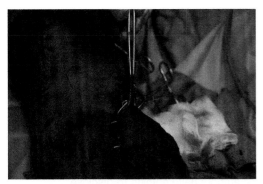

Fig. 6. PTA perforator flap elevated with subcutaneous vein dissected out for potential use as a lifeboat (held by forceps) in cases of venous congestion.

compression or tourniquet effect (see **Fig. 4**I). Dressings include light compression distal to the flap and splinting.

POSTOPERATIVE CARE AND EXPECTED OUTCOMES

The flap is monitored clinically postoperatively. There is no consensus regarding postoperative compression and dangle protocols, but elevation is paramount. The author's protocol is individualized; however, it generally consists of compression distal to the flap. Dangling begins on postoperative day 1 for 5 minutes every 4 hours, and is increased 5 minutes per session every 2 days. Limited ambulation is usually commenced by the first week. Recent investigation suggests benefit to including the flap in compression and demonstrated excellent outcomes by introducing progressively increased, intermittent compression on postoperative day 3 and ambulation on postoperative day 5; there was no diminution in perforator flow velocity or volume with a custom 30 to 35 mm Hg pressure garment applied.[28]

On systematic review, propeller flaps had a 26% overall complication rate in the lower extremity,[3] comparable to literature-reported rates for free tissue transfer (16%–38%).[10] Complications included 11% partial flap loss, 8% venous congestion, 4% epidermolysis, less than 2% hematoma, and 6.5% return to the operating room. Ultimately, flap failure occurred just 1% of the time, less than free tissue transfer (4%–19%).[3,29] Risk was not correlated with age, gender, etiology of wound, or flap size. Larger peroneal artery perforator flaps (>120 cm[2]) and flaps of the distal third extremity had more complications. Meta-analysis demonstrated comparable outcomes as

well, including flap failure (2.8% propeller vs 3.9% free flap) and overall complications (21.4% propeller vs 19.0% free flap). Propeller flaps had higher rates of partial necrosis, but less wound dehiscence and infection.[30]

MANAGEMENT OF COMPLICATIONS

A well-vascularized flap often appears hyperemic, but without the quick capillary refill more indicative of venous congestion. If the flap does suffer congestion, the surgeon should first rule out overly tight donor-site closure or compression secondary to fluid collection. Sutures may be opened to reduce tension and allow egress of fluid. If congestion persists, the flap undergoes operative interrogation, evaluating for twisting, compression, or excess tension of the pedicle. The flap can also be a derotated, further pedicle dissected, or utilized as an advancement flap. Finally, if there is truly an intrinsic flap issue, lifeboat veins may be anastomosed. Ultimately, flap necrosis is allowed to declare, and the surgeon may elect for debridement, dressing changes, skin graft, advancement, or free tissue transfer.

REVISION OR SUBSEQUENT PROCEDURES

Secondary orthoplastic procedures are also possible given the fasciocutaneous design. The reconstructive surgeon should be present for re-elevation of the flap. Unlike traditional bulky flap counterparts, PPFs also do not typically warrant recontouring. Nonetheless, similar revision procedures may be offered to the patient a year or more after the index operation including suction lipectomy for flap thinning, scar revision, and serial excision of donor-site skin graft.

CASE DEMONSTRATIONS

Case 1 (From **Fig. 1**A–E). SFA perforator emerging through vastus medialis for propeller coverage of peripatellar defect after tumor extirpation.

Case 2 (From **Fig. 2**A–C). LSGA perforator flap for reconstruction of a traumatic knee injury with long-term healing.

Case 3 (From **Fig. 4**A–I). Medial lower leg sarcoma defect reconstructed using PTA perforator flap measuring 20 × 7 cm raised on a middle third perforator emerging between the flexor digitorum longus and the soleus.

Case 4 (From **Fig. 5**A–C). Knee reconstruction using medial gastrocnemius flap with overlying skin paddle independently rotated as PPF based on an MSA perforator.

DISCUSSION

Successful propeller flap reconstruction relies on an understanding of perforator anatomy, identifying clinically robust perforators, and adhering to the principles of reliable flap design. Flaps are designed from untraumatized/previously nonirradiated tissues only. All perforators near the defect are initially preserved, and then selective clamping and/or adjunctive imaging modalities such as indocyanine green and thermography can help assess perforator reliability and facilitate decision making. A single, wide exploratory incision is extended from the defect according to preliminary flap design and consideration of a possible backup free flap recipient site. An elliptically shaped flap is elevated adjacent to the defect on the most optimal perforator, which is skeletonized for rotation. Lower extremity propeller flaps are most easily dissected subfascially, should be oriented longitudinally, and oversized for the defect. Rotation is commonly 90° to 180°. The donor site is closed primarily if possible; however, a low threshold for skin grafting is maintained to avoid flap congestion. The flap should be scrutinized throughout the operation and postoperatively for causes of venous congestion, and early corrective maneuvers should be performed. Problem solving maneuvers include derotation, further pedicle dissection, advancing the flap, or lifeboat vein anastomosis. A cautious dangle protocol is performed.

SUMMARY

Several propeller flap options are available as alternatives to conventional flaps in managing complex lower extremity defects, and their advantages are numerous. Each level of injury has preferable donor sites that can be used to design freestyle flaps according to perforator flap principles.

CLINICS CARE POINTS

- Subfascial dissection of propeller flaps is generally easier for identifying perforators as opposed to suprafascial dissection.
- Harvest begins with a single exploratory incision that can be converted for muscle flap harvest or free flap recipient site dissection as backup options if adequate perforators are absent.
- All perforators near the defect are initially preserved during harvest until committing to the most robust and opportunely located perforator.
- Selective clamping and/or adjunctive imaging modalities such as indocyanine green and

thermography can help assess perforator reliability.
- A superficial vein can be harvested for sue as a flap lifeboat.
- The threshold for skin grafting the donor site should be low to avoid pedicle constriction; mature skin grafts can be excised serially to improve long-term cosmesis.

DISCLOSURE

The authors have nothing to disclose.

REFERENCES

1. Mohan AT, Sur YJ, Zhu L, et al. The concepts of propeller, perforator, keystone, and other local flaps and their role in the evolution of reconstruction. Plast Reconstr Surg 2016;138(4):710e–29e.
2. Lecours C, Saint-Cyr M, Wong C, et al. Freestyle pedicle perforator flaps: clinical results and vascular anatomy. Plast Reconstr Surg 2010;126(5): 1589–603.
3. Gir P, Cheng A, Oni G, et al. Pedicled-perforator (propeller) flaps in lower extremity defects: a systematic review. J Reconstr Microsurg 2012;28(9): 595–601.
4. Pignatti M, Ogawa R, Hallock GG, et al. The "Tokyo" consensus on propeller flaps. Plast Reconstr Surg 2011;127(2):716–22.
5. Wong C, Saint-Cyr M, Mojallal A, et al. Perforasomes of the DIEP flap: vascular anatomy of the lateral versus medial row perforators and clinical implications. Plast Reconstr Surg 2010;125(3):772–82.
6. Saint-Cyr M, Schaverien M, Wong C, et al. The extended anterolateral thigh flap: anatomical basis and clinical experience. Plast Reconstr Surg 2009; 123(4):1245–55.
7. Saint-Cyr M, Wong C, Schaverien M, et al. The perforasome theory: vascular anatomy and clinical implications. Plast Reconstr Surg 2009;124(5): 1529–44.
8. Laungani AT, Christner J, Primus JA, et al. Study of the impact of the location of a perforator in the perfusion of a perforator flap: the concept of "angle of perfusion. J Reconstr Microsurg 2017;33(1):049–58.
9. Quaba O, Quaba A. Pedicled perforator flaps for the lower limb. Semin Plast Surg 2006;20(2):103–11.
10. Lee ZH, Stranix JT, Rifkin WJ, et al. Timing of microsurgical reconstruction in lower extremity trauma: an update of the godina paradigm. Plast Reconstr Surg 2019;144(3):759–67.
11. Sur YJ, Morsy M, Mohan AT, et al. Three-dimensional computed tomographic angiography study of the interperforator flow of the lower leg. Plast Reconstr Surg 2016;137(5):1615–28.

12. Pereira N, Hallock GG. Smartphone thermography for lower extremity local flap perforator mapping. J Reconstr Microsurg 2020;1(212). https://doi.org/10.1055/s-0039-3402032.

13. Mojallal A, Boucher F, Shipkov H, et al. Superficial femoral artery perforator flap: anatomical study of a new flap and clinical cases. Plast Reconstr Surg 2014;133(4):934–44.

14. Mohan AT, Zhu L, Morsy M, et al. Reappraisal of perforasomes of the superficial femoral, descending genicular, and saphenous arteries and clinical applications to locoregional reconstruction. Plast Reconstr Surg 2019;143(3):613E–27E.

15. Miyamoto S, Kayano S, Kamizono K, et al. Pedicled superficial femoral artery perforator flaps for reconstruction of large groin defects. Microsurgery 2014;34(6):470–4.

16. Zheng HP, Zhuang YH, Lin J, et al. Revisit of the anatomy of the distal perforator of the descending genicular artery and clinical application of its perforator "propeller" flap in the reconstruction of soft tissue defects around the knee. Microsurgery 2015;35(5):370–9.

17. Ratanshi I, McInnes CW, Islur A. The proximal superficial femoral artery perforator flap: anatomic study and clinical cases. Microsurgery 2017;37(6):581–8.

18. Nguyen AT, Wong C, Mojallal A, et al. Lateral supragenicular pedicle perforator flap: clinical results and vascular anatomy. J Plast Reconstr Aesthet Surg 2011;64(3):381–5.

19. Schaverien M, Saint-Cyr M. Perforators of the lower leg: analysis of perforator locations and clinical application for pedicled perforator flaps. Plast Reconstr Surg 2008;122(1):161–70.

20. Saint-Cyr M, Schaverien MV, Rohrich RJ. Perforator flaps: history, controversies, physiology, anatomy, and use in reconstruction. Plast Reconstr Surg 2009;123(4):132–45.

21. Satoh K, Sakai M, Hiromatsu N, et al. Heel and foot reconstruction using reverse-flow posterior tibial flap. Ann Plast Surg 1990;24(4):318–27.

22. Koshima I, Moriguchi T, Ohta S, et al. The vasculature and clinical application of the posterior tibial perforator-based flap. Plast Reconstr Surg 1992;90(4):643–9.

23. Cheng L, Yang X, Chen T, et al. Peroneal artery perforator flap for the treatment of chronic lower extremity wounds. J Orthop Surg Res 2017;12(1). https://doi.org/10.1186/s13018-017-0675-z.

24. Tee R, Jeng SF, Chen CC, et al. The medial sural artery perforator pedicled propeller flap for coverage of middle-third leg defects. J Plast Reconstr Aesthet Surg 2019;72(12):1971–8.

25. Luca-Pozner Vlad, Delgove Anais, Kerfant Nathalie, et al. Medial sural artery perforator flap for leg and knee coverage: extended skin paddle with 2 perforators. Ann Plast Surg 2020. https://doi.org/10.1097/SAP.0000000000002356.

26. Jakubietz RG, Schmidt K, Bernuth S, et al. Evaluation of the intraoperative blood flow of pedicled perforator flaps using indocyanine green-fluorescence angiography. Plast Reconstr Surg Glob Open 2019;1. https://doi.org/10.1097/gox.0000000000002462.

27. Dancey A, Blondeel PN. Technical tips for safe perforator vessel dissection applicable to all perforator flaps. Clin Plast Surg 2010;37(4):593–606.

28. Suh HP, Jeong HH, Hong JPJ. Is early compression therapy after perforator flap safe and reliable? J Reconstr Microsurg 2019;35(5):354–61.

29. Spector JA, Levine S, Levine JP. Free tissue transfer to the lower extremity distal to the zone of injury: indications and outcomes over a 25-year experience. Plast Reconstr Surg 2007;120(4):952–9.

30. Bekara F, Herlin C, Somda S, et al. Free versus perforator-pedicled propeller flaps in lower extremity reconstruction: what is the safest coverage? A meta-analysis. Microsurgery 2018;38(1):109–19.

Perforator-Plus Flaps in Lower Extremity Reconstruction

Ping Song, MD, Lee L.Q. Pu, MD, PhD*

KEYWORDS

• Perforator flap • Skin flap • Perforator-plus flap • Soft tissue reconstruction • Lower extremity

KEY POINTS

- The perforator-plus flap combines a perforator flap with a traditional skin rotation flap.
- Ubiquitous use of hand-held Doppler and other preoperative imaging techniques make the perforator-plus flap a viable option for soft tissue reconstruction.
- The flap is technically simple to perform and faster than traditional free flaps.
- It is a viable alternative option for soft tissue reconstruction once targeted perforators are identified.

INTRODUCTION

Lower extremity trauma remains a reconstructive challenge to plastic surgeons. Many such defects occur as a result of high-energy impact and are often associated with concomitant osseous and vascular injuries. The treatment concepts for traumatized lower extremities have evolved throughout modern times, with the most contemporary advances in the field of microsurgery. This has led to reliable use of free tissue transfer for coverage of the distal third of leg wounds, with current literature in agreement with this treatment algorithm.[1,2]

Even though free flaps are a readily available option for lower extremity soft tissue coverage, they may not be the best solution in every patient because of donor site morbidity and the surgeon's access and expertise to microvascular free tissue transfer. Research in the angiosome and perforasome concepts have introduced another reconstructive solution: the perforator flap.[3–6] However, classic perforator flaps are restricted by their sole vascular pedicle, which can limit the flap design because of concern over inadequate circulation, especially venous congestion and ultimate success of flap coverage.

The perforator-plus flap can be considered a modification of the classic perforator-based fasciocutaneous flap.[7] Instead of the skin paddle being supplied solely on the isolated perforator, the perforator-plus flap allows for an augmentation of the vascular supply to the perforating pedicle by keeping the skin paddle attached to a cutaneous base. Both the arterial inflow and venous outflow become more reliable. In exchange for a smaller arc of rotation, a larger and more robust skin flap can be designed. Although this flap does not replace free tissue transfer, it does offer reliable soft tissue coverage in appropriate wounds, with the added benefit of sparing the patient additional donor site complications and prolonged operating time. Additionally, it does not exclude from higher level of microvascular reconstruction.

INDICATIONS AND CONTRAINDICATIONS

The indications for perforator-plus flaps are the same as for any local or regional flaps as long as

Division of Plastic Surgery, Department of Surgery, University of California Davis Medical Center, University of California at Davis, 2335 Stockton Boulevard, Room 6008, Sacramento, CA 95817, USA
* Corresponding author.
E-mail address: llpu@ucdavis.edu

Clin Plastic Surg 48 (2021) 183–192
https://doi.org/10.1016/j.cps.2020.12.003
0094-1298/21/© 2020 Elsevier Inc. All rights reserved.

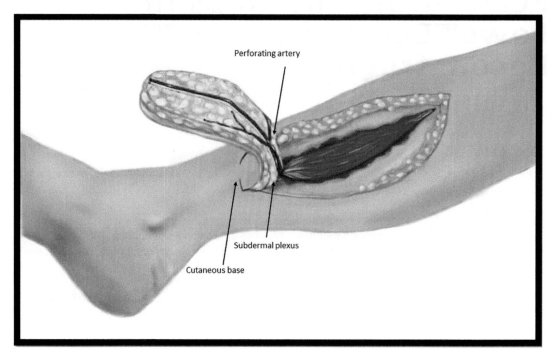

Fig. 1. A schematic diagram to illustrate the perforator-plus flap anatomy and design. Note the attached cutaneous base that allows a dual blood supply from the perforating vessel and the subdermal plexus.

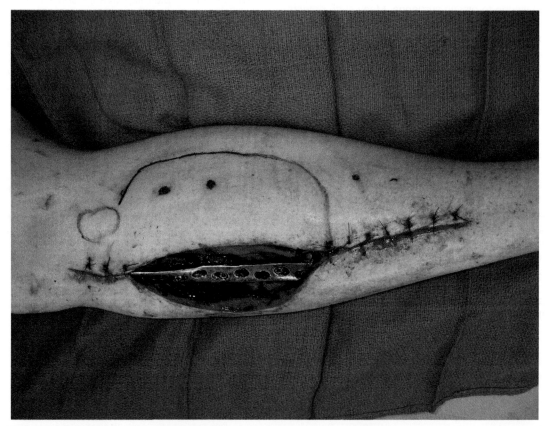

Fig. 2. An intraoperative view shows the outline of the flap, 2 identified perforators within the flap territory, and intact skin portion.

reliable perforators within the flap territory can be reliably identified and the flap itself is not within zone of injury. The common indications for perforator-plus flaps in the senior author's practice are any less extensive lower extremity soft tissue defects with exposed hardware or vital structures. This could be any acute or chronic wounds (up to 50 cm^2) in the lower extremity, but the timing of such a reconstruction depends on zone of injury and mechanism of injury. In general, definitive flap reconstruction is usually performed within 7 to 10 days after injury in the acute setting if the patient's medical condition is permissible.

The contraindications are poor local soft tissue compliance (ie, radiation changes, poorly controlled lymphedema); absolute limb salvage contraindications or patient desire for amputation; and no available local perforasomes secondary to zone of injury or prior surgery/scars; and large defects that require more soft tissue coverage than locally available flap tissue.

PREOPERATIVE EVALUATION AND SPECIAL CONSIDERATIONS

The patient is seen in consultation and the wound evaluated. The surgeon must take into account the acuity of the wound, the zone of injury, defect size, and defect components. Additionally in the acute setting, one must consider evolving tissue loss. Unlike free-tissue transfer, the use of a local perforator-plus flap relies on a reliable local soft tissue donor site.

The authors prefer the use of intraoperative Duplex scan in addition to a hand-held Doppler to accurately identify target perforators.[8] In general, at least 1 good perforator is needed for the design of such a flap. The ad hoc nature of this step can be considered free style, as it relies on the reconstructive surgeon's expertise to determine the planned approach. However, preoperative CT angiogram may also serve as adjunct to presurgical workup. This does not replace intraoperative Duplex or Doppler to pinpoint the exact locations of the cutaneous perforators. Because there may be several adjacent perforators, the flap design is finalized based on the most appropriate perforator and arc of flap rotation to maintain a skin bridge prior to the start of the flap dissection.

Ultimately, it is important to evaluate the defect in light of the patient's potential donor sites and the associated morbidity of free tissue transfer. However, if a perforator-plus flap is chosen as the first-line reconstructive option, it is imperative

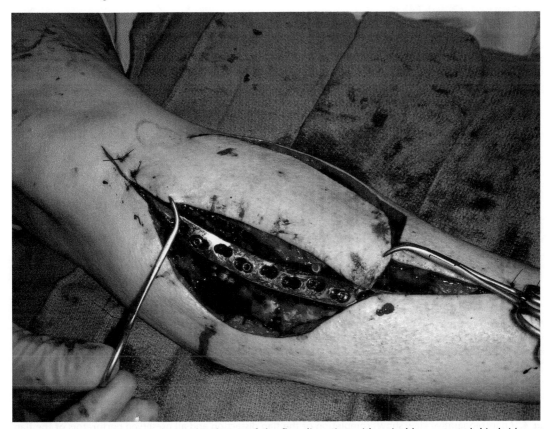

Fig. 3. An intraoperative view shows completion of the flap dissection with a sizable connected skin bridge.

to discuss with the patient the step-wise approach of possible regional, distant, or free tissue transfer as salvage options.

SURGICAL PROCEDURES
Pertinent Anatomy of the Flap

The perforator-plus flap receives its blood supply primarily from 1 or 2 or more musculocutaneous or septocutaneous perforators, the same as any other free style pedicled perforator flaps. It also receives an additional blood supply from the intact skin bridge, since both the arterial inflow and venous outflow can be augmented (**Fig. 1**). Depend on the width of the skin bridge, the flap itself may even survive based on the intact skin connection. With this kind of flap design, the perforator-plus flap would be more reliable, since an additional skin bride can serve as a supercharge that can minimize ischemia or venous congestion of the flap. Therefore, in exchange for a smaller arc of rotation, a larger and more robust skin flap can be designed.

Flap Design and Dissection

The flap design is essentially the same as a skin rotation flap. The flap is marked with a marking pen first, and at least 1 perforator within the flap territory is then identified with a duplex scan (**Fig. 2**). The information regarding the size, blood flow, and intramuscular course of each perforator can be obtained. All perforators are again confirmed by a hand-held Doppler before flap elevation. The incision is carried down to the level of the fascia, and a suprafascial dissection is completed to raise the skin paddle, keeping the most proximal portion attached to its cutaneous base. The width of such a skin connection really depends on the required arc of flap rotation (**Fig. 3**). During the flap dissection, attention is paid to identify and preserve the perforators (**Fig. 4**). Although intramuscular dissection of the perforator can be performed, it is usually not necessary, since the flap can be rotated and advanced to the defect without difficulty (**Fig. 5**). If necessary, intramuscular dissection of the perforator can be performed to improve arc of the flap rotation. This can be facilitated by use of a hand-held Doppler. A skin graft is often needed for the flap donor site as any other skin rotation flaps (**Fig. 6**).

No use of pneumatic tourniquets is needed in those cases. All skin edge bleeding can be

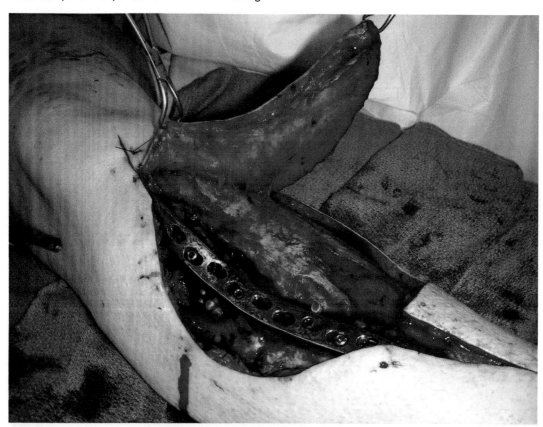

Fig. 4. An intraoperative view shows completion of the flap dissection and all preserved perforators of the flap.

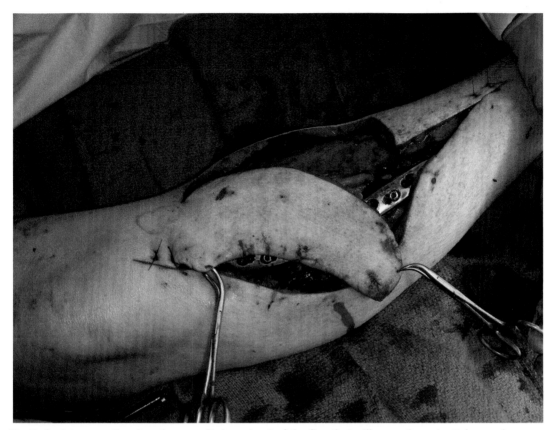

Fig. 5. An intraoperative view shows preliminary inset of the flap that will cover the potential wound.

controlled easily with an electric cautery. General anesthesia is used for patients in the senior author's practice, although regional block is certainly possible. The use of Duplex imaging does require assistance from our ultrasound technicians. It is important to coordinate with the vascular laboratory to ensure timing and prevent delays to the start of the case.

POSTOPERATIVE CARE AND EXPECTED OUTCOME

The postoperative care is often dictated by the region of the reconstruction. For example, a flap wound closure around the knee requires postoperative positioning to decrease tension across the suture lines. It is routine for 5 days of bedrest when skin grafts are utilized in addition to the perforator-plus flap. This allows time for the skin graft to begin revascularization. It is also important to provide immobilization of the limb, and the authors commonly use a soft knee immobilizer to accomplish this.

Elevation of the affected lower extremity in the postoperative period is also important. Even though the perforator-plus design allows for improved venous congestion, the authors believe elevation can augment the drainage of the flap. Weight-bearing status often is dictated jointly with orthopedic surgery colleagues. However, in simple soft tissue defects, return to weight bearing is allowed within 2 weeks, depending on follow-up clinical examinations.

In the authors' experience, venous congestion has not been encountered. Occasionally, there is partial separation of the incision at the distal edge of the flap suture line that can be treated successfully by readvancement of the flap. The authors have not observed any partial or total flap necrosis for nearly 20 perforator-plus flaps in their series. In the senior author's practice, the flap becomes a workhorse in selected patients who have a relatively less extensive skin defect of their lower extremity.

MANAGEMENT OF COMPLICATIONS

One common complication for all lower extremity reconstruction is the presence of venous congestion. If encountered in the immediate operating

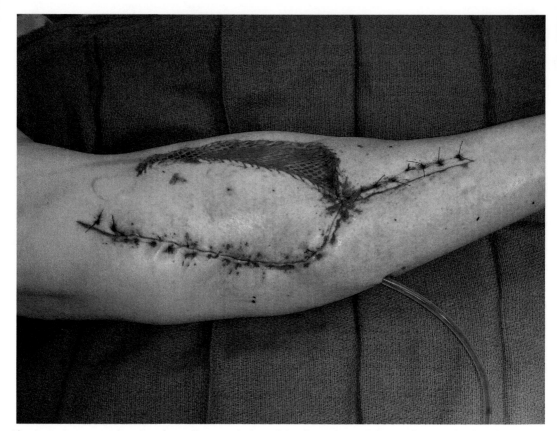

Fig. 6. An intraoperative view shows the completion of the flap inset and skin grafting to the flap donor site.

room setting, interrogation of the pedicle is warranted to ensure no kinking or twisting. If the venous congestion persists, or worsens, the perforator-plus flap can be inset back into the donor site. In case of significant postoperative venous congestion, application of topical nitroglycerin paste or medicinal leech therapy may be employed.

Any delayed wound separation of the flap from the wound can be successfully treated by local wound care. However, if there is exposure of vital underlying structures, readvancement of the perforator-plus flap is indicated. If hardware is exposed, it is advisable to contact the orthopedic surgery team and perform washout prior to readvancement and reinsetting of the flap. In the chance of complete flap failure, the surgeon must be able to proceed with a reconstructive procedure higher on the reconstructive ladder when indicated.

CASE DEMONSTRATIONS
Case 1

A 58-year-old woman presented with history significant for osteopetrosis complicated by chronic

nonunion and osteomyelitis of her left lower extremity. She underwent debridement and plating of her left tibia by an orthopedic trauma service (**Fig. 7**A). Because of significant leg atrophy, the gastrocnemius muscle was not an adequate candidate. An 11 × 5 cm perforator-plus flap was designed and used to cover the exposed hardware and fracture site (**Fig. 7**B). During the procedure, 2 large perforators were identified, and the flap was also based on those 2 perforators. The flap was inset under minimal tension with closure achieved to the opposing wound edge. The flap donor site was skin grafted. The patient experienced no flap problems and went on to successfully heal from her flap reconstruction (**Fig. 7**C).

Case 2

A 38-year-old woman presented with chronic renal failure had a wound brake down after her previous patella fracture repair (**Fig. 8**A). Although the size of her wound dehiscence was small, additional direct wound closure was thought to have high change of failure. After wound debridement, An 11 × 6 cm perforator-plus flap was designed and

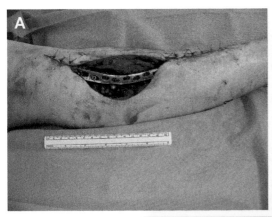
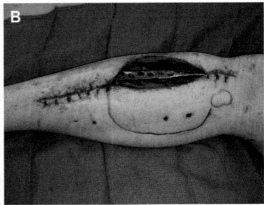
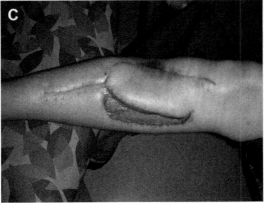

Fig. 7. (*A*) A 58-year-old woman with exposed hardware and fracture site of the left lower extremity. (*B*) An intra-operative view shows the design of the flap. (*C*) Results at 2 months follow-up. Successful flap closure was achieved.

used to close the wound (**Fig. 8**B). During the procedure, 1 perforator was identified, and the flap was also based on that perforator. The flap was inset nicely, and tension-free closure was achieved (**Fig. 8**C). The flap donor site was closed primarily with additional adjacent skin advancement. The patient experienced no flap problems and went on to successfully heal from her flap reconstruction (**Fig. 8**D).

Case 3

The patient was a 65-year-old man with a history of rheumatoid arthritis and on chronic steroids who underwent a right ankle arthroplasty and sub-talar fusion through an anterior incision. Unfortunately, he developed subsequent anterior wound dehiscence resulting in exposure of his extensor halluces longus tendon but no exposure of the hardware (**Fig. 9**A). Because of his medical conditions, the decision was made to perform a perforator-plus flap for his wound closure. The flap was designed and rotated laterally into the

anterior ankle defect (**Fig. 9**B). During the procedure, 1 perforator was identified in the flap based on the posterior tibial artery. The flap was easily inset into the defect without tension. The flap donor site was skin grafted in the usual fashion (**Fig. 9**C). The patient developed a fluid collection from the ankle joint under the flap, and a small site of flap edge separation was noted (**Fig. 9**D) After the initial drainage that was treated successfully with antibiotics per the orthopedic team, readvancement of the flap was performed by the authors' team. A perforator-plus flap was again elevated based on 2 perforators (**Fig. 9**E), and the flap donor site was skin grafted (**Fig. 9**F). The patient went on to heal without further wound complications (**Fig. 9**G).

DISCUSSION

The perforator-plus flap can be used successfully to cover a less extensive skin defect of the lower extremity in selected patients. The authors acknowledge that the perforator-plus flap does

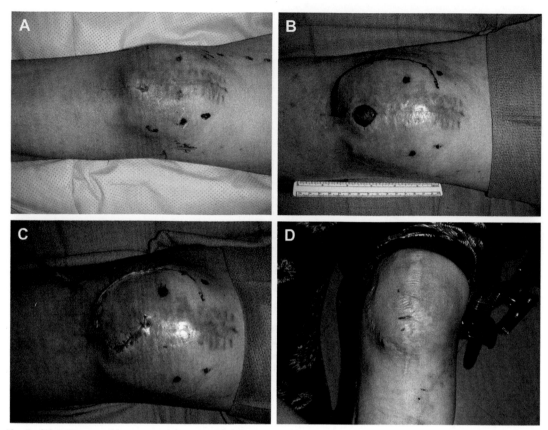

Fig. 8. (*A*) A 38-year-old woman with a wound dehiscence of her right knee. (*B*) An intraoperative view shows the design of the perforator-plus flap with perforators marked out after wound debridement. (*C*) An intraoperative view shows both flap closure and donor site closure. (*D*) Results at 14 months follow-up, and a successful flap closure was achieved.

not replace free tissue transfer; however, it can offer reliable soft tissue coverage in the appropriate wound if reliable perforators can be identified within the flap that is outside the zone of injury. This technique does not burn any reconstructive bridges and can be applied to centers without microsurgical resources. It has the added benefit of less donor site morbidity and shorter operating time than free tissue transfer; additionally, it may have fewer complications related to major surgical procedures in the lower extremity.

Experience has shown that the use of perforator-based flaps for lower extremity reconstruction is a viable option; however, they may face venous congestion and distal flap necrosis, or require delay procedure.[6] These observations are attributable to the anatomic constraints of the sole perforator artery and vein, as well as the degree of rotation that may cause suboptimal flow geometry with inset. In order to address these concerns, Mehrotra describes the use of a perforator-plus design that incorporates a fasciocutaneous flap based on a perforator, and augmented by a retained cutaneous base, achieving a dual blood supply from the perforator and subdermal plexus.[7] By keeping the base of the flap attached, the subdermal plexus helps improve venous outflow, and the perforating pedicle is limited from extreme degrees of twisting or kinking. Additionally, the subdermal plexus can also augment the arterial inflow and allow for a larger, more reliable cutaneous flap to be designed.

The authors emphasize the importance of adherence to the following principles to optimize outcomes. Meticulous identification of local perforator anatomy is by use of multimodality imaging in a free style fashion. Flap design is finalized based on the most appropriate perforator and arc of the flap rotation to maintain a skin bridge and to ensure tension-free closure. Additionally, design should be made to ensure readvancement is possible in case of distal flap separation. Care should be taken with dissection of the

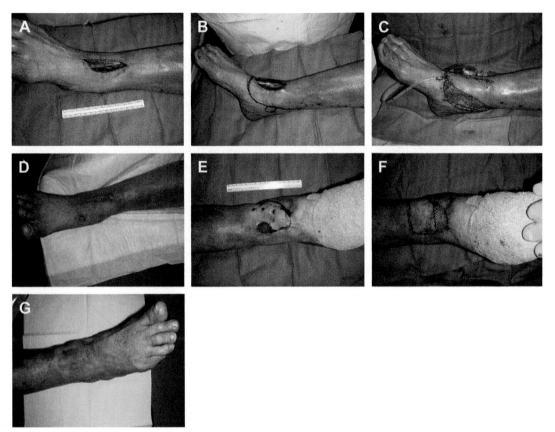

Fig. 9. (*A*) A 65-year-old man with right ankle hardware and tendon exposure after his ankle joint fusion. Note the extensor halluces longus tendon. (*B*) An intraoperative view shows the design of the perforator-plus flap with perforators marked out. The wound has also been debrided. (*C*) An intraoperative view shows inset of the flap and skin grafting to the donor site. (*D*) At 2 months postoperatively, the patient developed a wound dehiscence from chronic drainage under the flap. (*E*) An intraoperative view shows after debridement of the incision dehiscence and the planned readvancement with marked perforators. (*F*) An intraoperative view shows successful re-advancement and skin grafting of the donor site. (*G*) Results at 5 months after secondary procedure; no further complications were seen, and a successful wound closure was achieved.

fasciocutaneous or cutaneous perforator-plus flap and to avoid damage to the subdermal plexus. Observant postoperative care includes immobilization and bedrest if applicable to allow adequate reduction of leg swelling. Any signs of venous congestion can be managed with nonoperative methods (ie, local nitroglycerin paste or leech therapy). In addition, any incisional separation or flap tip necrosis can be successfully treated by readvancement of the flap.

SUMMARY

As the reconstructive pendulum has swayed toward microsurgery in recent decades, the period where one begins to re-embrace options for local fasciocutaneous flaps, especially in the era of perforator flap surgery may be hearing. Although the authors also recognize the role of regional

muscle flaps in lower extremity reconstruction,[9,10] a perforator-plus flap may also play a role in soft tissue reconstruction of the lower extremity, because it is a relatively simple procedure with almost no donor site morbidities except a scar. As continued knowledge and techniques in these arenas improve, plastic surgeons should also make room in their armamentarium for these nonmicrosurgical, reconstructive options.

CLINICS CARE POINTS

- A perforator-plus flap is more reliable than a perforator flap.
- Identification of perforators is the key for a successful flap elevation.
- Partial flap necrosis can be managed with additional flap re-advancement.

DISCLOSURE

The authors have no financial interest to declare in relation to the drugs, devices, and products mentioned in this article.

REFERENCES

1. Soltanian H, Garcia RM, Hollenbeck ST. Current concepts in lower extremity reconstruction. Plast Reconstr Surg 2015;136(6):815e–29e.
2. Hallock GG. Evidence-based medicine: lower extremity acute trauma. Plast Reconstr Surg 2013; 132(6):1733–41.
3. Koshima I, Soeda S. Inferior epigastric artery skin flaps without rectus abdominis muscle. Br J Plast Surg 1989;42:645–8.
4. Taylor GI, Palmer JH. The vascular territories (angiosomes) of the body: experimental study and clinical applications. Br J Plast Surg 1987;40:113–41.
5. Saint-Cyr M, Wong C, Schaverien M, et al. The perforasome theory: vascular anatomy and clinical implications. Plast Reconstr Surg 2009;124(5):1529–44.
6. Hallock GG. Lower extremity muscle perforator flaps for lower extremity reconstruction. Plast Reconstr Surg 2004;114:1123–30.
7. Mehrotra S. Perforator-plus flaps: a new concept in traditional flap design. Plast Reconstr Surg 2007; 119(2):590–8.
8. Dorfman D, Pu LL. The value of color Duplex imaging for planning and performing a free anterolateral thigh perforator flap. Ann Plast Surg 2014; 72(Supple 5):S6–8.
9. Pu LL. Successful soft-tissue coverage of a tibial wound in the distal third of the leg with a medial hemisoleus muscle flap. Plast Reconstr Surg 2005; 115(1):245–51.
10. Pu LL. Soft-tissue reconstruction of an open tibial wound in the distal third of the leg: a new treatment algorithm. Ann Plast Surg 2007;58(1):78–83.

Freestyle Local Island Pedicle Flap in Lower Leg Reconstruction

Seng-Feng Jeng, MD*, Marios Papadakis, MD, PhD, MBA,
Hsiang-Shun Shih, MD

KEYWORDS

• Freestyle flaps • Lower leg • Perforator-based flaps • Propeller flaps • Puzzle flaps

KEY POINTS

• The freestyle pedicled perforator flap is an advanced version of the island pedicle flap that can be elevated from various parts of the body to cover soft tissue defects.
• Intramuscular dissection can provide a longer pedicle and reach defects more easily.
• Precise preoperative planning and design, including a backup plan, are essential for the success of free style local perforator flaps.
• Careful patient selection allows for optimal reconstructive outcome with minimal donor site morbidity.

INTRODUCTION

The reconstructive choice of skin coverage and soft tissue defect in the lower leg depends mainly on its location and extent. In the past half century, the gastrocnemius and soleus muscle flaps have been commonly used for upper and middle third defects, but the lower third has to undergo microsurgical free flap transfer, because of the lack of both local muscle and skin flaps with adequate vascular pedicle length.

Conventionally, the vascular pedicle of a pedicled skin island flap depends only on the presence of a direct or a septal vessel that is, the terminal branch of a source vessel or a branch arising from a source vessel and running between muscles before reaching the skin.[1] However, there is a third type skin vessel, probably the most common one, known as the "myocutaneous perforator," which has an intramuscular course between its source artery and its entry to the skin.[2] Pedicled island flaps that depend on this type of skin vessels were often not useable in the past because of their limited pedicle length, which

did not allow the flap to reach far enough to lower third defects in the leg.[3] However, in the middle of 1990s, intramuscular dissection of the "myocutaneous perforator" from its surrounding muscle fibers became possible. The flap elevated using this technique, was named "perforator flap" by Koshima and Soeda.[4] Perforator flaps have since then revolutionized reconstruction from free skin flaps to "perforator"-based flaps. This development was made possible by the angiosome theory of Taylor and Palmer[5] and uses Doppler probes for vascular mapping on skin flaps.

Initially, the perforator flap was mostly harvested as a microsurgical free flap. Rapid accumulation of experience from pioneers,[6,7] as well as better understanding of the vascular territory of individual vessels, intervessel connections,[5] and perfusion characteristics of each clinically significant perforator,[8] led to revisits of many donor sites previously considered unusable for harvesting a cutaneous flap. It was found that, when intramuscular dissection is done, the pedicle becomes long enough that such flaps could indeed be raised. Hence, reconstructive microsurgery entered a

Department of Plastic and Reconstructive Surgery, E-Da Hospital, Yida Road, Jiaosu Village, Yanchao District, Kaohsiung City 82445, Taiwan
* Corresponding author.
E-mail address: jengfamily@hotmail.com

Clin Plastic Surg 48 (2021) 193–200
https://doi.org/10.1016/j.cps.2020.12.004
0094-1298/21/© 2020 Elsevier Inc. All rights reserved.

new era of perforator flaps. In 1983, Asko-Selja-vaara[9] introduced the concept of "freestyle free flap," which was subsequently materialized by Wei and Mardini[10] and Feng and colleagues[11] with several clinical series. Many small to moderate dimensioned skin flaps could be harvested from previously unknown areas, as long as the supplying vessel can be identified. The same principle is applicable to many local island skin flaps traditionally considered nonfeasible, particularly for small and moderate defect coverage.

This article focuses on local perforator-based island skin flaps and their indications, contraindications, and preoperative preparations, including vascular mapping, flap selection and design, and flap dissection techniques. Various types of flap transpositions were shown with clinical cases.

INDICATIONS AND CONTRAINDICATIONS

Indications for freestyle local flap for lower leg reconstruction include the following:

1. Small to moderate size defects of the lower leg.
2. Defects require like-with-like reconstruction, where local or regional flaps provide a superior aesthetic and functional match.
3. Raising a flap with anatomic anomalies, including no sizable perforators found during the dissection.
4. Patients who have undergone multiple flap procedures that have exhausted the typical donor sites.
5. Revision of previously transferred flap with difficult second or sequential reconstruction.

CONTRAINDICATIONS

1. Personal history of heavy smoking.
2. Extended trauma or profound infection of lower extremity
3. Previous radiotherapy around the defect.
4. Nonsizable perforator found during the dissection.

PREOPERATIVE EVALUATION AND SPECIAL CONSIDERATIONS

Freestyle flaps can be harvested from any location where a skin vessel is found. Defect-related parameters and donor site considerations can assist flap selection. The donor sites can be selected based on the "ideal" flap theory. Suitable freestyle flaps for lower leg reconstruction ideally meet following criteria: versatility in design, adequate tissue volume, good texture and color match, reliable large and long pedicle, straightforward flap dissection, and minimal donor site morbidity. To avoid damage of critical structures, such as major vessels or nerves, and to minimize donor site morbidity, knowledge of the anatomy of the lower limb, where the freestyle flap is to be elevated, is helpful. Ideally, a backup flap should also be available in the region where the incision is planned to facilitate conversion to the backup procedure when needed. In our experience, perforators larger than 0.5 mm can reliably be dissected and microanastomosed. Freestyle perforator flaps can be raised as local, regional, or free flaps.

Freestyle local flaps are considered more technically demanding and challenging than conventional flaps. The risk of flap failure decreases with a surgeon's increasing experience and comfort in techniques required for perforator flap dissection under loupe magnification or the microscope. However, disadvantages include the possibility of inaccurately mapping the location of a skin vessel and the inability to predict the pedicle length. For these reasons, surgeons always need a backup plan.

SURGICAL PROCEDURES
Preoperative Skin Vessel Identification

Landmark for a freestyle local flap is the localization of the Dopplered skin vessels. We use the Super Dopplex II model number MD2/SD2 (Huntleigh Diagnosis, Cardiff, UK) connected to a VP10 (10 MHz). Perforator identification is essential to prevent random flap raising and is usually based on the presence of an audible Doppler signal.[12] The more intense Doppler signal should be selected. The signal points should be preoperatively marked, ideally in the expected operative position to minimize discrepancies between audible signals and intraoperative findings.[13] In distal limbs, signals from superficial perforators may overlap with signals from the axial vessel. In such cases, direct pressure on the skin surface with the Doppler probe or moving of the probe at the long axis with its head held at the same point, will alter the perforator signal and help to distinguish it from the axial vessel signal.[14] Intraoperative exploration at the deep fascia plane through the wound edges of the defect or a noncommittal exploratory incision also can reveal suitable perforators supplying potential nearby local flaps, even without prior Doppler-aided mapping.[15]

Flap Design

Flap design depends on the number and locations of detected skin vessels, defect size, regional anatomy, and donor site availability. The originally selected skin vessel can be replaced by a more suitable one found intraoperatively, and the planned skin flap should follow the axiality of its source vessel whenever possible. The flexibility for modification of the size and shape of the skin flap should be maintained and a backup flap with common border should be prepared to cope with unexpected intraoperative findings or injury to the vascular pedicle. The backup flap also can be a free microsurgical flap. The final skin incision should be decided only after taking all skin vessels into consideration and choosing the most reliable one that is long enough to reach the defect. The flap can be advanced or rotated toward the defect, depending on the positional relationship between the pedicle and the defect. Taking care not to strangulate the dissected vascular pedicle, the skin flap can be rotated 180° to reach the defect (so-called "propeller flap").[13]

Dissection

The dissection can be performed in a suprafascial or a subfascial plane. The perforator is then skeletonized under loupe magnification down to the source vessel. Preserving a tissue cuff surrounding the perforator prevents pedicle stretching during harvesting. If more than one skin vessel is found, the best one is selected with various criteria, such as pulsatility, size, number and size of accompanying veins, proximity to the defect, subcutaneous course, and difficulty of donor site closure. Applying microclamps on minor pedicles could assist this decision. Preservation of more than one perforator is advisable, but rarely feasible because of restricted flap movement.

All vessel branches should be meticulously cauterized or ligated with hemoclips to achieve the best possible hemostasis, which allows the surgeon to clearly visualize all skin vessels and important structures. During the dissection, the vascular pedicle should be irrigated with normal saline and lidocaine solution to maintain moisture and always be under minimal tension so that the arterial pulsation can be observed throughout its entire length. If a tourniquet is used, complete exsanguination before tourniquet inflation should be avoided to ensure that blood vessels remain full to assist the dissection. Once a sizable skin vessel is detected by Doppler ultrasonography and confirmed intraoperatively, the freestyle flap can be harvested safely without fear of anatomic inconsistencies.[10]

POSTOPERATIVE CARE AND EXPECTED OUTCOME

Depending on the regions where the freestyle flap is harvested and the size and volume of the flap, the donor site is chosen in an area that matches the recipient site and has a favorable donor site location. The donor site is closed primarily or with skin grafting. Future procedures such as serial excision or tissue expansion allow for excising the skin graft if needed.

MANAGEMENT OF COMPLICATIONS

Freestyle propeller flaps are popular in lower extremity reconstruction; however, their reliability remains uncertain and they have relatively important complication rates. The main complication is venous congestion, which frequently leads to venous necrosis and sometimes total flap failure. Salvage procedures include venous supercharging or conversion into a free flap transfer using the microsurgical technique.

REVISION OR SUBSEQUENT PROCEDURES

The type of tissue transferred can be selected according to the requirements of the recipient site. Usually, freestyle flaps are harvested from the area around the defect, which has the same color, texture, pliability, and thickness. However, in case of bulky flaps, debulking procedures can be done at least 3 months after the flap reconstruction for optimal cosmetic results. These include staged excision, suction lipectomy, or 1-staged full-thickness skin grafting.

CASE DEMONSTRATIONS
Case 1

Freestyle local V-Y advancement flap for coverage of a chronic ulcer of the lateral retromalleolar region with underlying osteomyelitis: (1) the marking line indicates the initial flap design; (2) by means of a handheld Doppler device, an audible perforator was marked; the advancement flap is elevated; (3) flap advancement into the defect and tension-free wound closure; (4) long-term result with uneventful wound healing 6 months after the operation (**Fig. 1**).

Case 2

Freestyle local propeller flap to cover the donor site of a fibular flap: (1) flap design with preoperative marking of audible perforators (blue spots); the proximal skin paddle is designed to be rotated and serve as a propeller flap to cover the donor site defect; (2) after harvesting the fibula osteocutaneous flap, the defect was reconstructed with a propeller flap based on the muscular branch of the vessel; (3) flap rotation into the defect in a propeller fashion and tension-free wound closure; (4) long-term result with uneventful wound healing after the operation (**Fig. 2**).

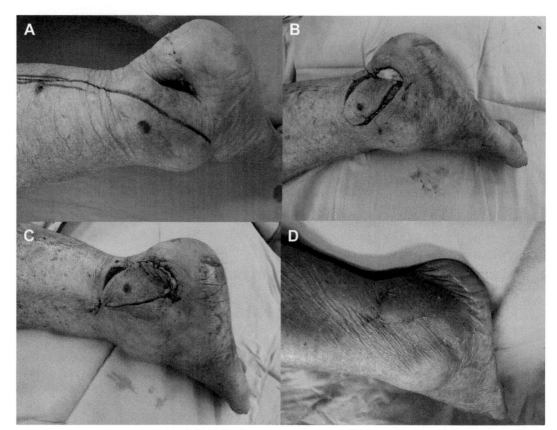

Fig. 1. Freestyle local V-Y advancement flap for coverage of a chronic ulcer of the lateral retromalleolar region with underlying osteomyelitis: (A) the marking line indicates the initial flap design; (B) by means of a handheld Doppler device an audible perforator was marked; the advancement flap is elevated; (C) flap advancement into the defect and tension-free wound closure; (D) long-term result with uneventful wound healing 6 months after the operation.

Case 3

Freestyle reversed anterolateral thigh (ALT) flap to cover an ulcered below-knee amputation stump with soft tissue defect 12 × 7 cm at the middle third of tibia. The flap was elevated and transferred as a regional flap: (1) flap design with preoperative marking of audible perforators (blue spots); (2) flap elevation with skeletonization of the pedicle based on reverse flow of lateral circumflex femoral vessels; the long arrow indicates the pivot point; (3) flap rotated into the defect and tension-free wound closure of donor site; (4) long-term result with uneventful wound healing 6 months after the operation (**Fig. 3**).

Case 4

Freestyle recycled flap to cover an adjacent anteromedial recurrent ulcer defect of the malleolar region: (1) flap design with preoperative marking of audible perforators within the previous ALT flap using Doppler ultrasonography; (2) flap elevation and dissection until the flap reaches the medial defect margin; (3) flap advancement into the defect in a V-Y fashion with primary tension-free wound closure of the donor site; (4) long-term result with uneventful wound healing (**Fig. 4**).

DISCUSSIONS
Freestyle Advancement Flaps

Fig. 1 demonstrates an advancement flap for coverage of a soft tissue defect of the lateral retromalleolar region with exposed bone with chronic osteomyelitis. A Doppler ultrasound detected a skin vessel signal adjacent to the defect, where vascular anatomy was largely unknown to the surgeon, and most of the time distal skin flap is less movable. A skin flap, oblique in design, was elevated and advanced to cover the defect. Compared with traditional rotation flaps, advancement flaps have several advantages, including safer blood supply, as they are not twisted on their axis, possible inclusion of more than 1 perforator, easy conversion into island pedicle skin flaps, and easier to close the donor site primarily.[13]

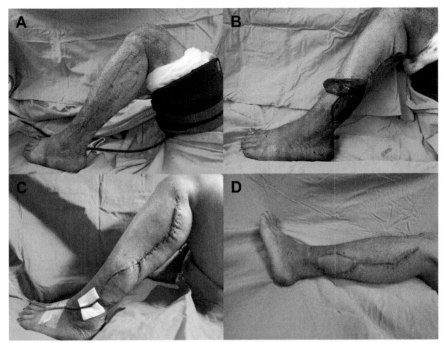

Fig. 2. Freestyle local propeller flap to cover the donor site of a fibular flap: (*A*) flap design with preoperative marking of audible perforators (*blue spots*); the proximal skin paddle is designed to be rotated and serve as a propeller flap to cover the donor site defect; (*B*) after harvesting the fibula osteocutaneous flap, the defect was reconstructed with a propeller flap based on the muscular branch of the vessel; (*C*) flap rotation into the defect in a propeller fashion and tension-free wound closure; (*D*) long-term result with uneventful wound healing after the operation.

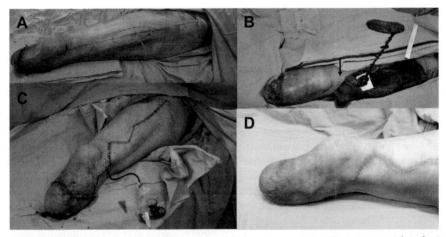

Fig. 3. Freestyle reversed ALT flap to cover an ulcerated below-knee amputation stump with soft tissue defect 12 × 7 cm at the middle third of tibia. The flap was elevated and transferred as a regional flap: (*A*) flap design with preoperative marking of audible perforators (*blue spots*); (B)flap elevation with skeletonization of the pedicle based on reverse flow of lateral circumflex femoral vessels; the long arrow indicates the pivot point, (*C*) flap rotated into the defect and tension-free wound closure of donor site; (*D*) long-term result with uneventful wound healing 6 months after the operation.

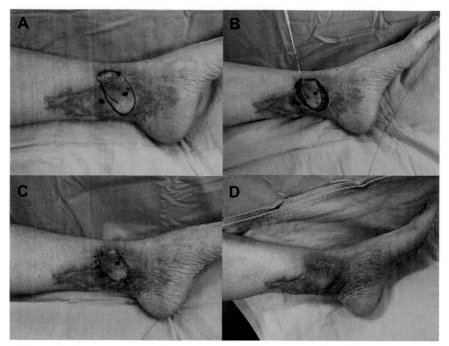

Fig. 4. Freestyle recycled flap to cover an adjacent anteromedial recurrent ulcer defect of the malleolar region: (*A*) flap design with preoperative marking of audible perforators within the previous ALT flap using Doppler ultrasonography; (*B*) flap elevation and dissection until the flap reaches the medial defect margin; (*C*) flap advancement into the defect in a V-Y fashion with primary tension-free wound closure of the donor site; (*D*) long-term result with uneventful wound healing.

However, advancement flaps are not indicated if the distance between the perforator and the nearest defect margin is shorter than the defect's diameter. In such cases, propeller flaps should be considered.

Freestyle Propeller Flaps

Propeller flaps are island flaps that reach the recipient site through an axial rotation.[16] It can be considered an extreme type of rotation flap. The typical propeller flap is longitudinally oriented and elevated from the donor site proximal to the defect. Ideally, its major axis is located on the projection of the source vessel.[17] The skin vessel represents the pivot point. Therefore, the closest one to the defect is preferred. The skin paddle's size should be at least equal to the defect's diameter plus the distance between the skin vessel and the nearest edge of the defect. Propeller flaps should be designed longer and wider than the defect to avoid tension during inset.[16]

Propeller flaps based on skin vessels deriving from the posterior tibial vessels are preferred for defects located in the Achilles region, whereas peroneal-based propeller flaps are usually used for lateral foot, lateral malleolus, and midfoot defects.

Even though the wound closure of the fibula flap donor site has been thoroughly studied and specific techniques and designs have been described,[18] many donor sites require skin grafting. Freestyle skin flaps can facilitate direct wound closure in some patients. The design of such a skin flap for the donor site closure should allow primary closure of its own donor site. **Fig. 2** demonstrates an example of a freestyle propeller flap to cover the donor site of a fibular flap (see **Fig. 2**).

Regional Freestyle Propeller Flaps

Knee defects can be covered with a distally based propeller ALT flap, the distal pivot point being placed approximately 10 cm proximal to the patella. A freestyle skin flap can be elevated from the adjacent area as a regional reversed flow flap,[19] for example, to cover a below-knee stump defect (see **Fig. 3**). Freestyle skin flaps also can be transferred as freestyle adipocutaneous flaps. There is no difference in flap survival between fasciocutaneous and adipocutaneous propeller flaps. The mean arc of rotation in propeller flaps of the lower leg is 160 to 180°, the most common being 180°. Rotation arcs of 90° also have been described, as some investigators associated an arc of 180° with higher complication rates. Most common complications are congestion due to pedicle torsion with compression of the venae comitantes around the artery.[20]

Freestyle Puzzle (Recycled) Flaps

The so-called freestyle puzzle flap refers to the concept of reelevating a previously transferred flap as a pedicled island flap for use either as a local flap or as a free flap for reconstruction of a new defect. Its indications are limited to patients who have undergone multiple flap procedures that have exhausted the usual donor sites, provided there is flap redundancy that allows partial flap elevation, without compromising primary closure of the donor site. The pedicle should be well-bedded and untouched in the adipofascial tissue.[11] One should wait at least 3 to 6 months before considering a flap as a potential puzzle flap donor to allow for adequate neovascularization and safe reliable dissection. Contraindications include previously irradiated, scarred, or severely infected flaps.

Feng and colleagues[11] were the first to report 2 successful pedicled puzzle flaps for lower leg reconstruction. They recommended skeletonization of the pedicle flap to maximize its local transfer. **Fig. 4** shows the use of a freestyle puzzle flap based on the pedicle of a prior free ALT flap to reconstruct a chronic wound of the adjacent soft tissue. The recycling concept has also been used to elevate pedicled flaps from previously transferred tensor fascia lata flap for reconstruction of recurrent trochanter pressure sores and from chimeric latissimus dorsi and serratus anterior free flap for foot and ankle reconstruction.

SUMMARY

In the past 2 decades, island pedicled local flaps have gradually gained popularity for reconstruction of lower leg defects, especially of the lower third, because of their ability to provide longer vascular pedicles through intramuscular dissection. The technique for harvesting perforator flaps facilitated the discovery of numerous new donor sites for skin flaps of small to moderate size. Moreover, it recruited new flap donor sites that were traditionally considered unusable. Further efforts from pioneer surgeons led to freestyle flaps, and now a skin flap can be raised anywhere a strong Doppler signal is detected, and locally used to reconstruct defects without microsurgery. This development is a new major weapon in the reconstructive arsenal, relieving concerns regarding vascular anatomic variations in flap surgery. The results of coverage using local island pedicle skin flaps are just as good if not better than those of microsurgical flaps.

CLINICS CARE POINTS

- Freestyle pedicle flaps can be harvested from any location of lower leg and foot where a skin vessel in which the size of perforators greater than 0.5mm are reliable enough for dissection is found.
- The donor sites could be selected, based on the "ideal" flap theory, versatile in its design. Suitable freestyle flaps for lower leg reconstruction ideally meet following criteria: versatility in design, adequate tissue volume, good texture and color match, straightforward flap dissection and minimal donor site morbidity.
- To elevate a freestyle pedicle flap, using the handheld ultrasound to map the perforator, one side of incision and retrograde dissection using the meticulous techniques.
- A back-up flap should also be available in the region where the freestyle flap is considered. The incisions should be planned to facilitate conversion to the back-up flap when needed.

ACKNOWLEDGMENTS

The authors thank Professor Fu-Chan Wei for his helpful suggestions to this article.

DISCLOSURE

The authors have nothing to disclose.

REFERENCES

1. Hallock GG. Complications of 100 consecutive local fasciocutaneous flaps. Plast Reconstr Surg 1991;88: 264–8.
2. Harii K, Ohmori K, Sekiguchi J. The free musculocutaneous flap. Plast Reconstr Surg 1976;57:294–303.
3. Song YG, Chen GZ, Song YL. The free thigh flap: a new free flap concept based on the septocutaneous artery. Br J Plast Surg 1984;37:149–59.
4. Koshima I, Soeda S. Inferior epigastric artery skin flaps without rectus abdominis muscle. Br J Plast Surg 1989;42(6):645–8.
5. Taylor GI, Palmer JH. The vascular territories (angiosomes) of the body: experimental study and clinical applications. Br J Plast Surg 1987;40(2):113–41.
6. Nakajima H, Fujino T, Adachi S. A new concept of vascular supply to the skin and classification of skin flaps according to their vascularization. Ann Plast Surg 1986;16(1):1–19.
7. Wei FC, Jain V, Celik N, et al. Have we found an ideal soft-tissue flap? An experience with 672

anterolateral thigh flaps. Plast Reconstr Surg 2002; 109:2219–30.

8. Saint-Cyr M, Wong C, Schaverien M, et al. The perforasome theory: vascular anatomy and clinical implications. Plast Reconstr Surg 2009;124(5): 1529–44.

9. Asko-Seljavaara S. Free style free flaps. Abstracts of the Seventh Congress of the International Society of Reconstructive Microsurgery. New York, June 19–30, 1983.

10. Wei FC, Mardini S. Freestyle free flaps. Plast Reconstr Surg 2004;114(4):910–6.

11. Feng KM, Hsieh CH, Jeng SF. Freestyle puzzle flap: the concept of recycling a perforator flap. Plast Reconstr Surg 2013;131(2):258–63.

12. Mardini S, Tsai FC, Wei FC. The thigh as a model for free style free flaps. Clin Plast Surg 2003;30(3): 473–80.

13. Brunetti B, Tenna S, Aveta A, et al. Freestyle local perforator flaps: versatility of the v-y design to reconstruct soft-tissue defects in the skin cancer population. Plast Reconstr Surg 2013;132(2):451–60.

14. Bhat S, Shah A, Burd A. The role of freestyle perforator-based pedicled flaps in reconstruction of delayed traumatic defects. Ann Plast Surg 2009; 63(1):45–52.

15. Lecours C, Saint-Cyr M, Wong C, et al. Freestyle pedicle perforator flaps: clinical results and vascular anatomy. Plast Reconstr Surg 2010;126(5): 1589–603.

16. Ioannidis S, Spyropoulou GA, Sadigh P, et al. Pedicled freestyle perforator flaps for trunk reconstruction: a reliable method. Plast Reconstr Surg 2015; 135(2):602–9.

17. Innocenti M, Menichini G, Baldrighi C, et al. Are there risk factors for complications of perforator-based propeller flaps for lower-extremity reconstruction? Clin Orthop Relat Res 2014;472(7):2276–86.

18. Pachón Suárez JE, Sadigh PL, Shih HS, et al. Achieving direct closure of the anterolateral thigh flap donor site-an algorithmic approach. Plast Reconstr Surg Glob Open 2014;2(10):e232.

19. Sadigh PL, Wu CJ, Shih HS, et al. Reverse anterolateral thigh flap to revise a below-knee amputation stump at the mid-tibial level. Plast Reconstr Surg Glob Open 2014;6(1):88.

20. Bekara F, Herlin C, Mojallal A, et al. A systematic review and meta-analysis of perforator-pedicled propeller flaps in lower extremity defects: identification of risk factors for complications. Plast Reconstr Surg 2016;137(1):314–31.

Free Flaps in Lower Extremity Reconstruction

Lee L.Q. Pu, MD, PhD

KEYWORDS

• Free flap • Free tissue transfer • Lower extremity • Reconstructive microsurgery • Limb salvage

KEY POINTS

- Free flap lower extremity reconstruction remains challenging to plastic surgeons.
- A comprehensive approach has been developed to ensure better clinical outcomes.
- Each step in the comprehensive approach has its unique considerations.
- A second free tissue transfer can also be performed successfully if the cause of the failure for the first free tissue transfer can be identified.
- There is a learning curve for free flap lower extremity reconstruction.

INTRODUCTION

Free tissue transfer to the lower extremity provides a critical means for limb salvage after orthopedic trauma or extensive tumor resection. With many recent advances in reconstructive microsurgery, a successful free tissue transfer can be achieved for soft tissue reconstruction of the lower extremity.[1,2] Frequently, free tissue transfer to the lower extremity may be the only option for limb salvage in patients with a complex traumatic wound.[3]

The overall success rate of free tissue transfer to the lower extremity is still lower than to the head and neck or breast, even from some of the best microsurgery centers in the country.[4–7] This may be due to several important factors. For example, massive edema of the leg is frequently present after trauma and abnormal or thrombogenic recipient vessels are a common problem secondary to peripheral vascular disease or traumatic injury. Therefore, the failure of free tissue transfer to the lower extremity remains relatively common and limb salvage for certain patients is still challenging to many plastic surgeons.

In this article, issues related to perioperative care of lower extremity free flap patients are discussed. The author's comprehensive approach of free tissue transfer to lower extremity is also described in detail (**Box 1**). With many recent advances in reconstructive microsurgery, it is possible that the clinical outcome of free tissue transfer to the lower extremity can be improved.

INDICATIONS AND CONTRAINDICATIONS

The classic indication for free flap lower extremity reconstructions in the author's practice is an extensive wound in the distal third of the leg. In addition, a free flap is frequently indicated for an extensive wound in the upper or middle third of the leg or in the foot and ankle. A free flap is also indicated for a more complex wound in the lower extremity or a large wound with composite tissue loss. The timing of a free flap lower extremity reconstruction usually depends on the patient's readiness and associated medical conditions. In general, a definitive soft tissue reconstruction is commonly performed within 7 to 10 days after initial consultation. However, with vacuum-assisted wound closure, the timing for such a reconstruction can be safely prolonged for to up to 3 weeks.

The contraindications for free flap lower extremity reconstruction in the author's practice are the following: The patient's general medical conditions cannot tolerate a lengthy procedure under general anesthesia; major vascular or nerve injury in the lower extremity; and a large composite

Division of Plastic Surgery, University of California, Davis, 2335 Stockton Boulevard, Room 6008, Sacramento, CA 95817, USA
E-mail address: llpu@ucdavis.edu

Clin Plastic Surg 48 (2021) 201–214
https://doi.org/10.1016/j.cps.2020.12.002

tissue loss in the lower extremity beyond possibility of soft tissue or bony reconstruction. In addition, significant loss of a muscle compartment, associated with a vessel injury, deep vein thrombosis, or a hypercoagulative state are relatively contraindications for a free flap surgery in the lower extremity.

PREOPERATIVE EVALUATION AND SPECIAL CONSIDERATIONS

When a patient is evaluated for free tissue transfer to the lower extremity, his or her medical condition should be evaluated carefully, especially if the patient has an associated injury from trauma. Just like any other surgeries, major surgical risks include previous heart attack, stroke, severe diabetes, uncontrolled hypertension, and significant hepatic or renal insufficiency. Many orthopedic trauma patients are commonly started on anticoagulation agents. Therefore, proper management of anticoagulation therapy for these patients perioperatively can be important to ensure a successful free tissue transfer. It may also be critical to screen certain patients for a hypercoagulable state if they have a history of recurrent vessel thrombosis or embolism or a recent splenectomy, because patients with a hypercoagulable state are very poor candidates for free tissue transfer. An appropriate hematologic consultation may be needed for those patients.

There are several issues that need to be considered for a free flap selection. In general, soft tissue requirement, availability of the flap tissue, and adequate length and size of the flap pedicle are the first 3 important considerations. It has been the author's philosophy that a vein graft should be avoided if possible, for free tissue transfer to

the lower extremity because of the added complexities and risks of venous anastomotic thrombosis. It is also important to select a flap that has minimal donor site morbidities. Sometimes, a surgeon's familiarity with the flap may also be an important factor in flap selection. The commonly used flaps for lower extremity reconstructions in the author's practice are the anterolateral thigh perforator (ALT) flap, or latissimus dorsi, rectus abdominus, and gracilis muscle flaps. The ALT flap has recently been used more frequently in soft tissue reconstruction of the lower extremity, representing a paradigm shift in the flap selection, because most microsurgeons including the author are now familiar with the ALT flap and the flap dissection becomes more successful, even it is still technically challenging.[8] Other perforator flaps can also be selected based on the surgeon's preference and familiarly with the flap.

SURGICAL PROCEDURES
Recipient Vessels Selection

When one considers the selection of recipient vessels, the surgeon should pay attention to both the artery and the vein because it is common that the flap loss is due to venous thrombosis. Therefore, an adequate size and quality of the vein without proximal obstruction is equally important as the artery to serve as a recipient vessel. Avoiding the "zone of the injury" is another important consideration for selection of recipient vessels in free flap lower extremity reconstruction. Lower extremity angiography or computed tomography angiography have been used routinely in the author's practice as a baseline test to evaluate recipient vessels, especially for orthopedic trauma patients. If the surgeon has any suspicion about potential trauma to recipient vessels or deep venous thrombosis, the accompanied vein should also be evaluated separately by duplex scan or venography.

For lower extremity free tissue transfer, it has been the author's preference that one should try to perform an end-to-end anastomosis if possible, even for the artery. This can be true if the anterior tibial artery or dorsalis pedis artery is chosen as a recipient vessel because an end-to-end arterial microanastomosis is considered technically easier by most surgeons, although there are no clear data to show that an end-to-end anastomosis would have better outcomes than end-to-side anastomosis.

As indicated, the descending branch of the lateral circumflex femoral artery and vein or the anterior tibial artery and vein can be dissected free and used as recipient vessels in a turnover fashion for free tissue transfer to the difficult areas of the lower extremity, such as in the distal thigh or around knee (**Fig. 1**). In that way, microvascular anastomoses for both artery and vein can be performed without difficulty and vein grafts can be avoided.[9,10]

Flap Dissection

To ensure a relatively quick and easy flap dissection, the surgeon should know as much as possible about the detailed vascular anatomy of the flap before its dissection. This is particularly true for most perforator flaps. In the author's practice, a duplex scan is routinely used for the preoperative mapping of the perforators, as well as the pedicle of the perforator flap before the flap dissection. In this way, the size and the number of the perforators that can be selected for the flap, the course of potential intramuscular dissection, and even the depth of the flap's pedicle are evaluated.[11] With this critical information in mind, a perforator flap, such as an ALT flap, can be elevated smoothly and safely. For an ALT flap dissection, the combination of retrograde and antegrade dissections of the pedicle can be performed for an easy flap dissection once the skin paddle of the flap is elevated (**Fig. 2**).

Flap Preparation

The pedicle preparation of the flap can also be an important step in free tissue transfer. Once the pedicle of the flap is divided, it is the author's preference that the artery of the pedicle is flushed with a higher concentration of heparinized saline (100 U/mL). In this way, the microvascular system of the flap may be loaded with heparin so that future thrombosis within the flap may be prevented

without the systemic administration of heparin.[12] The pedicle vessels of the flap is prepared under loop magnification. It is the author's preference that the surgical preparation of the pedicle vessels be done mostly with surgical loops so that a lengthy preparation of the pedicle vessels under an operating microscope can be avoided.

In general, no systemic heparinization is needed for a routine free tissue transfer to the lower extremity in the author's practice, although systemic heparin is still used by some surgeons before clamping vessels. Occasionally for the patient with severe peripheral vascular disease, heparinized saline may be perfused distally before the clamping of the recipient artery.

Microvascular Anastomosis

Microvascular anastomosis is a critical step for the success of free tissue transfer. After intense flap dissection and preparation of the recipient vessels, the surgeon should consider taking a break before the next intense part of the procedure (the microvascular anastomosis). It is the author's belief that taking a short break (about 10–15 minutes) greatly enhances the microsurgeon's performance for microvascular anastomosis under a microscope. There are also additional advantages for the patient while the surgeon takes a break. For example, the flap is allowed to rest and perfuse normally after flap dissection to restore normal perfusion, and the recipient vessels can be rested and recovered from vasospasm. In addition, hypothermia or hypovolemia, a common condition when a patient has been under general anesthesia for a longer period of time, can be corrected by the anesthesiologist while the surgeon is taking a break. Because of this break, the surgeon, the

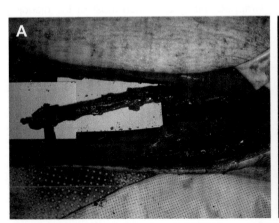 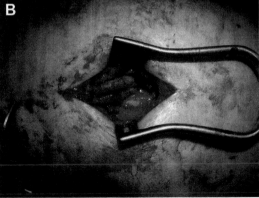

Fig. 1. (*A*) An intraoperative view shows the anterior tibial vessels are dissected free and can be used as recipient vessels after their turnover toward the knee. (*B*) An intraoperative view shows completion of end-to-end arterial and venous microanastomoses of a free flap around the knee with this approach.

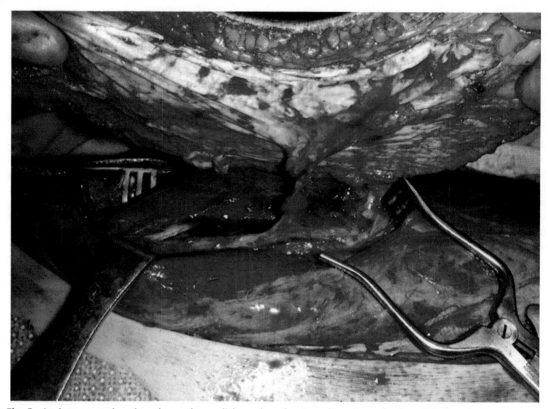

Fig. 2. An intraoperative view shows the pedicle and perforators dissection of a free ALT flap that can be performed from both retrograde and antegrade directions.

patient, the flap, and the recipient vessels are all in optimal conditions and, thus, the success of microvascular anastomosis can almost be guaranteed.

Before microvascular anastomosis, the surgeon should take time to set up the vessels. It is the author's preference that a double-armed microvascular clamp is used to aid an end-to-end arterial microanastomosis (**Fig. 3**). For an end-to-side arterial microanastomosis, an adequate size and shape of an arteriotomy over the recipient artery should be performed to ensure a successful end-to-side arterial microanastomosis (**Fig. 4**). The author prefers to use an 8-0 nylon suture for routine arterial microanastomosis when the size of the pedicle artery is greater than 1.5 mm, resulting in fewer sutures needing to be placed to the anastomosis.

For venous microanastomosis, it is the author's preference that a coupler device is routinely used for an end-to-end venous anastomosis (**Fig. 5**). The author has always been able to find proper size of both pedicle and recipient veins for venous microanastomosis with the device. The coupler device has an excellent patency rate from the study of large clinical series even for the lower extremity free tissue transfer.[13] It is

fast and easy to learn and is shown not to leak once the anastomosis has been completed. It makes venous microanastomosis much more enjoyable without struggling. It also has an additional advantage because the ring of the device may be able to prevent external compression to the anastomotic site.

Once the microclamps are released, it is the author's preference that the arterial anastomosis is wrapped with gauze since most of the bleeding can be stopped with this maneuver. It is seldom necessary to place additional sutures unless there is a high flow of bleeding from the arterial anastomotic site. In that case, a 9-0 nylon suture is used to repair the leak site.

Flap Inset

For a flap inset, it is important to avoid any tension or compression to the arterial and venous microanastomoses. The author prefers to place horizontal mattress sutures for the flap inset so that a more cosmetically pleasing result can be achieved.[14] This can be done for either muscle flap or fasciocutaneous flap. A closed suction drain should be placed away from both microvascular anastomoses (**Figs. 6** and **7**).

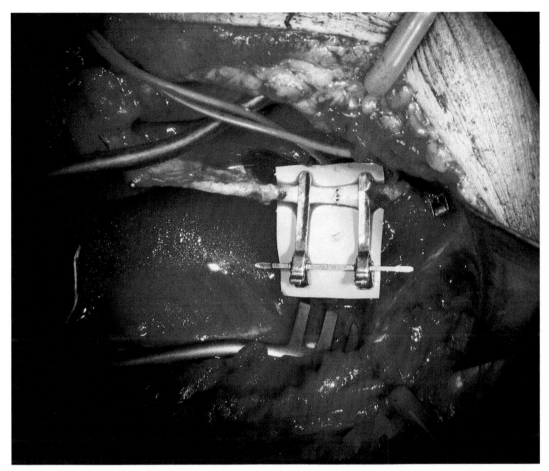

Fig. 3. An intraoperative view shows an end-to-end arterial microanastomosis under an operating microscope. The anastomosis is precisely performed with 8-0 nylon in an interrupted fashion after a proper preparation of both pedicle and recipient arteries.

POSTOPERATIVE CARE AND EXPECTED OUTCOMES

A standard postoperative care protocol for free tissue transfer to the lower extremity is important and practical. This protocol would ensure that everyone on the microsurgical team is on the same page for patient care. It is the author's opinion that protocol-driven postoperative care will be able to provide a better postoperative care after a free flap for the lower extremity reconstruction, especially in a resident training program. **Box 2** summarizes the author's standard protocol for immediate postoperative care for free tissue transfer to the lower extremity.[12,15]

Because the flap is always in a dependent position, intermediate postoperative care for free tissue transfer to the lower extremity can be unique, but also critical. It is agreeable that dangling should be done for each patient so that the flap can tolerate venous congestion when it is placed in a dependent position. Unfortunately, there is no unified dangling protocol that is universally acceptable.[15] **Box 3** summarizes a standard dangling protocol used by the author. The protocol itself has been used widely by the author and his trainees with good success. Recently, wrapping in combination with dangling has been proposed by other surgeons to speed up the process of flap maturation.[16]

Besides ensuring adequate healing of the flap, the contour of the flap in the lower extremity can also become an issue during further follow-up. It has been common that the bulkiness of the flap needs to be revised so that a better contour of the lower extremity can be achieved. It is the author's preference that a minimum of 6 months' waiting period should be expected before a debulking procedure can be considered, especially for a skin-grafted muscle flap. Within the 6 months postoperatively, an elastic wrapping to the flap site can be placed to improve swelling of the flap.

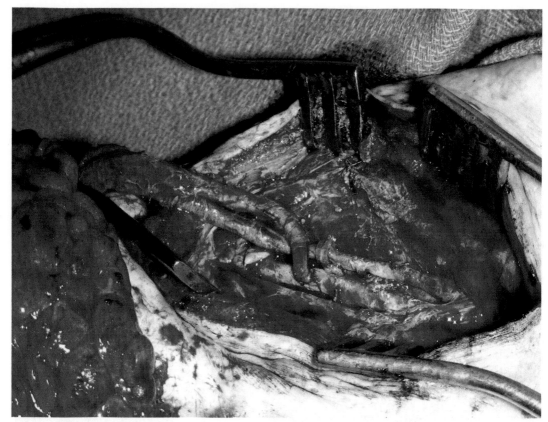

Fig. 4. An intraoperative view shows an end-to-side arterial microanastomosis. The anastomosis is precisely performed with 8-0 nylon in an interrupted fashion after the adequate size and shape of an arteriotomy over the recipient artery is made.

Between 2001 and 2019, more than 200 consecutive lower extremity free tissue transfers were performed by the author for soft tissue reconstruction of a thigh, leg, ankle, or foot wound primarily after orthopedic trauma. The majority of the free flaps in the author's practice were free ALT flaps, free latissimus dosi muscle flaps, free gracilis muscle flaps, and free rectus abdominis muscle flaps. In addition, free-style free perforator flaps and free fibula vascularized bone grafts were also performed. The overall successful rate was about 98%. Flap loss was commonly related to the patient's medical conditions such as perioperative hypotension, thrombocytosis, and deep venous thrombosis. There was no flap loss that was related to any technical issues of the microvascular anastomosis. All patients were discharged home once they tolerated dangling according to the protocol.

MANAGEMENT OF COMPLICATIONS

Complications such as hematoma under the flap, flap dehiscence, distal flap necrosis, and partial loss of skin graft over the muscle flaps, as well as flap donor site problems such as seroma, wound separation, or skin edge necrosis, can be managed successfully with good clinical judgment and well-executed reoperations. The successful outcome of the free tissue transfer to the lower extremity can still be achieved if most parts of the flap have survived.

If the first free flap goes on for a complete loss, the surgeon should be prepared to perform a second free tissue transfer if the cause of the flap failure is critically analyzed. After careful preoperative planning and preparation, meticulous intraoperative execution, and proper postoperative care, the second free tissue transfer can be performed successfully, and limb salvage can still be achieved for those patients.[17]

REVISIONS AND SUBSEQUENT PROCEDURES

In general, flap elevation can safely be performed for subsequent orthopedic procedures after 6 weeks and flap debulking can be performed to improve the contour of the flap after 6 months.[13]

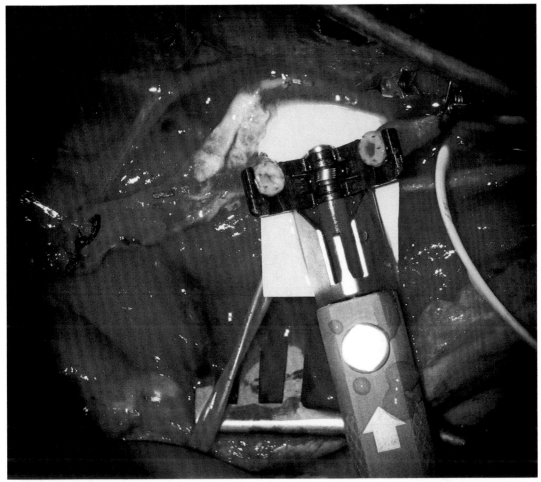

Fig. 5. An intraoperative view shows an end-to-end venous microanastomosis with a coupler device before its completion under an operating microscope. The coupler device is precisely placed to each end of pedicle and recipient veins after a proper preparation.

For a muscle flap, it has been the author's preference that a tangential incision of excess flap tissue can be performed. Once adequate excision of excess flap tissue is done, additional skin grafts are placed to the rest of the flap. In this way a better contour of the leg or foot can be achieved (**Fig. 8**). For a fasciocutaneous flap, suction-assisted lipectomy should be performed first to remove excess adipose tissue of the flap. Additional skin resection is often necessary to achieve better contour of the flap (**Fig. 9**).

CASE REPORTS
Case 1

An 18-year-old man had a complex soft tissue wound measuring 30 × 10 cm over his right lateral thigh and knee with the exposed femur fracture site after being hit by a light train (**Fig. 10**A). Because no suitable adjacent recipient vessel

was available, the descending branch of the lateral circumflex femoral vessel in the distal thigh was explored and dissected free and served as a recipient vessel (**Fig. 10**B). A contralateral ALT flap with a 30 × 10 cm skin paddle was harvested (**Fig. 10**C) and microvascular anastomoses for both artery and vein were performed in an end-to-end fashion without difficulty (**Fig. 10**D). The flap was inset into the defect and a portion of the wound was also closed with a split-thickness skin graft (**Fig. 10**E). The patient's wound healed nicely with well-vascularized flap tissue over his distal femur fracture site (**Fig. 10**F).

Case 2

A 29-year-old man had significant left proximal tibia bone loss and open knee injury from an explosion. He had a large (22 × 10 cm) upper tibial wound extending to the knee after patella

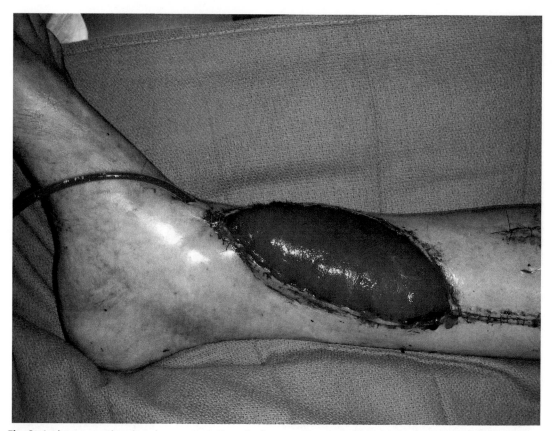

Fig. 6. An intraoperative view shows completion of a free gracilis muscle flap inset into the right distal leg wound before placement of a skin graft. An acceptable contour of the flap is achieved in the operating room.

reconstruction (**Fig. 11**A). An external fixator was placed to stabilize his fractures and bony defect was filled with antibiotic beads (**Fig. 11**B). A free latissimus dorsi muscle flap was selected and harvested to provide good soft tissue coverage of the wound. With the patient in a near prone position, the popliteal vessels were explored and used as recipient vessels for both arterial and venous end-to-side microanastomoses. The flap was inset to cover the entire wound and the muscle flap was covered with a split thickness skin graft (**Fig. 11**C). His extensive knee wound healed without complications. Autologous bone grafting was performed 3 months later after the flap elevation (**Fig. 11**D). The patient was eventually able to ambulate fully without assistance and had an aesthetically pleasing result during follow-up (**Fig. 11**E).

Case 3

A 43-year-old man had a mangled left lower extremity after a motorcycle collision. He was hemodynamically unstable and underwent splenectomy for splenic laceration and subsequently developed acute pulmonary embolism. He had a near circumferential left Gustillo IIIC middle and distal one-third leg wound with transection of the posterior tibial artery and vein in the middle leg. His peroneal artery was also not patent (**Fig. 12**A, B). A medial gastrocnemius flap was performed first to cover the middle third leg wound and during that procedure, both the transected posterior tibial artery and vein were explored and found useable for future microvascular anastomoses (**Fig. 12**C). Two days after, a contralateral free latissimus dorsi muscle flap was performed to cover the distal third leg wound, using both posterior tibial artery and vein stumps as recipient vessels (**Fig. 12**D). The free latissimus dorsi flap surgery was uneventful.

On postoperative day 4, the patient had fever and hypotension owing to an infected hematoma of the left knee. It was noted that both the arterial and venous anastomoses were thrombosed. After embolectomy and redo arterial and venous microvascular anastomoses, both the pedicle artery and vein were patent; however, both microanastomoses were thrombosed again within 1 hour. At this point, the flap became unsalvageable. A temporary vacuum assisted closure device was placed

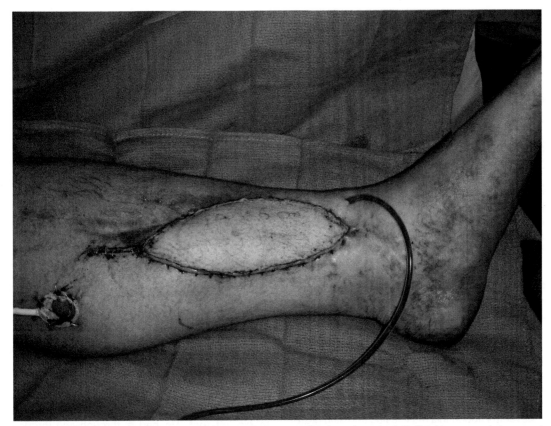

Fig. 7. An intraoperative view shows completion of a free ALT flap inset into the left distal leg wound. An acceptable contour of the flap is also achieved in the operating room.

Box 2
A standard protocol for immediate postoperative care after free tissue transfer to the lower extremity

Aspirin 325 mg suppository per rectum in the recovery room, then 81 mg/d by mouth for 3 months

Lactated Ringer's solution intravenously at ±125 mL/h for 3 days and keep urine output greater than 50 mL/h

Dextran-40 intravenously at 25 mL/h for the first 3 days, half at day and off at day 5 (for difficult and complicated free tissue transfer only)

Warm unit to flap site

Flap check with Doppler/clinical examination every hour for the first 24 hours, then every 4 hours for 4 days (alternative: Cook implantable Doppler monitoring for first 5 days)

Bed rest for first 3 days and may get out of bed at day 4

Physical therapy as per operating surgeon

Box 3
A dangling protocol for intermediate postoperative care after free tissue transfer to the lower extremity

At 1 week postoperatively: Start dangling if flap has no complications

   5 minutes every hour for first and second days

   10 minutes every hour for third and fourth days

   15 minutes every hour for fifth and sixth days

At 2 weeks postoperatively

   If patient tolerates dangling, discharges home with elastic wrap but remains leg elevated as much as possible and no weight bearing

At 3 weeks postoperatively

   Start progressive weight bearing with ACE wrap protection for up to 3 months

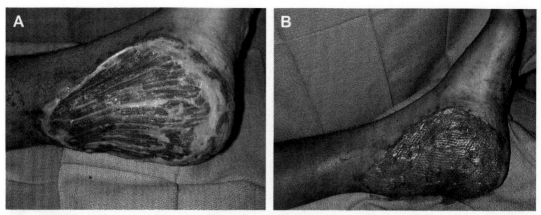

Fig. 8. (*A*) An intraoperative view shows completion of a skin-grafted free latissimus dorsi muscle flap debulking in the left foot and ankle. The excess flap tissue is tangentially excised under tourniquet control. (*B*) The raw surface of the flap is then placed with new split-thickness skin grafts.

(**Fig. 12**E). When looking into the failure of his first free tissue transfer, we noted his platelet count to have a coincidental peak that exceeded more than 1,000,000 platelets/μL at the time of his flap exploration. After appropriate consultation, an apheresis service was used to aid in the perioperative management of thrombocytosis. After the first apheresis session, platelet counts reached a nadir of 197,000/mm³, and the patient underwent a free rectus abdominis muscle flap and skin grafting to his left lower extremity, again using the posterior tibial artery stump and vein stump as recipient vessels (**Fig. 12**F, G). Two additional apheresis sessions were performed postoperatively. The second free flap encountered no

additional complications except an additional skin grafting procedure. His leg wound completely healed after his second free flap reconstruction (**Fig. 12**H). He subsequently healed his fracture site after bone grafting by our orthopedic trauma team (**Fig. 12**I).

Case 4

A 35-year-old man sustained a gun shoot wound to his left foot. He had a through-and-through complex wound (12 x 6 × 4 cm) and a comminuted fracture of the first metatarsal with a 5-cm bony defect and complete destruction of the first metatarsophalangeal joint (**Fig. 13**A-1, A-2). A free gracilis muscle flap was selected to provide soft

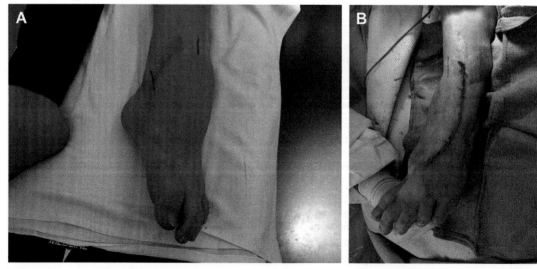

Fig. 9. (*A*) An intraoperative view shows a well-healed free ALT flap in the left foot and ankle. (*B*) The completion of the flap debulking procedure. The excess subcutaneous flap tissue is removed via liposuction and the excess skin of the flap is excised directly.

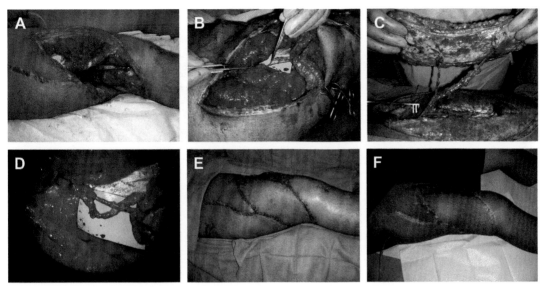

Fig. 10. (*A*) A large complex soft tissue defect in the distal lateral thigh and knee with exposed distal femur fracture site. (*B*) An intraoperative view shows an excellent arterial inflow from the descending branch of the lateral circumflex femoral artery. (*C*) An intraoperative view shows completion of both end-to-end arterial and venous microvascular anastomoses under an operating microscope. (*D*) An intraoperative view shows completion of a free ALT flap dissection based on 2 perforators. (*E*) An intraoperative view shows completion of the flap reconstruction and skin grafting. (*F*) Results at the 1-month follow-up show a well-healed wound and good soft tissue coverage.

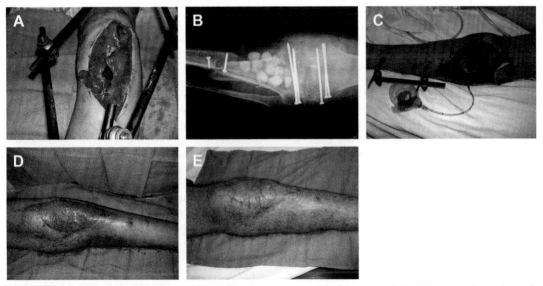

Fig. 11. (*A*) A large upper tibial wound extending to the knee with the exposed tibial fracture site and patella reconstruction site. (*B*) A radiograph shows the proximal tibial fracture and bony defect that is filled with antibiotic beads. (*C*) One week after a free latissimus dorsi muscle flap reconstruction to his knee and proximal tibial wound. (*D*) Results at 3.5 months follow-up before autologous bone grafting. (*E*) Results at 7.5 months follow-up after the free flap reconstruction and 4 months after autologous bone grafting.

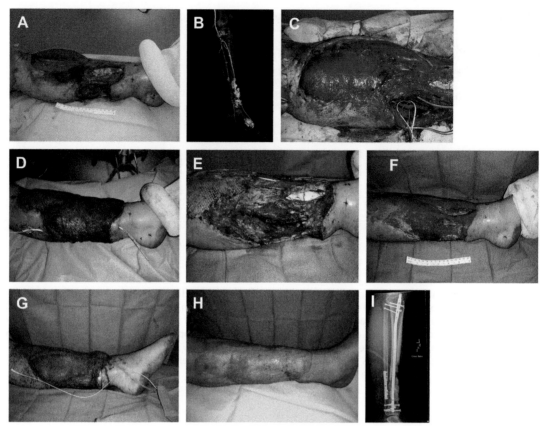

Fig. 12. (*A*) The initial presentation of the left lower extremity wound at time of our consultation. (*B*) Preoperative computed tomography angiogram shows the transected posterior tibial artery. In addition, the peroneal artery is also transected. (*C*) An intraoperative view shows completion of a medial gastrocnemius muscle flap and explored both stumps of the posterior tibial artery and vein (wrapped with vessel loops). (*D*) An intraoperative view shows completion of free latissimus dorsi muscle flap reconstruction (first free tissue transfer). (*E*) An intraoperative view shows appearance of the leg after debridement of necrotic free latissimus dorsi flap. (*F*) An intraoperative view shows the appearance of the leg before the second free flap reconstruction. (*G*) An intraoperative view shows the completion of free rectus abdominis muscle transfer (second free tissue transfer). (*H*) Results at 11 months after the second free rectus abdominis muscle flap reconstruction. (*I*) Follow-up radiographs shows appropriate healing of the fracture site 30 months after bone grafting.

tissue coverage of his wound after initial bony fixation with K-wires. End-to-end arterial and venous microvascular anastomoses were performed between the pedicle vessels and dorsalis pedis artery and vein. A skin graft was also placed over the muscle flap (**Fig. 13**B). He had an uncomplicated postoperative course. His definitive bony reconstruction was performed at 6 weeks after a successful free tissue transfer when the flap was elevated (**Fig. 13**C, D). At follow-up, he had healed well at the both flap site and the bone graft site (**Fig. 13**E-1, E-2, F). He had resumed normal ambulation without problems.

DISCUSSION

To ensure success for every free tissue transfer to the lower extremity, the author has developed a comprehensive approach that includes patient selection, flap selection, selection of recipient vessels, flap dissection, flap preparation, microvascular anastomosis, flap inset, immediate postoperative care, intermediate postoperative care, and further follow-up care (see **Box 1**). Every single step in this comprehensive approach is critical to the success for free tissue transfer to the lower extremity, in contrast with some beliefs that only the microvascular anastomosis is important. If each step in this comprehensive approach is not conducted properly, failure of free tissue transfer to the lower extremity is likely to occur. This can be true from the patient selection (ie, with hypercoagulable state) to the further follow-up care when the flap debulking is not performed properly.

The etiologic factors associated with failure of free tissue transfer, in general, can be

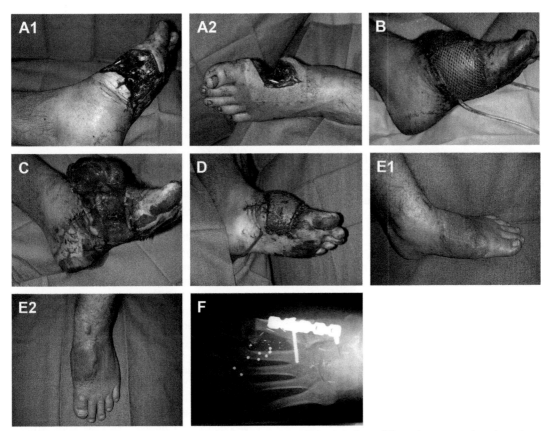

Fig. 13. (*A*) A composite wound after initial debridement of the left foot. (*B*) An intraoperative view shows completion of a free gracilis muscle flap with skin graft. (*C*) Intraoperative view shows completion of an iliac bone graft in 6 weeks after elevation of the gracilis muscle flap. (*D*) An intraoperative view shows complete coverage of the bone graft with the gracilis muscle flap again. (*E*) Results at 14 months after the bone graft. (*F*) Follow-up radiographs shows appropriate healing of the bone graft site 8 months after the procedure.

multifactorial. Khouri has[18] classified them into 3 categories: preoperative factors, operative factors (ie, preanastomotic, anastomotic, and postanastomotic), and postoperative factors. Because the failure of free tissue transfer to the lower extremity is relatively common compared with the head and neck or breast and the consequences of such a failure is usually amputation,[1–6] the surgeon should be prepared to perform the second free tissue transfer if the first one has failed. After a careful preoperative planning and preparation, meticulous intraoperative execution, and proper postoperative care, the second free tissue transfer can be successful and limb salvage can still be achieved for these patients. A strategy for reoperative free flaps after failure of a first flap is summarized as follows: (1) reconsideration of the need for vascularized free tissue transfer; (2) a sensitive psychosocial approach to the patient and family; (3) an analysis of the cause of the first flap failure; and (4) a change in the microsurgical strategy.[19]

A comprehensive approach to lower extremity free tissue transfer has been proposed by the author.[20] This approach represents the best summary of a reconstructive microsurgeon's successful experience. There are many justifications or reasoning behind each step in the protocol. Some justifications are based on the best available knowledge in each specific topic the author has learned, as well as based on his clinical experience.

The dangling protocol described in **Box 3** was developed by the author based on the recommended protocol in the literature and his clinical experience.[14] In general, the dangling can be started 1 week postoperatively if both arterial and venous anastomoses have been uneventful. For a lower extremity free flap with initial signs of venous congestion or a difficult anastomosis, the dangling should be postponed to even 2 weeks postoperatively. Once the patient tolerates more than 15 minutes of dangling, he or she can safely be discharged home with clear follow-up instructions.

SUMMARY

With adequate microsurgical skill, good surgical judgment, well-instructed and step-by-step intra-operative execution, and a protocol-driven practice, a free flap reconstruction in the lower can be performed successful with minimal complications. Attention should also be paid to many unique issues related to free flap lower extremity reconstruction such as recipient vessel selection, avoiding the zone of injury, effective dangling protocol, even just its learning curve.

CLINICS CARE POINTS

- Systemic anticoagulation is not necessary during lower extremity free flap reconstruction.
- Taking time for preparation of pedicle and recipient vessels is important for successful micro-vascular anastomoses.
- Proper dangling during post-op care is critical after lower extremity free flap reconstruction.
- Subsequent revision surgery may be necessary for an optimal outcome.

DISCLOSURE

The author has no financial interests in any of the drugs, products, or devices mentioned in this article.

REFERENCES

1. Pu LLQ, Stevenson TR. Principles of reconstruction for complex lower extremity wounds. Tech Orthopedics 2009;24:78–87.
2. Heller L, Levin SL. Lower extremity microsurgical reconstruction. Plast Reconstr Surg 2001;108:1029–41.
3. Pu LLQ, Medalie DA, Rosenblum WJ, et al. Free tissue transfer to a difficult wound of the lower extremity. Ann Plast Surg 2004;53:222–8.
4. Fischer JP, Wink JD, Nelson JA, et al. A retrospective review of outcomes and flap selection in free tissue transfers for complex lower extremity reconstruction. J Reconstr Microsurg 2013;29:407–16.
5. Yu P, Chang DW, Miller MJ, et al. Analysis of 49 cases of flap compromise in 1310 Free Flaps for head and neck Reconstruction. Head Neck 2009;31:45–51.
6. Massey MF, Spiegel AJ, Levine JL, et al. Perforator flaps: recent experience, current trends, and future directions based on 3974 microsurgical breast reconstructions. Plast Reconstr Surg 2009;124:737–51.
7. Roehl KR, Mahabir RC. A practical guide to free tissue transfer. Plast Reconstr Surg 2013;132:147–158e.
8. Nazerali RS, Pu LLQ. Free tissue transfers to the lower extremity: a paradigm shift in flap selection for soft tissue reconstruction. Ann Plast Surg 2013;70:419–22.
9. Dorfman DW, Pu LLQ. Using the descending branch of the lateral circumflex femoral artery and vein as recipient vessel for free tissue transfer to the difficult areas of the lower extremity. Ann Plast Surg 2013;70:397–400.
10. Zeiderman MR, Bailey CM, Arora A, et al. Anterior tibial vessel turnover as recipient vessel for complex free tissue transfer around the knee. J Plast Reconstr Aesthet Surg 2020;73(10):1897–916.
11. Dorfman DW, Pu LLQ. The value of Color duplex imaging for planning and performing a free anterolateral thigh perforator flap. Ann Plast Surg 2014;72:S6–8.
12. Conrad MH, Adams WP. Pharmacologic optimization of microsurgery in the new millennium. Plast Reconstr Surg 2001;108:2088–96.
13. Medina ND, Fischer JP, Fosnot J, et al. Lower extremity free flap outcomes using an anastomotic venous Coupler device. Ann Plast Surg 2014;72:176–9.
14. Marek CA, Pu LLQ. Refinements of free tissue transfer for optimal outcome in lower extremity reconstruction. Ann Plast Surg 2004;52:270–5.
15. Rohde C, Howell BW, Buncke GM, et al. A recommended protocol for the immediate postoperative care of lower extremity free-flap reconstructions. J Reconstr Microsurg 2009;25:15–20.
16. Ridway EB, Kutz RH, Cooper JS, et al. New insight into an old paradigm: wrapping and dangling with lower-extremity free flaps. J Reconstr Microsurg 2010;26:559–66.
17. Song P, Patel N, Pu LLQ. Re-operation of lower extremity microsurgical reconstruction when facing post-splenectomy thrombocytosis. Plast Reconstr Surg Glob Open 2019;7:e2492–6.
18. Khouri RK. Avoiding free flap failure. Clin Plast Surg 1992;19:773–80.
19. Baumeister S, Follmar KE, Zenn MR, et al. Strategy for reoperative free flaps after failure of a first flap. Plast Reconstr Surg 2008;122:962–71.
20. Pu LLQ. A comprehensive approach to lower extremity free tissue transfer. Plast Reconstr Surg Glob Open 2017;5:e1228.

Free-Style Free Perforator Flaps in Lower Extremity Reconstruction

Matthew R. Zeiderman, MD, Lee L.Q. Pu, MD, PhD*

KEYWORDS

• Free-style flap • Perforator flap • Free flap • Supermicrosurgery • Lower extremity • Reconstruction
• Free tissue transfer

KEY POINTS

- The Free-style free perforator flap can be a good option for lower extremity reconstruction.
- Free-style free flaps serve a valuable role when aberrant anatomy is encountered.
- Donor site morbidity is minimized with the versatile nature of free-style perforator flaps.
- Preoperative identification of perforators and their course may help to facilitate surgical dissection of the flap.
- The reconstructive surgeon should have knowledge of free-style flaps and be skilled at perforator dissection.

INTRODUCTION

Perforator flap surgery has greatly grown in popularity since first description by Koshima and Soeda in the 1980s.[1] Their early innovation lead to the description of perforator flaps, advancing microsurgical reconstruction beyond fasciocutaneous and musculocutaneous free flaps. Perforator flap surgery reduces donor site morbidity by sparing underlying muscle and may allow for a more aesthetically pleasing reconstructive result. Much of the early innovation in traditional and free-style perforator flaps has been pioneered by colleagues in Asia.[1–5] This was taken further when Wei and Mardini described the concept of a free-style free flap in 2004, in which a cutaneous perforator was identified with Doppler ultrasonography in the desired donor tissue and dissected retrograde to the source vessel.[3] This surgical innovation has been made possible by advanced knowledge of perforator anatomy.

A landmark anatomic study by Taylor and Palmer in 1987 described over 350 major perforating vessels sized 0.5 mm or larger throughout the body, leading to the angiosome concept.[6] The vascular territory of these perforators and their dynamic interplay with other nearby perforators via linking vessels are complex.[7] Detailed anatomic studies have built on these findings, showing that each perforator has its own vascular territory, described as the perforasome theory.[7] The perforasome theory proposes that a skilled surgeon can design a skin flap from almost any part of the body where a suitable perforator can be identified.[7,8] The primary limiting factors are the diameter and length of the source vessel. Free-style pedicled flaps can also be used for reconstructive surgery based on the same perforasome theory, and similarly are limited by location of the pivot point perforator relative to the defect.[8,9] However, the use of perforator flaps for free tissue transfer has overshadowed their utility as pedicled flaps. For

Division of Plastic Surgery, Department of Surgery, University of California Davis Medical Center, University of California at Davis, 2335 Stockton Boulevard, Room 6008, Sacramento, CA 95817, USA
* Corresponding author.
E-mail address: llpu@ucdavis.edu

Clin Plastic Surg 48 (2021) 215–223
https://doi.org/10.1016/j.cps.2020.12.001
0094-1298/21/© 2020 Elsevier Inc. All rights reserved.

example, traditional fasciocutaneous perforator flaps such as an anterolateral thigh perforator (ALT) flap have been shown to be useful in lower extremity reconstruction.[10–12] This article highlights the utility of free-style free perforator flaps in lower extremity reconstruction. With adequate knowledge and surgical skill for free-style perforator flaps, the surgeon can also achieve an equally good outcome for lower extremity soft tissue coverage when those flaps are used as an alternative to a classic free perforator flap.

INDICATIONS AND CONTRAINDICATIONS

Use of a free-style free perforator flap can be indicated for any lower extremity wound that requires reconstruction with a microvascular fasciocutaneous free flap. This technique is particularly useful when preoperative identification of vessels for traditional flaps such as the ALT perforator flap using handheld Doppler, duplex sonography, or other imaging modalities does not identify perforators of good caliber in the usual location.[13] Because the thigh is a good donor site as a free skin or fasciocutaneous flap, a free-style free perforator flap can be designed in the same flap donor site of an ALT flap as long as a large and reliable perforator can be identified. Using principles of free-style perforator flaps, aberrant anatomy encountered during perforator flap dissection still allows for successful flap elevation after intramuscular pedicle dissection. Obviously, free-style free flaps should not be attempted if a suitable perforator cannot be identified or if the donor site does not have adequate tissue. Other contraindications for a free-style free perforator flap are the same as other free flap lower extremity reconstruction.

The timing for a free-style free perforator flap lower extremity reconstruction is the same as other free flap reconstruction in the lower extremity. Besides the patient's readiness and associated medical conditions, a definitive soft tissue reconstruction is commonly performed within 7 to 10 days after initial consultation. With vacuum-assisted wound closure, the timing for free-style free perforator flap reconstruction can be prolonged to up to 3 weeks.

PREOPERATIVE EVALUATION AND SPECIAL CONSIDERATIONS

Preoperative evaluation for a free-style free perforator flap is the same as for most lower extremity microvascular soft tissue reconstructions. The wound must be thoroughly debrided of all infected and necrotic tissue and ready for soft tissue coverage. Suitable recipient vessels outside the zone of injury should be identified with preoperative duplex sonography, computed tomography (CT) angiogram, or formal angiogram. The size of the defect and bulk required are measured. Flap donor site is selected based on minimizing donor site morbidity, tissue quality, and expected aesthetic outcome. For lower extremity reconstruction, the thigh is commonly used, as it typically provides the most reliable source of soft tissue with minimal donor site morbidity.

Traditionally, a handheld Doppler probe is used to identify perforators in the region of interest.[3] However, it is the senior author's preference is to use color duplex sonography preoperatively to measure a perforator's vessel caliber and map its 3-dimensional course.[13,14] Once the perforator of adequate size and even the status of its blood flow can be identified and the 3-dimensional course of a perforator's anatomy is known, such a perforator can be used to design a free-style free perforator flap. The septocutaneous or musculocutaneous course of that perforator is also identified preoperatively, which may help to save time or to limit extent of the flap dissection. This enables easier dissection and is particularly useful in the obese patient in whom the perforator may have a long subcutaneous course. Color duplex sonography is a cheap, effective method to reliably identify a perforator for a free skin perforator flap or free-style free perforator flap.

Pedicle length must be strongly considered when designing a free-style free flap. Ideally, the flap will be designed on a perforator that is far away from the source vessel.[3] By doing so, the shortest pedicle will be the straight distance between the identified perforator and the source vessel. For example, in the thigh, this source vessel can be the superficial femoral artery or the profound artery.

Flap design is based on the location of the perforator(s) identified. Ideally, more than one perforator should be included in the flap design. The flap axis should be designed in the same orientation as that of the perforator linking vessels.[7] This is axially in the extremities and along the axiality of muscles perpendicular to the midline on the posterior trunk and chest.[7]

It is recommended that a conventional perforator flap such as an ALT flap be dissected first. Such a flap likely has more consistent perforators and is reliable for a safe flap dissection. If those typically more consistent perforators of the flap are found to be too small or insufficient blood flow, any larger sized perforator within the flap territory could be explored. It may serve as the perforator for a free-style free perforator flap even if it is

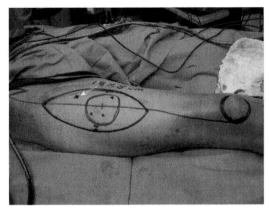

Fig. 1. An intraoperative view shows the design of a free ALT flap and the potential design of a free-style free perforator flap. Three perforators are identified in the usual location, but a large perforator (*arrow*) has also been identified outside the usual location of an ALT flap.

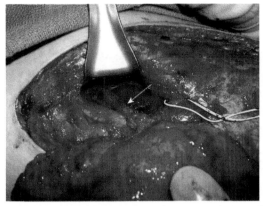

Fig. 3. An intraoperative view shows completion of the flap's pedicle dissection (*arrow*) after a retrograde intramuscular dissection from the perforator. The pedicle can then be divided once the adequate length and diameter of the pedicle vessels are determined.

not centrally located. A free-style free perforator flap should not be thought of as improvisation, but as an additional option in the microsurgeon's armamentarium.

In the obese patient, it is the senior author's preference to use a traditional free muscle flap with split-thickness skin graft in the management of complex lower extremity wounds. Although free muscle flaps atrophy and conform to the tissue, any perforator flaps in obese patients are difficult to perform and indeed require multiple debulking and revision procedures after initial flap reconstruction.

SURGICAL PROCEDURES

The free-style free perforator flap is the next level of flap choice for reconstruction of a lower

extremity wound and may need additional surgical skill for the flap dissection. Certain reliable imaging studies for the perforator's anatomy can be helpful, because the length of intramuscular dissection and the potential diameter of the pedicle can be estimated prior to the flap dissection. In that way, the surgeon can estimate whether the free-style free perforator flap can be harvested as a free skin flap for free tissue transfer. The common donor site is still in the thigh for most patients.

In the senior author's practice, preoperative mapping of perforators with a color duplex scan is performed first, and at least 1 good perforator can be identified. Such a perforator may not even be centrally located if it is within the flap territory and has a good blood flow. The skin paddle of the free-style free perforator flap can be marked as the same as an ALT flap (**Fig. 1**). The suprafascial dissection is performed first to explore the

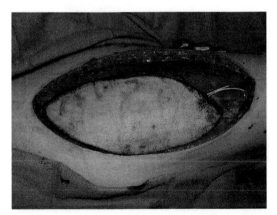

Fig. 2. An intraoperative view shows an elevated skin paddle of a free-style free perforator flap.

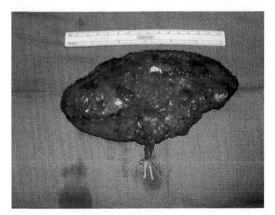

Fig. 4. An intraoperative view shows completion of the flap dissection.

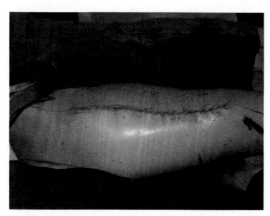

Fig. 5. An intraoperative view shows primary closure of the flap donor site.

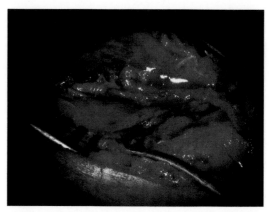

Fig. 7. An intraoperative view shows completion of an end-to-side arterial microanastomosis and an end-to-end venous microanastomosis with a coupler device under an operating microscope.

perforator (Fig. 2). If the perforator appears to be larger (>1 mm in diameter) with good flow, sometimes with visible pulsation, further dissection around the perforator can be performed. During the perforator dissection, more attention should be paid for intramuscular dissection. Because it is unknown where the perforator would go inside a deep muscle, intramuscular dissection of the perforator can be tricky and difficult. The surgeon should be patient during the flap dissection and put proper traction on the perforator so that the intramuscular dissection of the perforator can be facilitated (Fig. 3). Once the adequate pedicle length is achieved and the diameter of the pedicle is adequate for microvascular anastomosis, the pedicle can be divided, and a free-style free perforator flap dissection is completed (Fig. 4). If the thigh is chosen as a donor site, the size of the skin island can be as large as 25 × 8 cm for subsequent primary closure (Fig. 5). The average

length of the pedicle is about 10 cm, but this can be tailored as long as the recipient vessel can be reached. However, the diameter of the pedicle can be quite small, and the surgeon who performs a free-style free perforator flap should feel comfortable performing microsurgery for the size of the vessel less than 1.5 mm in diameter (Fig. 6). Often, an end-to-side arterial microvascular anastomosis is performed for such a small size of the pedicle artery from the flap. However, an end-to-end venous microvascular anastomosis can still be performed with a proper size of venous coupler (Fig. 7).

POSTOPERATIVE CARE AND EXPECTED OUTCOME

The postoperative care is the same as for any free flap lower extremity reconstruction, with

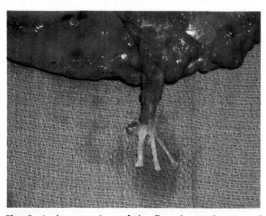

Fig. 6. A close-up view of the flap shows the size of the pedicle artery (center) and 2 accompanied veins. One vein is larger and can be used for end-to-end venous microanastomosis.

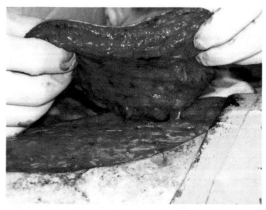

Fig. 8. An intraoperative view shows the potential thickness of a free-style free perforator flap from the thigh in a Caucasian female patient.

postoperative flap monitoring and implementation of a dangle protocol per surgeon preference. Postoperative complications are managed the same as for an ALT or other perforator flap. Free-style free perforator flaps typically have smaller pedicle diameters than traditional free perforator flaps and may be more prone to develop complications at the site of microvascular anastomosis. So far, this difficulty has been handled well by the senior author, and no complications related to microvascular anastomoses have been encountered. In addition, the authors have not seen any partial flap necrosis of the skin paddle while the flap survives.

Between 2009 and 2019, free-style free flaps were performed in 10 patients by the senior author for soft tissue reconstruction of a knee, leg, or foot wound following orthopedic trauma. There was no total or partial flap loss, and successful soft tissue reconstruction was achieved in all patients who were discharged home once they tolerated dangling.

MANAGEMENT OF COMPLICATIONS

Complications such as delayed flap site healing are managed successfully with local wound care or repeat operation. Satisfactory outcome of the free flap lower extremity reconstruction can still be achieved. The authors have not encountered any donor site complications in their series.

REVISIONS OR SUBSEQUENT PROCEDURES

Need for subsequent revisional surgery for flap contouring or debulking is ideally decreased with the use of a free-style free perforator flap because of increased ability to choose an optimal donor site. However, patient habitus or wound location may necessitate flap revision for an optimal aesthetic and functional outcome.

The contour of the flap in the lower extremity during follow-up can be an issue, because the thigh tissue in some Caucasian patients may be relatively thicker (**Fig. 8**). It has been common that the bulkiness of the flap needs to be revised so that a better contour of the lower extremity can be achieved. It is the senior author's preference that a minimum of 6 months' waiting period should be expected before a debulking procedure can be considered. Unlike a free muscle flap, the bulkiness of the flap would not shrink any further after 6 months, and debulking procedure via liposuction and skin resection can be performed relatively sooner. Again, because a free-style free perforator flap is a fasciocutaneous flap, conventional liposuction can be performed first to remove excess adipose tissue of the flap. Additional skin

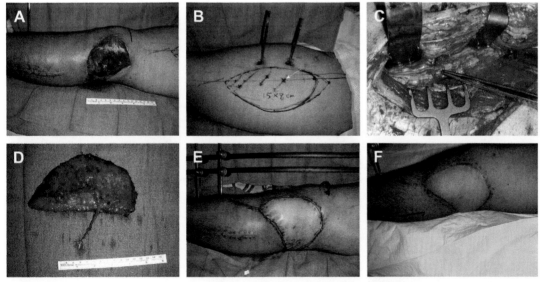

Fig. 9. (*A*) An intraoperative view showing a 13 × 9 cm soft tissue wound in the left lateral knee with the exposed fracture site and knee joint. (*B*) A standard design of a reversed ALT perforator flap for possible coverage of the lateral knee wound. A large perforator (*arrow*) was identified within the skin paddle. (*C*) In this patient, the pedicle of the reversed ALT flap was found injured by a pin during the flap dissection. (*D*) An intraoperative view showing a successfully elevated free-style free perforator flap based on the perforator identified previously. (*E*) An intraoperative view showing the completion of the free-style free perforator flap reconstruction to the lateral knee. (*F*) The result at 4 months follow-up.

resection may be necessary to achieve better contour of the flap in the leg or foot.

CASE DEMONSTRATIONS
Case 1

A 26-year-old Asian man sustained a gunshot wound to his left lateral knee. He had a 13 × 9 cm soft tissue wound over the left lateral knee with an exposed fracture site and knee joint (**Fig. 9**A). An external fixator was also placed to stabilize his fracture. Initially, a 15 × 9 cm reversed ALT flap was planned for his soft tissue coverage (**Fig. 9**B). Unfortunately, the distal descending branch of the lateral circumflex femoral vessels was injured by a pin placed by the orthopedic trauma service (**Fig. 9**C). However, before the senior author discarded the flap, a sizable perforator that was not joined to the descending branch of the lateral circumflex femoral vessels was identified. Therefore, the decision was made to perform a free-style free perforator flap that included the same skin paddle. After a tedious intramuscular dissection of the perforator, an almost 10 cm-long pedicle was dissected out successfully, and the diameter of the pedicle was determined to be adequate for successful microvascular anastomoses (**Fig. 9**D). After a successful end-to-side arterial microanastomosis to the anterior tibial artery and end-to-end venous microanastomosis to the vein with a coupler device, the flap was transferred

to cover the lateral knee wound (**Fig. 9**E). The patient did well postoperatively and tolerated flap dangling well. During the follow-up, he had a well-healed soft tissue wound and subsequently had a bone graft procedure 6 months later (**Fig. 9**F).

Case 2

A 48-year-old Hispanic man sustained a deep burn to his right leg. He had a 20 × 15 cm wound in his leg with exposed distal tibia and tendons (**Fig. 10**A) Several perforators within the flap territory were identified, and a 25 × 12 cm ALT flap was designed (**Fig. 10**B). During the flap dissection, 2 perforators that were in the usual location of an ALT flap were found to be small and less reliable, but 2 larger and reliable perforators were found more proximal to the previously identified 2 perforators in an unusual location but still in the flap territory. After a tedious intramuscular dissection, an adequate length and diameter of the flap pedicle were determined, and the flap was elevated as a free-style free perforator flap (**Fig. 10**C). Both end-to-end microvascular anastomoses were performed between the flap pedicle and the anterior tibial vessels, and the flap was successfully transferred to his leg wound. The flap donor site was partially closed, and additional closure was performed with a skin graft (**Fig. 10**D). He did well postoperatively and was discharged home after tolerating flap dangling. During

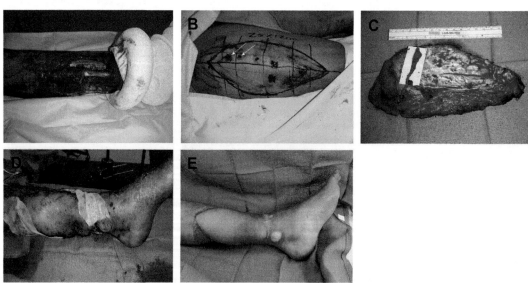

Fig. 10. (A) An intraoperative view showing a 20 × 15 cm soft tissue wound in the distal leg with the exposed fracture site and tendons. (B) A standard design of an ALT perforator flap for possible coverage of the left distal leg wound and 2 large perforators (arrows) were also identified outside usual location of an ALT flap but within the skin paddle. (C) An intraoperative view showing a successfully elevated free-style free perforator flap based on those 2 perforators identified previously. (D) An intraoperative view showing the completion of the free-style free perforator flap reconstruction to the distal leg. (E) The result at 4 months follow-up.

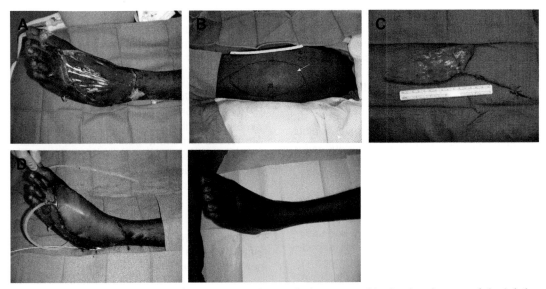

Fig. 11. (*A*) An intraoperative view showing a 15 × 9 cm soft tissue wound in the dorsal aspect of the left foot with the exposed fracture site, reconstruction plate, and tendons. (*B*) A standard design of an ALT perforator flap for possible coverage of the left dorsal foot wound and 1 additional perforator (*arrow*) were identified outside the usual location but within the skin paddle. (*C*) An intraoperative view showing a successfully elevated free-style free perforator flap based on the perforator identified previously. (*D*) An intraoperative view showing completion of the free-style free perforator flap reconstruction to the dorsal foot wound. (*E*) The result at 3 months follow-up.

follow-up, the free-style free flap site healed well, and the patient was fully ambulating without problems (**Fig. 10**E).

Case 3

A 30-year-old African American man had a large (15 × 9 cm) left dorsal foot wound with exposed extensor tendons and reconstruction plate following a motor vehicle accident (**Fig. 11**A). A perforator within the skin paddle in the usual location was identified and a 15 × 8 cm ALT flap was designed (**Fig. 11**B). During the flap elevation, the perforator, however, was found to be small and less reliable but a larger and reliable perforator was found more proximally to the previously identified perforator in an unusual location of an ALT flap but still in the flap territory. After a tedious intramuscular dissection, an adequate length and diameter of the flap pedicle was determined, and the flap was elevated as a free-style free perforator flap (**Fig. 11**C). Both end-to-end microvascular anastomoses were performed between the flap pedicle and the anterior tibial vessels, and the flap donor site was closed primarily (**Fig. 11**D). The patient did well postoperatively and was discharged home after tolerating flap dangling. During follow-up, the free-style free flap site healed well, and the patient was fully ambulating without problems (**Fig. 11**E).

DISCUSSION

Free-style free perforator flaps have expanded the reconstructive microsurgeon's options for providing patients the best functional and aesthetic result while minimizing donor site morbidity when performing lower extremity reconstruction.[15,16] Free-style selection of perforators allows design of small-to-medium sized flaps from most anatomic locations. Perforators can be identified preoperatively using pencil Doppler, colored duplex sonography, CT angiography, magnetic resonance angiography, or formal angiogram.[13,17] The senior author prefers color duplex sonography, because it is accessible, inexpensive, and noninvasive, and allows assessment of perforator diameter and course.[13,14]

Sound knowledge of traditional perforator flap anatomy and how to raise traditional perforator flaps is essential. The concept of a free-style flap does not decrease the importance of traditional perforator flaps; free-style free perforator flaps increase flexibility for the experienced microsurgeon and serve as a back-up when aberrant anatomy is encountered as demonstrated in **Figs. 10** and **11**. Further, knowledge of perforator anatomy and common locations is essential when designing flaps to best suit the reconstructive need. This helps the surgeon select the appropriate flap for the patient's needs with a high success rate.

When elevating a free-style free perforator flap, a sizable perforator with unknown anatomic course but within the flap territory may be identified. Intramuscular perforator dissection is performed until the length (8–10 cm) and diameter (1.2–1.5 mm) of the pedicle are thought to be adequate for arterial and venous microvascular anastomoses. The pedicle is then divided, and the flap dissection is completed. However, tedious and difficult intramuscular dissection of the perforator and pedicle and need to perform microvascular anastomosis in less than 1.5 mm of the vessel may be expected.

The technical challenging of performing intramuscular dissection of the perforator for a free-style free perforator flap should not be underestimated. Experience and technical skill for perforator dissection and supermicrosurgery are essential for successful flap harvest and microvascular anastomosis. With adequate experience, perforator-to-perforator, end-to-end supermicrosurgical anastomosis can be performed successfully in lower extremity reconstruction.[15]

A surgical dissection of the perforator and potential microvascular anastomosis of a free-style free perforator flap can be challenging for reconstructive surgeons. Thus, the learning curve for surgeons performing free-style free perforator flaps can be steep. The surgeon must be trained in the approach to raising a free-style free perforator flap and have proficient supermicrosurgical skills. Preoperative perforator identification and mapping of its course allow dissection closer to the known perforator and increase operative efficiency.

A free-style free perforator flap can be a good alternative to some of the conventional free perforator flaps if the surgeon has become skillful in performing a perforator flap dissection and microvascular anastomosis of small vessels. It is recommended that a conventional free perforator flap should be dissected first, because such a flap would have much more consistent perforators and be more reliable for a safe flap dissection. If these more consistent perforators of the flap are found to be too small or with less blood flow, any larger size of the perforator could be explored and may be used as a free-style free perforator flap.

SUMMARY

Improved knowledge of perforator anatomy has allowed for better understanding and design of free-style perforator flaps, whether pedicled or free. With appropriate planning and execution, free-style free perforator flaps can be performed safely and successfully. The flaps can be a good alternative to conventional free perforator flaps for lower extremity reconstruction. However, experience and skill are needed in order to successfully perform free-style free perforator flaps.

CLINICS CARE POINTS

- Preoperative knowledge of available perforators in a specific region can be critical.
- Surgical skills for perforator flap dissection are needed to perform free- style free perforator flaps.
- Supermicrosurgical skills are also needed for microanastomoses.

DISCLOSURE

The authors have no financial interest to declare in relation to the drugs, devices, and products mentioned in this article.

REFERENCES

1. Koshima I, Soeda S. Inferior epigastric artery skin flaps without rectus abdominis muscle. Br J Plast Surg 1989;42(6):645–8.
2. Pu LL. Learning from our international colleagues: a US plastic surgeon's perspective. Ann Plast Surg 2013;70(4):470–5.
3. Wei FC, Mardini S. Free-style free flaps. Plast Reconstr Surg 2004;114(4):910–6.
4. Wei FC, Jain V, Celik N, et al. Have we found an ideal soft-tissue flap? An experience with 672 anterolateral thigh flaps. Plast Reconstr Surg 2002;109(7):2219–26 [discussion: 2227–30].
5. Song YG, Chen GZ, Song YL. The free thigh flap: a new free flap concept based on the septocutaneous artery. Br J Plast Surg 1984;37(2):149–59.
6. Taylor GI, Palmer JH. The vascular territories (angiosomes) of the body: experimental study and clinical applications. Br J Plast Surg 1987;40(2):113–41.
7. Saint-Cyr M, Wong C, Schaverien M, et al. The perforasome theory: vascular anatomy and clinical implications. Plast Reconstr Surg 2009;124(5):1529–44.
8. Lecours C, Saint-Cyr M, Wong C, et al. Freestyle pedicle perforator flaps: clinical results and vascular anatomy. Plast Reconstr Surg 2010;126(5):1589–603.
9. Mohan AT, Sur YJ, Zhu L, et al. The concepts of propeller, perforator, keystone, and other local flaps and their role in the evolution of reconstruction. Plast Reconstr Surg 2016;138(4):710e–29e.
10. Abdelfattah U, Power HA, Song S, et al. Algorithm for free perforator flap selection in lower extremity reconstruction based on 563 cases. Plast Reconstr Surg 2019;144(5):1202–13.
11. Cho EH, Shammas RL, Carney MJ, et al. Muscle versus fasciocutaneous free flaps in lower extremity

traumatic reconstruction: a multicenter outcomes analysis. Plast Reconstr Surg 2018;141(1):191–9.

12. Yazar S, Lin CH, Lin YT, et al. Outcome comparison between free muscle and free fasciocutaneous flaps for reconstruction of distal third and ankle traumatic open tibial fractures. Plast Reconstr Surg 2006; 117(7):2468–75 [discussion: 2476–7].

13. Dorfman D, Pu LL. The value of color duplex imaging for planning and performing a free anterolateral thigh perforator flap. Ann Plast Surg 2014;72(Suppl 1):S6–8.

14. Blondeel PN, Beyens G, Verhaeghe R, et al. Doppler flowmetry in the planning of perforator flaps. Br J Plast Surg 1998;51(3):202–9.

15. Hong JP. The use of supermicrosurgery in lower extremity reconstruction: the next step in evolution. Plast Reconstr Surg 2009;123(1):230–5.

16. Song JW, Ben-Nakhi M, Hong JP. Reconstruction of lower extremity with perforator free flaps by free-style approach in pediatric patients. J Reconstr Microsurg 2012;28(9):589–94.

17. Pratt GF, Rozen WM, Chubb D, et al. Preoperative imaging for perforator flaps in reconstructive surgery: a systematic review of the evidence for current techniques. Ann Plast Surg 2012;69(1): 3–9.

The Superficial Circumflex Iliac Artery Perforator Flap in Lower Extremity Reconstruction

Joon Pio Hong, MD, PhD, MMM

KEYWORDS

- Superficial circumflex iliac artery perforator (SCIP) flap • Lower extremity reconstruction
- Microsurgery • Thin flap

KEY POINTS

- The superficial circumflex iliac artery perforator flap is one of the thinnest flaps available based on the perforator from the superficial circumflex iliac artery.
- One must understand the anatomy of the perforators, as the flap can be elevated on either the medial (superficial) or lateral (deep) branch or both.
- The design of the flap will vary depending on the branch used: medial branch will provide a medium or large-sized flap based on the perforator pattern (anchoring vs axial), whereas lateral branch will have an axial pattern allowing to harvest a flap extending into the flank.
- The flap can be harvested as a chimeric flap with lymph nodes, bones, and part of a muscle.
- It has a very well-hidden donor scar.

INTRODUCTION

Free flap approach is inevitable when defects are complex exposing essential structures such as tendons, bones, nerves, and joints. In the lower extremity this region remains to be the lower leg, ankle, and foot. Even for a moderate-size defect, local solutions will not be enough and free flaps will be required to cover the defect. Once free flap is planned, multiple other challenges arise. In the age where aesthetic outcome is as important as function, one must consider a thin flap for the anterior surface of the tibia, as this region is naturally thin and consider a flap with a skin paddle resembling the natural skin surface. Donor site morbidity such as potential loss of muscle function or a large scar can also be an issue. It is within this regard that the superficial circumflex iliac artery

perforator (SCIP) flap deserves attention to reconstruct defects for lower extremity.[1–3]

The SCIP flap is an evolution from groin flap. The groin flap, supplied by the superficial circumflex iliac artery (SCIA), is one of the first free flaps successful in reconstruction. This flap was first described as a pedicle flap by McGregor and Jackson and then introduced as a free flap by Daniel and Taylor.[4,5] This flap was the workhorse flap during the early period of microsurgery as required for lower extremity reconstruction provides a hidden scar and a large cutaneous tissue. However, its use for lower extremity slowly faded away, as introduction of muscle flaps was perceived to function better in extremities against infection and because the short pedicle of the groin flap made it difficult to use when longer pedicle was needed. Other disadvantages of groin

Conflict of interest: All the authors of this article do not have any conflict of interest to declare in relation to the content of this article.
Department of Plastic Surgery, Asan Medical Center, University of Ulsan, 88 Olympicro 43 gil Songpagu, Seoul 05505, Korea
E-mail address: joonphong@amc.seoul.kr

Clin Plastic Surg 48 (2021) 225–233
https://doi.org/10.1016/j.cps.2020.12.005
0094-1298/21/© 2020 Elsevier Inc. All rights reserved.

flap were variable arterial anatomy, donor/recipient vessel size disparity, bulky flap in obese patients, and donor site seroma collection.[1,6–9]

It was not till Koshima and colleagues[10] revisited the groin flap and modified it as a skin flap elevated above the deep fascia based on the SCIP that the groin region as a free flap regained recognition. The SCIP flap was able to overcome some disadvantages such as bulkiness and variable arterial anatomy by using the free-style free flap approach.[11,12] But even with these evolved technique and concept, the SCIP flap was still challenging to use due to the short pedicle, small vessel caliber, relative bulkiness especially in obese patients, and donor site morbidity such as lymphorrhea. Further modifications were made where Hong and colleagues harvested the flap on the superficial fascia making the flap thinner (super-thin flaps) while avoiding injuries to the lymphatic system, which is located on the deep fat below the superficial fascia, thus minimizing lymphorrhea.[1–3,13–15] Further studies clarified the superficial (medial) branch and deep (lateral) branches of SCIA as well as the venous outflow, which helped to achieve better design, vascular supply, harvest multiple composition, and understand the limit of the flap.[2,16,17] Although both medial and lateral branch stems from the SCIA, it can be seen as 2 different flaps based on each perforating branch, as it provides very distinctive and unique characters. In this article, the author reviews the surgical elevation technique, benefits, and indications of the SCIP flap for lower extremity reconstruction.

INDICATIONS AND CONTRAINDICATIONS

The indications for the SCIP flap will be for defects that need to use the merits of the flap. The most commonly applied indication will be for lower extremity defects that require a thin flap coverage especially in the anterior surface of the leg and the ankle region. The SCIP flap has replaced the anterolateral thigh (ALT) flap as our workhorse flap for simple resurfacing of the leg. When a large flap has to be harvested, using the lateral branch allows to harvest the skin extending to the abdominal flank region. If lymph node is required to treat lymphedema or prevent potential development of lymphedema on the contralateral limb, harvesting 1 or 2 lymph nodes with the skin paddle may be indicated. Soft tissue defects with small bone gaps of the leg or foot that needs simultaneous bone and skin coverage is another good indication. The use of skin flaps for chronic osteomyelitis has been shown to have no difference in outcome and the same

can be said for the SCIP flap. When a small dead space is noted, part of the flap can be deepithelialized to obliterate the dead space.[18]

The main contraindications for the SCIP flap would be defects that need a long pedicle to reach the recipient vessels. Although one can safely perform vessel grafts to extend the pedicle length, the chances for complication may increase and require more surgical time. Another contraindication would be when the groin region has prior surgery potentially altering the anatomic structure of the SCIA. The vascular structure can be confirmed by using the Duplex ultrasound, but the multiple scars in this region can have a negative effect on the circulation of the flap. A relative contraindication would be defects that exceed the coverage potential of the SCIP flap and unable to close primarily. Although one can perform skin grafts for the donor defect, it would be less ideal to use the advantages of the flap. The authors also recommend to avoid harvesting the SCIP flap on the side that underwent percutaneous angiograms or angioplasty before surgery. When hematoma is collected, it makes identifying the perforators very difficult.

PREOPERATIVE EVALUATION AND SPECIAL CONSIDERATIONS

Using an SCIP flap helps to (1) obtain a thin flap, (2) have reliable perforator anatomy (medial and lateral branches) and superficial vein, (3) have the capability to either elevate a small or a large flap (from 4 × 3 cm to 12 × 35 cm), (4) have a primarily closed hidden donor scar, and (5) elevate as a composite flap (including lymph nodes, iliac bone, and part of Sartorius muscle). The disadvantages of using SCIP flap include (1) a relatively short pedicle and (2) small perforator artery diameter (**Table 1**).

Preoperative ultrasound Doppler is used to mark the potential perforators of the SCIP flap. In 95% of the SCIP flaps, the medial perforators of the SCIA penetrate the deep fascia within an oval of 4.2 × 2 cm (vertical × horizontal) with the center of the oval point located 4.5 cm lateral and 1.5 cm superior from the superolateral corner of the pelvic tubercle.[19] The medial perforating branch then can be divided into 2 distinctive patterns. The axial pattern (44%) shows the perforator runs in an axial pattern on the superficial fat passing the anterior superior iliac spine (ASIS) reaching the flank region, whereas the anchoring pattern (56%) displays the perforator reaching the subdermal plexus without further branching.[19] This anatomy becomes relevant especially when longer SCIP flaps need to be harvested, for which the axial pattern would be

Table 1
Pros and cons of the superficial circumflex iliac artery perforator flap

Pros	Cons
Well-concealed donor site	Smaller vessel lumen
Thin and pliable skin flap—allows single-stage resurfacing	Short pedicle
Septocutaneous pedicle (medial branch)	Learning curve to elevate as thin flap
Expedient harvest	Supermicrosurgery technique required for certain defects
Composite with lymph node and bone	
Medium to large skin dimension	

safer to use. The deep branch can be detected on the lateral region of the axis drawn from the pubic tubercle to the ASIS. It usually travels laterally beneath the deep fascia and often with an intramuscular pathway perforating the deep fascia on the lateral aspect (deep branch) near the ASIS. The computed tomography angiogram allows to visualize the medial (deep) and lateral (superficial) branches with accuracy, allowing safer design especially in respect to size of the flap.[19] Recently, the use of ultrasound has helped to define not only the exact location but also the pathway of the perforator and the superficial vein as well with high accuracy. One should remember that the SCIP flap can be designed based on either the medial and lateral perforators or both when needed (**Fig. 1**). **Table 2** shows the points to consider when selecting either the medial or lateral branch of the SCIA of the SCIP flap.

SURGICAL PROCEDURE
Flap Harvest Using a Freestyle Approach

The medial branch is always a direct cutaneous perforator having an easy dissection, whereas the lateral branch travels underneath the deep fascia often needing dissection near or in the Sartorius muscle, making the dissection more complicated than the medial branch. The lateral branch is usually an axial pattern perforator traveling toward the flank allowing to take a larger skin paddle.

Required dimensions of the SCIP flap are outlined as per the defect. The flap is first elevated along the inferior and lateral borders under loupe magnification, as this approach allows to best identify the superficial fascia lying between the superficial and deep fat. This is a distinct white film-like layer, and elevation of the flap on or above this plane avoids injury to the lymphatic system, which is found in the deeper adipose tissue.[1,2,14,15] This plane is also avascular, allowing a bloodless field needed to identify the perforators piercing this plane. Once any reliable perforator is identified near the Doppler marked region, the rest of the flap can be elevated. Multiple other perforators can be further identified during the elevation. When multiple perforators are dissected, one can decide which branch (perforator) best serves the reconstructive purpose and then skeletonize

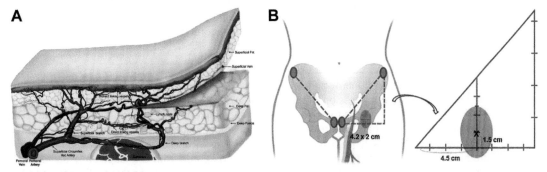

Fig. 1. The medial and lateral perforator originating from the SCIA. Note that the medial branch is a direct cutaneous perforator, whereas the lateral branch travels under the deep fascia, traveling passed the Sartorius muscle, and perforating near the ASIS (anterior superior iliac spine) and then axially toward the flank (*A*). Although the point that the lateral branch perforates deep fascia is variable, the medial perforator usually perforates the deep fascia about 4.5 cm laterally and 1.5 cm superiorly from the lateral margin of the pubic tubercle (*B*).

Table 2
Comparison between the flaps based on medial versus lateral perforating branches of the superficial circumflex iliac artery

Medial (Superficial) Branch	Lateral (Deep) Branch
Septocutaneous perforator	Muscular path included
Short pedicle	Relatively longer pedicle
Topographically constant perforator	Nonconstant perforator
Two distinct types of perforator • Axial pattern • Anchoring pattern	Mostly axial pattern perforator
Medium size skin paddle (anchoring type) Large size skin paddle (axial pattern)	Large size skin paddle
Expedient harvest	Slower harvest
Composite with lymph node	Composite with bone and muscle

Note that flaps can be based on both medial and lateral branch as well.

toward the source vessel passing the deep fascia.[2] The deep fascia can be incised to obtain a longer pedicle length and a larger vessel diameter. If one needs to take part of the iliac bone, a branch toward the crest from the lateral (deep) branch can be identified and elevated together.[16,20,21] The lymph node can be elevated together with the SCIP flap to provide lymphatic drainage for lymphedema patients. The lymph nodes are usually located near the superficial (medial) branch under the superficial fascia in the deep adipose tissue. A superficial vein running from the ASIS toward the pubis is normally identified and preserved. The accompanying vein of the medial branch often drains into the superficial vein, thus only one vein needs to be harvested. In cases where there is a small or absent superficial vein, the accompanying vein of the perforator is usually of a larger caliber. Whenever the donor vessels are small, dissection should be performed under the microscope. When designing a smaller flap, freestyle approach can be used to confirm the perforator reaching the skin. The average time for flap harvest is 45 minutes (range, 30–60 minutes). **Fig. 2** shows the overall approach to the elevation of the SCIP flap.

Donor Site Management

A pinch test is recommended to confirm primary closure of the donor site during the design of the flap. Usually, a flap of width 8 cm is able to achieve primary closure. However, one can take a wider flap and close the defect primarily with the hip flexed and gradually extend over the postoperative period. During the closure, the superficial fascia layer is plicated together with absorbable 2/0 sutures and a negative drain placed before the dermis and skin sutures. This is important to obliterate the dead space to prevent seroma formation.

POSTOPERATIVE CARE AND EXPECTED OUTCOME

A postoperative vasodilator (10 µg of lipoprostaglandin E_1, Eglandin; Welfide, Seoul, Korea) mixed in 5% dextrose is systemically infused over 4 hours for 5 days after the operation.[22] Low-molecular-weight heparin (Fraxiparine; Sanofi-Aventis, Paris, France), 3800 IU, when required is injected subcutaneously for 5 days. The flap is monitored by subjective means or objectively using the duplex ultrasound measuring the flap pedicle flow velocity. For lower extremity cases, pressure bandages and garments (30–60 mm Hg) are applied from day 4 to 6 to reduce edema and mold the flap,[23] which also enables early ambulation by day 5. If incisional negative pressure therapy was used for the donor site, it is removed on day 4 or 5.[24] The patients are usually discharged from the hospital within 5 to 10 days unless there are other medical problems. The overall success rate of the SCIP flap is very high, being a very reliable flap. The SCIP flap has now become the main workhorse flap being performed about 50% of all lower extremity reconstruction cases that needs soft tissue coverage.

MANAGEMENT OF COMPLICATIONS

As with any flap, the complications can be from either recipient site, donor site, or both. The biggest complications in regard to the recipient site is flap in distress. The salvage procedure is same compared with any flap. Early salvage will lead to better chance of salvage. Seroma and hematoma collection can also be seen within weeks, and proper evacuation followed by compression will most likely provide an adequate solution.[23] As for the donor site, the classic groin flap as

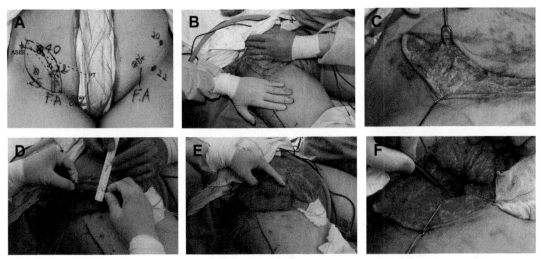

Fig. 2. The design of the flap is shown. Note that there are 3 systems in the groin; SCIA (superficial circumflex iliac artery), SIEA (superficial inferior epigastric artery), and the pudendal artery system. The SCIP flap design should be made along the axis between the groin crease and the ASIS (anterior superior iliac spine) where the SCIA usually travels. Using the handheld Doppler, the medial and lateral perforators can be identified and marked (*A*). The elevation begins from the lateral inferior margin with traction, as the superficial fascia will be most evident (*B*). Once the superficial fascia plane is found, the elevation proceeds from lateral to medial and caudal to cephalic until the perforators are seen (*C*). Note that the superficial vein is included in the flap (*D*). The lateral branches are identified first followed by the medial branch (*E*). After dissecting both medial and lateral branches, one can determine which perforator to use or can use both (*F*).

well as early SCIP flaps showed complications such as lymphorrhea. Because of the anatomic position of the lymphatic system, when the SCIP flap is harvested including the deeper adipose tissue, injury to the lymphatic system can occur leading to lymphorrhea especially when meticulous coagulation is not performed. One can avoid this complication by elevating the flap on or above the superficial fascia as a super-thin flap. However, if this complication does occur resembling the lymphorrhea after lymph node dissection in patients with cancer, prolong drainage is needed. Now with the introduction of supermicrosurgery and lymphovenous anastomosis, one can find the leaking lymphatics and anastomose to the vein allowing the lymphatics to drain into the vein resolving the problem.[25] In flaps that harvested wide flaps, donor site scar can be a problem seldom resulting from healed wound after dehiscence. However, conservative care for scars should suffice.

REVISION OR SUBSEQUENT PROCEDURES

In late phase, bulky flaps can be noted. If the flap is elevated on the superficial fascia as a super-thin flap, it usually will not require debulking. However, in obese patients, secondary debulking may be required depending on patient's need.[2]

CASE DEMONSTRATIONS
Case 1

Fig. 3 shows a 54-year-old man is presented with a long-standing drainage from the bone as well as unstable scarring around the chronic osteomyelitis of the left tibia. After complete debridement and part of the tibia debrided, exposed tendon and bone and defect of the skin is noted. A 15 × 6 cm SCIP flap was designed based on the medial branch. The Duplex ultrasound showed an axially traveling cutaneous vein. The flap was connected to the anterior tibial artery in end-to-side manner and the vein connected to the accompanying vein. After 3 weeks, the flap was reelevated from the margin for a secondary bone graft procedure. Note the pliable skin allowed an easy elevation than closure. The patient at 12 months show good contour of the flap without recurrence of the bone infection.

Case 2

Fig. 4 shows a 52-year-old female patient is presented with a lymphedema of the right leg lasting the last 7 years. The contralateral left leg showed normal contour, and the decision was made to harvest an SCIP flap with lymph nodes. After harvesting an 11 × 5 cm SCIP with one lymph node based on the medial perforating branch of the

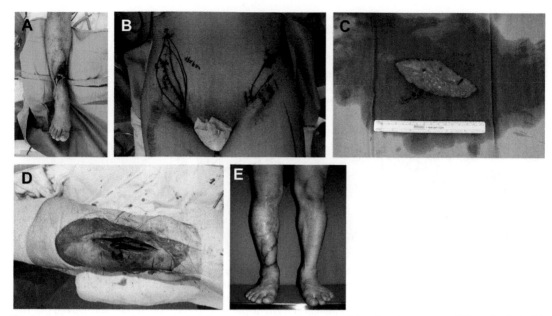

Fig. 3. A 54-year-old man is presented with an unstable scarring around the chronic osteomyelitis of the left tibia (*A*). After complete debridement of bone and soft tissue, a 15 × 6 cm SCIP flap was designed based on the medial branch to cover the bone gap and the soft tissue defect (*B*). The Duplex ultrasound showed an axially traveling cutaneous vein (*C*). The flap was connected to the anterior tibial artery in end-to-side manner and the vein connected to the accompanying vein. After 3 weeks, the flap was reelevated from the margin (*D*). Note the pliable skin allowed an easy elevation then closure during the bone graft procedure. The patient at 12 months show good contour of the flap without recurrence of the bone infection (*E*).

SCIA, the flap was transferred to the anterior aspect of the right ankle and anastomosed to anterior tibial artery and vein. The postoperative result at 1 month shows well-taken flap and well-concealed donor site scar.

DISCUSSION

The paradigm of reconstruction has shifted from the concept of climbing the ladder approach to providing the most complete solution resembling to reach the accurate floor by the elevator.[26] The key to success using the elevator approach is to provide necessary components in minimal stages. Chimeric flaps can provide multiple tissues to reconstruct complex defects and provide the best functional and aesthetic result. The SCIP flap can provide multiple components that may be needed for reconstruction such as lymph nodes and bones in addition to a large skin paddle. In the lower extremity, lymphedema, if it is unilateral, can be treated by harvesting the SCIP flap with 1 or 2 lymph nodes usually located close to the medial branch. When a small bone flap is needed, piece of the iliac crest can be included while using the lateral branch. Thus, the SCIP flap serves as a good chimeric flap for the lower extremity reconstruction. However, a good portion of lower

extremity reconstruction involves resurfacing over vital structures that are exposed. The skin on the anterior tibial region is naturally thin, and the SCIP flap being able to provide a thin flap, may be ideal for resurfacing that needs thin skin for coverage. A reasonably thin flap can be elevated without defatting procedure and seldom requires liposuction after reconstruction when elevated on the superficial fascial plane.[2] Recent publications show that the use of SCIP flap is catching on in the western hemisphere where more obese patients can be seen but still provides the advantages of being a pliable and thin flap.[27] Using this thin skin flap often sparks a debate whether or not it provides efficient outcome for osteomyelitis. As long as the principle of good debridement, obliteration of dead space, and coverage is performed, publications show that the composition of the covering tissue, whether it be muscle or skin, does not have a statistical difference in outcome.[18]

Regarding the skin paddle, flap extending to 12 × 32 cm can be harvested based on both or the lateral branch perforator. It is this character that the workhorse flap for resurfacing has changed from ALT to the SCIP flap. In our practice, the ALT is considered when (1) there is need for a long pedicle or to use the pedicle as a flow through

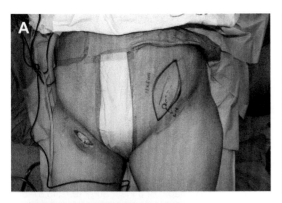

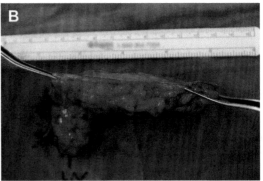

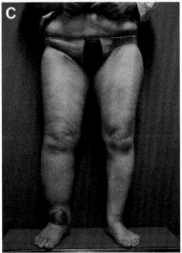

Fig. 4. A 52-year-old female patient is presented with a lymphedema of the right leg lasting the last 7 years. The contralateral left leg showed normal contour, and the decision was made to harvest an SCIP flap with lymph nodes (*A*). After harvesting an 11 × 5 cm SCIP with one lymph node based on the medial perforating branch of the SCIA, the flap was transferred to the anterior aspect of the right ankle and anastomosed to anterior tibial artery and vein (*B*). The postoperative result at 1 month shows well-taken flap and well-concealed donor site scar (*C*).

artery, (2) a deep fascia is needed to reconstruct the tendons, when a large muscle component is needed as a chimeric flap, (3) a sensate flap is needed using the cutaneous nerve, and (4) the groin is injured limiting the use of SCIP flap. In selecting the perforator flap for reconstruction, we consider 5 factors: the patient position on the operating table, flap size, flap composition, flap thickness, and pedicle length. According to this algorithm to reconstruct the lower extremity, the SCIP flap was the most commonly used in our practice where causes for reconstruction were trauma, cancer reconstruction, chronic wounds, and chronic osteomyelitis.[28]

One of the advantages in using the SCIP flap is the ease of pedicle dissection especially in using the medial (superficial) branch.[19] Majority is a direct cutaneous type allowing a quick dissection. However, when using the lateral (deep) branch, the dissection may be more difficult, as part of the pedicle may have a muscular pathway.[16,17] Nevertheless, dissection in the muscle portion is still relatively short. From our experience, most of the SCIP flap is based on the medial branch, as the need for a moderate- to small-sized flaps are more common in lower extremity reconstruction, making this flap a workhorse flap.

The challenges for using the SCIP flap are the initial learning curve, including to identify the superficial fascial plane and the ability to dissect and isolate the perforators followed by manipulating relatively short pedicles. For surgeons starting to work with this flap, patient selection should begin with leg, foot, forearm, and hand, where potential recipient artery and veins are superficially located, before moving on to the regions where recipient vessels are located deep and supermicrosurgery techniques (perforator to perforator) may be needed. In order to overcome the short pedicle of the flap, especially when using the medial branch of the SCIA, distal end branches, often perforators, from the axial artery and vein can be used as recipient vessels to accommodate the short pedicle. Using perforator to perforator supermicrosurgery in the lower extremity has shown to be safe and effective as using any major arteries and veins.[3,13] However, one must understand the limitation of the perforator vessel as a recipient, as the requirement of perfusion will be greater in large composite flaps. The only prerequisite in selecting the right recipient vessel is that it must have a strong pulse and a positive spurt test. The merits of this approach are that it minimizes the sacrifice of a major vessel, which is useful in limb salvage of a limb with only 1 remaining major vessel and in diabetic patients in whom the perforators are often the only vessels spared from the macrovascular disease.[2] Every flap has its pros and cons; such modifications allow us to maximize the potential of the SCIP flap.

SUMMARY

The SCIP flap is evolved from the groin flap, which was one of the early free flaps. In order to maximize the advantages of the SCIP flap, one must understand the anatomy and the relative character of the 2 perforators, medial and lateral branch, from the SCIA. In the reconstruction for the defects of the lower extremity, the SCIP flap provides advantage of being a thin flap, able to be harvested as a composite flap, and use of large skin dimension while having a well-hidden donor site scar. Despite these advantages, the relatively short pedicle still remains a challenge where long pedicle flaps are needed. One should select the flaps based on the recipient defect condition along with surgeons' experience, knowledge, and preference.

CLINICS CARE POINTS

- Identification of the target plane of elevation is the key to achieve the right SCIP flap variant.
- Best efforts should be made to close the donor site primarily.

REFERENCES

1. Hong JP, Sun SH, Ben-Nakhi M. Modified superficial circumflex iliac artery perforator flap and supermicrosurgery technique for lower extremity reconstruction: a new approach for moderate-sized defects. Ann Plast Surg 2013;71:380–3.
2. Goh TL, Park SW, Cho JY, et al. The search for the ideal thin skin flap: superficial circumflex iliac artery perforator flap–a review of 210 cases. Plast Reconstr Surg 2015;135:592–601.
3. Hong JP. The use of supermicrosurgery in lower extremity reconstruction: the next step in evolution. Plast Reconstr Surg 2009;123:230–5.
4. McGregor IA, Jackson IT. The groin flap. Br J Plast Surg 1972;25:3–16.
5. Daniel RK, Taylor GI. Distant transfer of an island flap by microvascular anastomoses. A clinical technique. Plast Reconstr Surg 1973;52:111–7.
6. Chuang DC, Colony LH, Chen HC, et al. Groin flap design and versatility. Plast Reconstr Surg 1989; 84:100–7.
7. Chuang DC, Jeng SF, Chen HT, et al. Experience of 73 free groin flaps. Br J Plast Surg 1992;45:81–5.
8. Hahn SB, Kim HK. Free groin flaps in microsurgical reconstruction of the extremity. J Reconstr Microsurg 1991;7:187–95 [discussion: 197–8].
9. Cooper TM, Lewis N, Baldwin MA. Free groin flap revisited. Plast Reconstr Surg 1999;103:918–24.
10. Koshima I, Nanba Y, Tsutsui T, et al. Superficial circumflex iliac artery perforator flap for reconstruction of limb defects. Plast Reconstr Surg 2004;113:233–40.
11. Hsu WM, Chao WN, Yang C, et al. Evolution of the free groin flap: the superficial circumflex iliac artery perforator flap. Plast Reconstr Surg 2007;119:1491–8.
12. Wei FC, Mardini S. Free-style free flaps. Plast Reconstr Surg 2004;114:910–6.
13. Hong JP, Koshima I. Using perforators as recipient vessels (supermicrosurgery) for free flap reconstruction of the knee region. Ann Plast Surg 2010;64:291–3.
14. Choi DH, Goh T, Cho JY, et al. Thin superficial circumflex iliac artery perforator flap and supermicrosurgery technique for face reconstruction. J Craniofac Surg 2014;25:2130–3.
15. Suh YC, Hong JP, Suh HP. Elevation technique for medial branch based superficial circumflex iliac artery perforator flap. Handchir Mikrochir Plast Chir 2018;50:256–8.
16. Yoshimatsu H, Steinbacher J, Meng S, et al. Superficial circumflex iliac artery perforator flap: an anatomical study of the correlation of the superficial and the deep branches of the artery and evaluation of perfusion from the deep branch to the sartorius muscle and the iliac bone. Plast Reconstr Surg 2019;143:589–602.
17. Yoshimatsu H, Yamamoto T, Iida T. Deep branch of the superficial circumflex iliac artery for backup. J Plast Reconstr Aesthet Surg 2015;68:1478–9.
18. Hong JPJ, Goh TLH, Choi DH, et al. The efficacy of perforator flaps in the treatment of chronic osteomyelitis. Plast Reconstr Surg 2017;140:179–88.
19. Suh HS, Jeong HH, Choi DH, et al. Study of the medial superficial perforator of the superficial circumflex iliac artery perforator flap using computed tomographic angiography and surgical anatomy in 142 patients. Plast Reconstr Surg 2017;139:738–48.
20. Fuse Y, Yoshimatsu H, Yamamoto T. Lateral approach to the deep branch of the superficial

circumflex iliac artery for harvesting a SCIP flap. Microsurgery 2018;38:589–90.

21. Yoshimatsu H, Iida T, Yamamoto T, et al. Superficial circumflex iliac artery-based iliac bone flap transfer for reconstruction of bony defects. J Reconstr Microsurg 2018;34:719–28.

22. Jin SJ, Suh HP, Lee J, et al. Lipo-prostaglandin E1 increases immediate arterial maximal flow velocity of free flap in patients undergoing reconstructive surgery. Acta Anaesthesiol Scand 2019;63:40–5.

23. Suh HP, Jeong HH, Hong JPJ. Is early compression therapy after perforator flap safe and reliable? J Reconstr Microsurg 2019;35:354–61.

24. Peter Suh HS, Hong JP. Effects of incisional negative-pressure wound therapy on primary closed defects after superficial circumflex iliac artery perforator flap harvest: randomized controlled study. Plast Reconstr Surg 2016;138:1333–40.

25. Yamamoto T, Yoshimatsu H, Koshima I. Navigation lymphatic supermicrosurgery for iatrogenic lymphorrhea: supermicrosurgical lymphaticolymphatic anastomosis and lymphaticovenular anastomosis under indocyanine green lymphography navigation. J Plast Reconstr Aesthet Surg 2014;67:1573–9.

26. Gottlieb LJ, Krieger LM. From the reconstructive ladder to the reconstructive elevator. Plast Reconstr Surg 1994;93:1503–4.

27. Berner JE, Nikkhah D, Zhao J, et al. The versatility of the superficial circumflex iliac artery perforator flap: a single surgeon's 16-year experience for limb reconstruction and a systematic review. J Reconstr Microsurg 2020;36:93–103.

28. Abdelfattah U, Power HA, Song S, et al. Algorithm for free perforator flap selection in lower extremity reconstruction based on 563 cases. Plast Reconstr Surg 2019;144:1202–13.

The Anterolateral Thigh Perforator Flap
Its Expanding Role in Lower Extremity Reconstruction

Chung-Chen Hsu, MD[a], Charles Yuen Yung Loh, MBBS, MS, MSc, MRCS[b], Fu-Chan Wei, MD[a],*

KEYWORDS

- Anterolateral thigh flap • ALT flap • Lower extremity reconstruction • Chimeric flap • Perforator flap

KEY POINTS

- The use of preoperative anterolateral thigh (ALT) flap perforator mapping helps facilitate the design of a skin flap.
- There are currently expanding indications for the versatile ALT flap for lower extremity reconstruction.
- ALT flap variation allows the incorporation of a chimeric flap design for lower limb defect reconstruction.
- It is not only available as a free flap but also can be raised as a pedicled ALT flap to provide a large arc of coverage for soft tissue reconstruction.
- ALT flap with 2 or more perforators can be used as split flaps or several independent flaps.

INTRODUCTION

The anterolateral thigh (ALT) flap is one of the most versatile flaps in a reconstructive surgeon's armamentarium. It is considered one of the more contemporary flaps in this era as reconstruction preferences change throughout the times. Its variations in design and tissue components in terms of a fasciocutaneous or chimeric flap with multiple components, including muscle and fascia, serve to reconstruct a myriad of defects. The ALT flap also has a lower donor site morbidity and can be harvested in the supine position, obviating any position change, which is convenient for most procedures.[1]

In lower extremity reconstruction, gaining optimal coverage quickly and safely is only the basic function of an ALT flap. The main pedicle, termed the descending branch of the lateral circumflex femoral artery (LCFA) and vein, allows a long and similar size match in vessel reconstruction of the lower limb. The various tissue types in the lower limb can be replaced with similar tissues in the ALT flap, which can be harvested with skin and fat alone or with muscle, fascia, and bone together. Volume for dead-space obliteration can be easily performed with the ALT flap. The fascia lata included in the ALT flap can be rolled to replace tendinous gaps in the lower extremity, such as the Achilles tendon. The iliac crest bone attached to the ALT flap or tensor fascia lata could be harvested simultaneously for 1-stage lower leg open fracture reconstruction that requires both soft tissue and bone components.

INDICATIONS AND CONTRAINDICATIONS

The ALT flap is indicated when there is a need for large surface area or volume defect reconstruction with vascularized tissue in the lower extremity.

[a] Department of Plastic and Reconstructive Surgery, Linkou Medical Center, Chang Gung Memorial Hospital, Chang Gung University, 5 Fu-hsing Street, Gueishan, Taoyuan 333, Taiwan, ROC; [b] Addenbrooke's Hospital, Hills Road, Cambridge CB2 0QQ, UK
* Corresponding author.
E-mail address: fuchanwei@gmail.com

Clin Plastic Surg 48 (2021) 235–248
https://doi.org/10.1016/j.cps.2020.12.008
0094-1298/21/© 2020 Elsevier Inc. All rights reserved.

When recipient vessels are a distance away, the ALT flap can be used with a long pedicle and large flap based on a distal perforator for greater length. The ALT flap is also a good option when multiple tissue types are required. It is an ideal flap for its versatility of inset and components that can be used to replace missing tissue for several purposes, including dead-space obliteration, the creation of a tendon gliding surface, tendon or ligament reconstruction, 1-stage soft tissue and bone defect reconstruction, a flow-through flap for major artery reconstruction, for coverage of a functioning rectus femoris muscle flap, or even for aesthetic soft tissue augmentation.

However, the contraindications are the same as for any free flap, including patients with severe comorbidities, extensive atherosclerotic disease,[2] and a dirty wound bed. When the donor site has been used before leaving no proximal stump of the descending branch of the lateral circumflex femoral vessels, the ALT flap should not be attempted. The ALT flap is also not preferred when extensive scar formation on the territory of the ALT flap is seen either from previous surgery or from trauma.

PREOPERATIVE EVALUATION AND SPECIAL CONSIDERATIONS
Preoperative Perforator Mapping

Handheld Doppler preoperative determination of perforators is generally reliable in the ALT flap, but they can vary in location during dissection.[3] Computed tomography (CT) angiography for ALT flap perforator mapping is useful for chimeric flap design but is not always necessary in experienced hands because of concern of radiation exposure and resource consumption.[4] Duplex ultrasonography is now another useful noninvasive choice for preoperative assessment of pressure and diameter of the perforators as well as their flow rate and course, which aids in dissection and flap design.[5]

Split Anterolateral Thigh Flap

The ALT flap can be split into various flaps depending on the perforators included in the flap. As such, this flap can be fashioned into a multitude of shapes all arising from the same pedicle, facilitating efficient use of the flap[6,7] (**Fig. 1**).

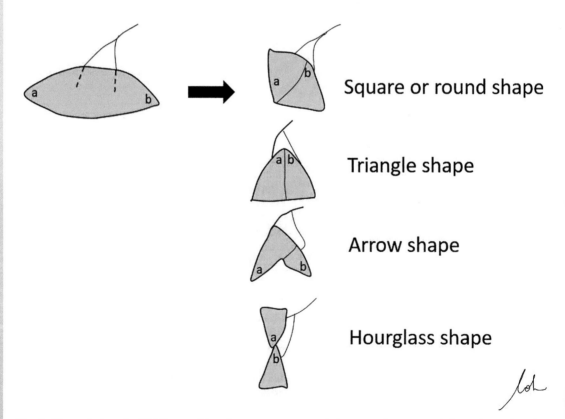

Fig. 1. The variations in ALT flap stacking for an assortment of shapes to fit various defects. (*Modified from* Chang NJ, Waughlock N, Kao D, et al. Efficient design of split anterolateral thigh flap in extremity reconstruction. Plast Reconstr Surg. 2011;128(6):1242-9; with permission.)

One Donor Site, 2 or more Free Flaps

The length of the descending branch of lateral circumflex also allows division of 1 ALT flap into 2 or more ALT flaps, each with its own separate perforators. The trick is ligation of the main trunk immediately distal to the bifurcation of the proximal perforator to get longer pedicle length for the distal flap. These techniques all allow minimizing donor site morbidity and maximizing flap output from a single donor site, which is not always possible with other flaps[8] (**Fig. 2**).

Timing of Flap Reconstruction

Marko Godina established the principle of early flap coverage for traumatic lower extremity injuries. Early free flap coverage performed within 3 days of injury has a lower flap failure rate and infection rate than the delayed free flap reconstruction (4–90 days) group. Based on a retrospective review of 358 free flap reconstructions, Lee and colleagues[9] updated Godina's paradigm, and the ideal early flap reconstruction can be safely performed within 10 days of injury without an adverse effect on outcomes. Reconstruction at an early stage has the benefit of less scarring and fibrosis around the vessels, which can make it more difficult for vessel dissection and lumen expansion. However, patients with trauma may present to the reconstructive surgeon at any time after their injury or after their earlier unsuccessful reconstruction, hence, surgeons should not be confined by those time lines. In our experience, timing may not be that critical, provided the surgeon is knowledgeable about time-related pathophysiology of the damaged tissue and is able to perform adequate debridement. A high flap success rate can still be expected even in the subacute phase. Immediate emergency flap reconstruction is defined as simultaneous flap coverage performed immediately following debridement after injury. It is indicated in cases where cover over an exposed critical organ (vessel, nerve, tendon, or bone) is required or to create a flow-through revascularization of the limb at the same time. Adequate debridement is the key point to achieving success in immediate emergency flap reconstruction.[10]

SURGICAL PROCEDURES FOR EXPANDING INDICATIONS
Dead-Space Obliteration

The presence of dead space can be filled with fluids that are easily infected. The ALT skin flap itself or vastus lateralis (VL) muscle can be used to fill large defects and obliterate dead space. The VL muscle is often supplied by the muscular branches of the same descending branch of the lateral circumflex pedicle.[1,11] The design with separated skin paddle and a VL muscle part could increase the flap inset freedom and avoid inadvertently damaging the perforator during its harvest, especially when the muscle is cut to the appropriate size. If further bulk is required, deepithelialization of the skin paddle can be performed and tucked into the defect. Inserting of drains into the dead space that is to be obliterated helps reduce any buildup of fluids, which can be a nidus of infection and compromise vascularity of the flap postoperatively (**Fig. 3**).

Creation of Tendon Gliding Surface

Tendons are unique because they serve a function that requires them to glide with the excursion of their respective muscle bellies. Skin grafting onto exposed tendon is also not feasible in most cases because take is not guaranteed, especially with

One donor site two flaps

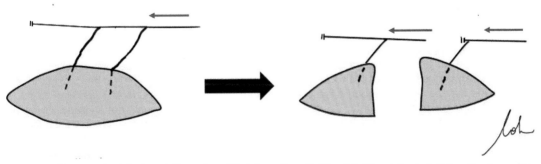

Fig. 2. ALT flaps can be split into 2 flaps. (*Modified from* Chou E, Ulusal B, Ulusal A, et al. Using the descending branch of the lateral femoral circumflex vessel as a source of two independent flaps. Plast Reconstr Surg. 2006;117(6):2059-63; with permission.)

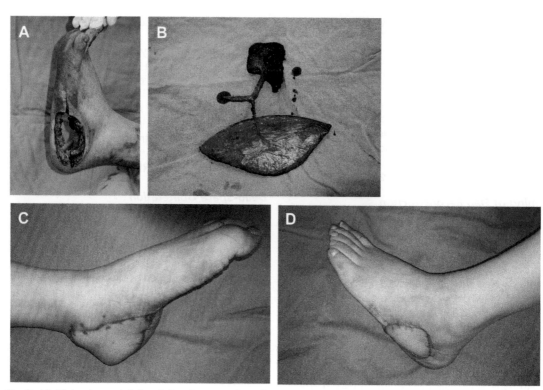

Fig. 3. (*A*, *B*) A calcaneal defect following resection of a sarcoma was reconstructed with a chimeric ALT flap for dead-space obliteration and resurfacing. (*C*, *D*) At 3-month follow-up.

denuded paratenon. The other problem with skin grafting onto tendons is that the graft is adherent and scars up, causing the tendons to stick and in turn reduce their function without appropriate glide and excursion. As such, the fascial component of an ALT fasciocutaneous flap that is vascularized can act as a barrier on top of the exposed tendons to minimize adhesions formed postoperatively. This approach in turn reduces the need for subsequent tenolysis to achieve a desirable function (**Fig. 4**). This ALT fasciocutaneous flap harvest can be designed in a more lateral aspect of the regular ALT territory to include a larger piece of fascia lata.

Tendon or Ligament Reconstruction

The fascia lata component of the ALT flap (ALT fasciocutaneous flap) can be rolled to form a tendonlike structure for large tendon defect reconstruction. It can be used for reconstructing the anterior tibialis and the Achilles tendon in the lower extremity. Planning with a template to design the ALT flap in the position of the pedicle and length of the fascia lata for tendon reconstruction has to be done preoperatively because the rolled fascia has to be placed under the optimal tension and right orientation to prevent pedicle compression by the reconstructed tendon. The fascia remains

revascularized and bleeding when the flap is debulked at a later stage. Full restoration of ankle movement is also possible with this technique[12] (**Fig. 5**). The patellar ligament and anterior tibialis tendon are crucial for knee and ankle extension and can also be reconstructed with an ALT fasciocutaneous flap with rolled fascia (**Fig. 6**).

Distally Based Pedicled Anterolateral Thigh Flap

Distally based pedicled ALT flaps are useful in preserving lower limb length and providing vital soft tissue coverage, including over the entire knee. When amputations, for example, occur for various reasons and bone is exposed, to prevent an above-knee amputation with exposed knee joint, a pedicled ALT flap can be useful with a reverse flow based on the distal runoff. A fasciocutaneous ALT flap can reach the knee joint distally.[13] Retrograde or reverse-flow ALT flap has similar arterial pressures to an antegrade ALT flap and, as such, arterial perfusion is usually not an issue.[14] However, venous congestion is a commonly encountered problem with reverse-flow ALT flaps, which may need venous supercharge to the great saphenous vein on the medial side of the thigh (**Fig. 7**). The larger the ALT flap taken, the more severe the degree of venous congestion to be expected.

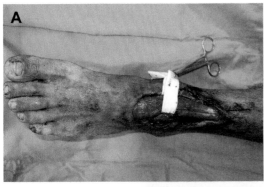
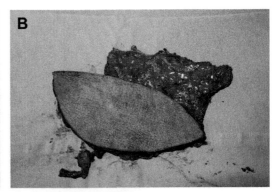
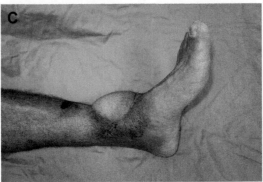

Fig. 4. (*A, B*) Exposed extensor tendons reconstructed with a free ALT flap containing vascularized fascia lata to allow for tendon gliding. (*C*) At 3-month follow-up.

Venous congestion can last 3 to 7 days postoperatively. If no intervention is performed, partial necrosis can be expected in the skin paddle.[15]

Designing the reverse-flow ALT flap paddle is also crucial depending on the origin and location of the chosen perforator. If the perforator arises from the transverse branch of the LCFA, extensive dissection is necessary in the proximal thigh to get to the connection point between the transverse branch and descending branch. The donor site morbidity is thus higher because of the damage to the muscle and its motor nerves and arteries

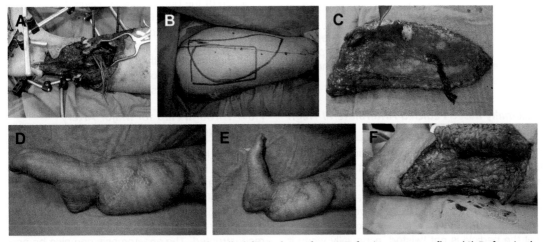

Fig. 5. Achilles tendon reconstruction with rolled fascia lata of an ALT fasciocutaneous flap. (*A*) Defect in the Achilles tendon. (*B*) Extension of fascia lata component beyond the ALT posterior margin was used as a graft. (*C*) Fascia lata rolled and connected to the stump of the Achilles tendon. (*D, E*) Good motion arc of the ankle at 2-year follow-up. (*F*) Well-vascularized fascia lata (new Achilles tendon) seen 2 years postoperatively during a debulking procedure.

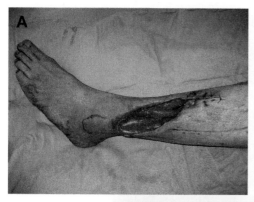
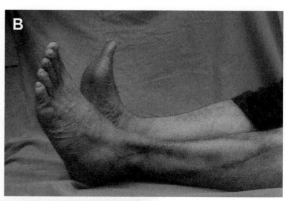
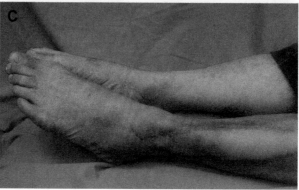

Fig. 6. Anterior tibialis and extensor hallucis longus tendon reconstruction with rolled fascia component of the ALT fasciocutaneous flap. (*A*) Crush injury with soft tissue and tendon defect. (*B, C*) The final result at 2-year follow-up with a weakened extension but functional ankle. The patient was able to ambulate without the need for a crutch.

supplying the surrounding muscle. Shifting to free flap is recommended in this scenario. If the chosen perforator is located distal in the thigh and is close to the knee, a propeller-style flap can be designed with a longer proximal flap segment for rotation distally because mobility for the advancement of the vascular pedicle is limited. If the perforator is located on the descending branch of the LCFA and is proximal, the proximal end of the pedicle can be detached with the flap advanced and inset distally as planned[16] (**Fig. 8**).

Proximally Based Pedicled Anterolateral Thigh Flaps

Proximally based pedicled ALT flaps also have their role in reconstructing defects in the lower abdomen, groin, or perineal area.[17] Using the LCFA point of origin as the center, the ALT flap can be harvested and inset to cover any defect within that arc radius. Care is taken to ensure that the pedicle is not twisted, especially when it is passed under the rectus femoris muscle to get more arc of rotation for defect coverage. For extra length, the pedicle to the rectus femoris may have to be sacrificed (**Fig. 9**).

One-Stage Soft Tissue and Bone Defect Reconstruction

Vascularized iliac bone can be harvested with ALT flap as a chimeric flap for simultaneous reconstruction of the bone and soft tissue defect in the lower extremity. The tensor fascia lata is included to preserve the blood supply to the iliac crest.[18] This approach allows 1-stage total reconstruction, which can decrease the risk of infection in the use of large amounts of nonvascularized bone grafts or cadaveric bone grafts (**Fig. 10**).

Flow-Through Flap for Major Artery Reconstruction

Ischemic lower extremity can be rescued or improved in its circulation with an ALT flow-through flap. Because both proximal pedicle and distal runoff have good diameter for microanastomosis, segmental defects in the anterior tibial artery or posterior tibial artery can be reconstructed. The anastomosis can also be performed out of the zone of trauma. This approach is particularly useful when revascularization and coverage reconstruction are needed at the same time. Segmental vascular defects of up to 15 cm

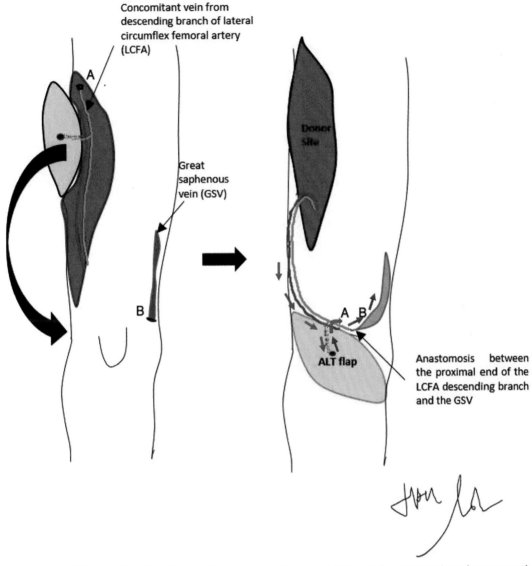

Fig. 7. The pedicled ALT flap for a knee defect reconstruction in a right leg with anastomosis to the great saphenous vein for supercharging venous drainage of dismally based pedicled ALT flap. (*Courtesy of* C. Hsu, MD, Taoyuan, Taiwan and C.Y.Y. Loh MBBS, MS, MSc, MRCS Cambridge, UK.)

in length can be bridged with the run-through ALT flap.[6] However, the length of the descending branch may be insufficient for revascularization of longer vascular defects in the lower leg. It may be prudent to use a vein graft at times to achieve revascularization (**Fig. 11**).

Simultaneous Coverage and Functional Muscle Reconstruction

Because the rectus femoris is also nourished by the descending branch of the LCFA, the rectus femoris can be included in the harvest of ALT

flap to serve as a functional muscle transfer. In anterior compartment muscle loss of the lower limb, the patients become unable to extend their ankles and toes, so this approach is useful for simultaneous functional and coverage reconstruction. Harvesting the skin paddle as an en bloc myocutaneous flap with rectus femoris muscle underneath is not advisable. Instead, a combined flap design with separate branches to rectus femoris muscle and skin is a more reliable and versatile design for flap inset. Neurotization is performed when the nerve to the rectus femoris is coapted to the remnant key motor nerve in the anterior

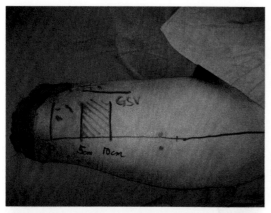
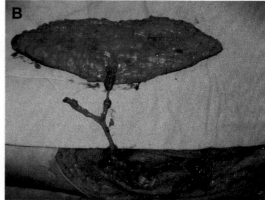
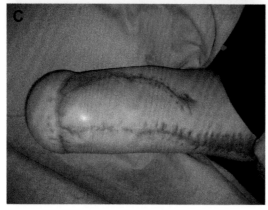

Fig. 8. (*A*) Distally based pedicled ALT flap for coverage of exposed bone from knee disarticulation. (*B*) Super-charging antegrade drainage to the greater saphenous vein (GSV) on the medial side of the knee for venous augmentation. Artery flow (*red arrow*), venous drainage (*blue arrow*), GSV. (*C*) Flap inset. However, shifting to free flap is recommended to avoid extensive dissection, which shall cause higher donor site morbidity as well as risks of uncertain artery perfusion or quality of venous return.

compartment of the lower limb. The pedicle to the rectus femoris can arise separately away from the descending branch of the LCFA and hence may need to have a second vascular anastomosis with another connecting vessel (**Fig. 12**).

Aesthetic Soft Tissue Augmentation and Resurfacing

The ALT flap can also be used for soft tissue augmentation and replacement of severe scarring in the lower limbs resulted from crush injuries (**Fig. 13**).

POSTOPERATIVE CARE AND EXPECTED OUTCOME

Postoperatively monitoring of the flap is performed in a dedicated flap unit with the patient on a strict bed-rest regime for the first 3 days until endotheli-alization of the anastomosis stabilizes. A dangling protocol is initiated after the third day with gradual increase in time with the limb dependent. Walking

is then commenced with the aid of physiothera-pists, and, depending on the underlying bone injury, weight bearing is then commenced. If at any time the flap becomes compromised, the au-thors have a low threshold for taking the flap back for reexploration, especially within the first 3 days.[19] Broad-spectrum antibiotics are given with stewardship guided by our microbiologists and cultures sent. Compression garments are gradually applied when wounds are healed.

Lin and colleagues[18] presented a series of 44 flap reconstructions based on the LCFA system. On top of achieving wound coverage, the recon-struction goals also included complex procedures, such as anterior compartment functioning muscle transfer and tibia and calcaneus bone reconstruc-tions. The success rate of these free flaps was 97.7%. Four flaps underwent reexplorations and 1 subsequently failed.[19] In the other series of 46 ALT flaps for lower extremity reconstructions, most of the flaps were designed in a pedicled fashion (63%) for the defects on hip/buttock, groin,

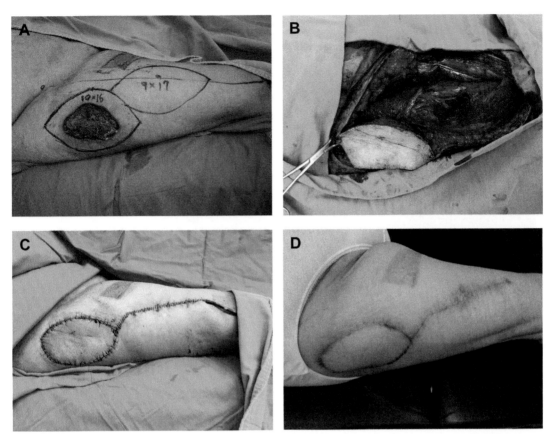

Fig. 9. Right thigh soft tissue tumor after excision with skin graft coverage. Wider excision was performed of a neurofibrosarcoma and a pedicled ALT fasciocutaneous flap was used for wound closure. (*A*) Flap design: a line from the anterior superior iliac spine to the lateral margin of the patella bone is marked as the axis of the flap. A flap measuring 9 × 17 cm was designed based on a perforator with a clear Doppler signal detected near the midpoint of the line. (*B*) Flap inset: the pedicle was dissected until the flap could be moved to cover the defect. (*C*). Immediate postoperative view. (*D*) A smooth lateral thigh contour was seen at 6-month follow-up.

thigh, knee, lower leg, and foot/ankle. The overall total flap failure rate was 4%, and 8 flaps (17%) needed reoperation for pedicle crisis, including compression or twisting.[20]

MANAGEMENT OF FLAP VARIATION

The ALT flap is known for its varied anatomy, and reconstructive microsurgeons should learn techniques to adapt to the scenario. When perforators to the ALT flap do not arise from the descending branch of the LCFA, intraflap anastomoses of the separate perforator may be required. When 2 perforators are chosen with 1 arising from the descending branch of the LCFA and the other from the transverse branch, the one from the transverse branch can be divided and microsurgically anastomosed to another branch of the main descending circumflex femoral artery for the flap supercharge. If

pedicles or perforators to various components, such as the VL and the skin paddle, arise from separate main pedicles, intraflap technique could be used to create a neochimeric ALT flap suited to the reconstructive needs. Intraflap anastomosis also has the advantage of decreasing the donor site morbidity because of saving motor nerves and muscle nutrient arteries during 1 component pedicle dissection of a chimeric flap. The incidence of unreliable or absent perforators was 4.8% in the ALT flap.[17] If no perforator or an unsuitable perforator is identified from the descending branch, perforators from an oblique or transverse branch are explored. When fascia is needed, a tensor fascia lata flap is the next best choice. If there is still a lack of a suitable perforator, the dissection can be extended medially to identify perforating vessels of the anteromedial thigh flap. Another option is to harvest a distant flap (free-style

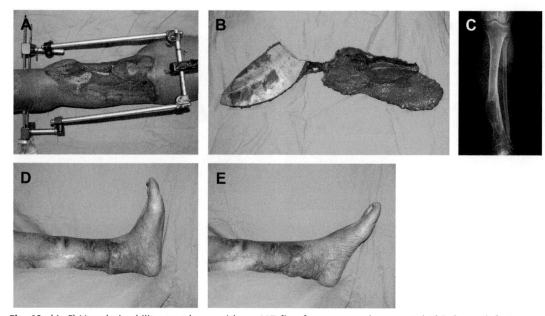

Fig. 10. (*A, B*) Vascularized iliac crest bone with an ALT flap for compound segmental tibia bone defect reconstruction of the tibia. (*C–E*) Primary healing of the soft tissue and bone defect seen on follow-up. (*Courtesy of C. Lin, MD, Taipei, Taiwan.*)

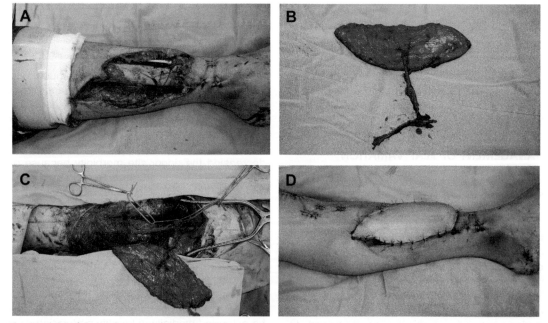

Fig. 11. (*A*) Left lower leg open fracture with bone exposure. An ALT fasciocutaneous flap was harvested for soft tissue defect coverage. (*B, C*) The descending branch of the lateral circumflex pedicle was about 10 cm in length to bridge the posterior tibial artery defect. (*D*) Immediate postoperative view.

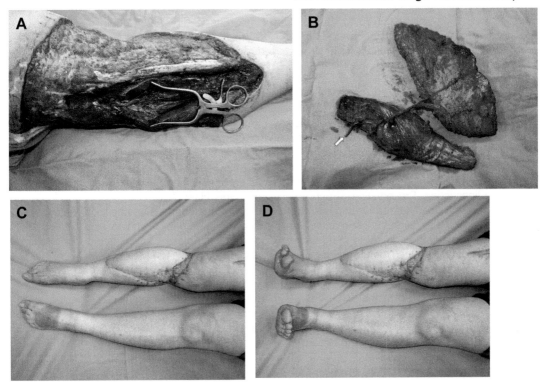

Fig. 12. Functional rectus femoris muscle transfer with an ALT flap for anterior compartment reconstruction in the lower limb. (*A*) Defect in the anterior compartment. (*B*) ALT flap harvested with the rectus femoris muscle and its motor nerve. The motor nerve is marked (*arrow*) (*C, D*) Functional result achieved at 3-year follow-up.

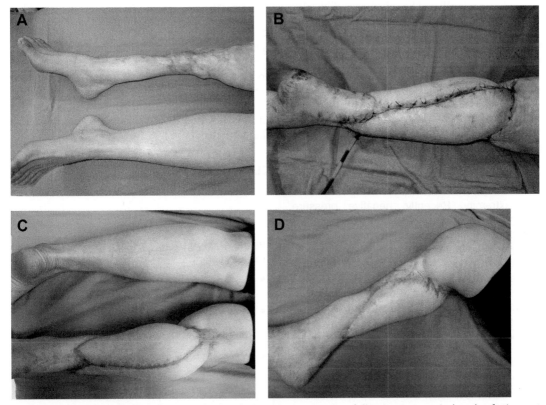

Fig. 13. Double free ALT flaps for lower limb soft tissue augmentation following trauma-induced soft tissue atrophy since childhood. (*A*) Right lower limb muscle and soft tissue atrophy. (*B*) Second-stage lateral side augmentation with a second free ALT flap. (*C, D*) The final result at 1-year follow-up.

perforator flap) or profunda femoral artery perforator flap when the contralateral thigh is not available.[21,22]

REVISION OR SUBSEQUENT PROCEDURES

At follow-up, if the flap remains bulky, a secondary debulking procedure is performed at a later date after several months. This secondary procedure can be performed either by elevating a part of the flap and debulking the flap under direct vision or via liposuction. Preservation of perforators is preferred but does not matter at this stage as long as 50% of the skin edge is left intact. Care is taken to avoid inadvertent injury to the pedicle of the flap. Removal of any metalwork can be done in conjunction with orthopedic colleagues, again with preservation of the pedicle, and debulking can be performed at the same time if required.

On the foot or dorsal ankle, thinner flaps are always required. The ALT flaps applied to this specific zone in the lower limb result in a thicker skin layer of the ALT flap despite multiple debulking procedures to remove almost all the initial subcutaneous fat. A 1-stage debulking procedure with full-thickness skin graft from the original flap introduced by Lin and Quing[23] can provide thin skin coverage and reliable long-term outcome. Under tourniquet control, direct excision of the subcutaneous tissue and fat, and even tangential excision of the muscle part if a myocutaneous ALT flap was used, can be performed. The skin graft is then fixed onto the raw surface and covered with a tie-over dressing for 9 days. A splint is used to keep the ankle joint immobilized.

DISCUSSION

Adequate debridement and a clean wound bed are the basic requirements of flap reconstruction in the lower extremity. Recently, negative pressure wound therapy has been touted as a more comfortable wound dressing, providing a better environment for granulation tissue growth. Nevertheless, early flap reconstruction is still the preferred strategy. During every debridement procedure, the defect size, location, and missing tissue components should be recorded for preoperative planning.

If a pedicled flap is needed, the perforator location can affect the potential flap arc of mobility or can decrease the pedicle tension by advancing or rotating the flap based on these carefully chosen perforator locations. If a free flap is indicated, optimal recipient vessel choice is important.

Physical examination, ultrasonography Doppler study, or CT angiography can help determine recipient vessel availability. However, the final selection must be decided intraoperatively by dissecting the closest vessel adjacent to the defect until good spurting of blood is visualized. In subacute or late-stage reconstruction of the lower limb, fibrosis around the vessel may impair vessel dissection. In such cases, the authors prefer to start the vessel dissection from the trauma zone distally to healthy proximal tissues until the vessel end is identified.[24]

Use of a template is another useful aid in facilitating the ALT flap design. A single nylon stitch on the template could avoid inadvertently mistaking the wrong side up in planning the flap design. The authors also mark on the template the possible direction for vessel anastomosis to facilitate inset. On the template, the location of perforators, muscle, or rolled fascia can be marked to make the orientation clear in designing the split or chimeric flap. This method allows us to reduce complications caused by poor flap component inset.

SUMMARY

The ALT flap is a workhorse flap of the lower extremity. The flap can be designed as a local island pedicle flap or free flap. In addition, many tissue components in the flap can be raised from the same vascular pedicle, which makes it versatile for surface or dead-space obliteration, and tendon, ligament, bone, or major artery reconstruction. Reconstructive surgeons have to be familiar with ALT flap anatomy and management of flap variation to push the applications of this flap to the limit.

CLINICS CARE POINTS

Pearls when ALT flap is used in lower extremity reconstruction:

- Avoid using previously injured donor sites when elevating an ALT flap.
- Accurate mapping of audible Doppler sounds and marking them with different sized dots depending on their loudness.
- Select appropriate dots to design the flap, taking into consideration pedicle length of reach and arc of rotation/advancement as a local flap or appropriate length and vessel diameters as a free flap.

- Use loupe or microscope magnification all the time, especially for dissection of the intramuscular portion of the vascular pedicle.
- Meticulously cauterize or ligate all visible small branches from the pedicle for perfect hemostasis.
- Always keep the pedicle moist with warm normal saline and 2% xylocaine to avoid desiccation and vasospasm.
- Confirm adequate circulation to the entire flap before being transferred to the defect or division of the pedicle as a free flap.
- Avoid twisting, kinking, or compression during flap inset.
- Perform the arterial anastomoses before venous anastomoses to ensure smooth pedicle inset.

Pitfalls when using the ALT flap for lower extremity reconstruction:

- Possible vascular anatomic variation of the pedicle, including the absence of any accompanying artery or vein.
- Not being able to be reliably thin this flap intraoperatively, making the flap slightly bulkier during inset in some locations, such as the foot and ankle.

DISCLOSURE

The authors have nothing to disclose.

REFERENCES

1. Lin YT, Lin CH, Wei FC. More degrees of freedom by using chimeric concept in the applications of anterolateral thigh flap. J Plast Reconstr Aesthet Surg 2006;59(6):622–7.
2. Saint-Cyr M, Wong C, Buchel EW, et al. Free tissue transfers and replantation. Plast Reconstr Surg 2012;130(6):858e–78e.
3. Stekelenburg CM, Sonneveld PM, Bouman MB, et al. The hand held Doppler device for the detection of perforators in reconstructive surgery: what you hear is not always what you get. Burns 2014;40(8):1702–6.
4. Shen Y, Huang J, Dong MJ, et al. Application of computed tomography angiography mapping and located template for accurate location of perforator in head and neck reconstruction with anterolateral thigh perforator flap. Plast Reconstr Surg 2016;137(6):1875–85.
5. Dorfman D, Pu LL. The value of color duplex imaging for planning and performing a free anterolateral thigh perforator flap. Ann Plast Surg 2014;72(Suppl 1):S6-S8.
6. Chang NJ, Waughlock N, Kao D, et al. Efficient design of split anterolateral thigh flap in extremity reconstruction. Plast Reconstr Surg 2011;128(6):1242–9.
7. Tsai FC1, Yang JY, Mardini S, et al. Free split-cutaneous perforator flaps procured using a three-dimensional harvest technique for the reconstruction of postburn contracture defects. Plast Reconstr Surg 2004;113(1):185–93.
8. Erh-Kang C, Betul U, Ali U, et al. Using the descending branch of the lateral femoral circumflex vessel as a source of two independent flaps. Plast Reconstr Surg 2006;117(6):2059–63.
9. Lee ZH, Stranix JT, Rifkin WJ, et al. Timing of microsurgical reconstruction in lower extremity trauma: an update of the godina paradigm. Plast Reconstr Surg 2019;144(3):759–67.
10. Hsu CC, Lin YT, Lin CH, et al. Immediate emergency free anterolateral thigh flap transfer for the mutilated upper extremity. Plast Reconstr Surg 2009;123(6):1739–47.
11. Koshima I, Kawada S, Etoh H, et al. Flow-through anterior thigh flaps for one-stage reconstruction of soft-tissue defects and revascularization of ischemic extremities. Plast Reconstr Surg 1995;95(2):252–60.
12. Ehrl D, Heidekrueger PI, Schmitt A, et al. The anterolateral thigh flap for achilles tendon reconstruction: functional outcomes. Plast Reconstr Surg 2019;143(6):1772–83.
13. Lin CH, Zelken J, Hsu CC, et al. The distally based, venous supercharged anterolateral thigh flap. Microsurgery 2016;36(1):20–8.
14. Pan SC, Yu JC, Shieh SJ, et al. Distally based anterolateral thigh flap: an anatomic and clinical study. Plast Reconstr Surg 2004;114(7):1768–75.
15. Lin CH, Hsu CC, Lin CH, et al. Antegrade venous drainage in a reverse-flow anterolateral thigh flap. Plast Reconstr Surg 2009;124(5):273e–4e.
16. Wong CH, Goh T, Tan BK, et al. The anterolateral thigh perforator flap for reconstruction of knee defects. Ann Plast Surg 2013;70(3):337–42.
17. Zelken JA, AlDeek NF, Hsu CC, et al. Algorithmic approach to lower abdominal, perineal, and groin reconstruction using anterolateral thigh flaps. Microsurgery 2016;36:104–14.
18. Lin CH, Wei FC, Lin YT, et al. Lateral circumflex femoral artery system: warehouse for functional composite free-tissue reconstruction of the lower leg. J Trauma 2006;60(5):1032–6.
19. Chen KT, Mardini S, Chuang DC, et al. Timing of presentation of the first signs of vascular compromise dictates the salvage outcome of free flap transfers. Plast Reconstr Surg 2007;120(1):187–95.
20. Nosrati N, Chao AH, Chang DW, et al. Lower extremity reconstruction with the anterolateral

thigh flap. J Reconstr Microsurg 2012;28(4): 227–34.

21. Lu JC, Zelken J, Hsu CC, et al. Algorithmic approach to anterolateral thigh flaps lacking suitable perforators in lower extremity reconstruction. Plast Reconstr Surg 2015;135(5):1476–85.

22. Wei FC, Mardini S. Free-style free flaps. Plast Reconstr Surg 2004;114(4):910–6.

23. Lin TS, Quing R. Long-term results of a one-stage secondary debulking procedure after flap reconstruction of the foot. Plast Reconstr Surg 2016; 138(4):923–30.

24. Yazar S, Lin CH. Selection of recipient vessel in traumatic lower extremity. J Reconstr Microsurg 2012; 28:199–204.

The Medial Sural Artery Perforator Flap in Lower Extremity Reconstruction

Cheng-Hung Lin, MD[a],*, Yun-Huan Hsieh, MBBS, MS (PRS)[b],
Chih-Hung Lin, MD[c]

KEYWORDS

- Medial sural artery perforator flap • Lower extremity reconstruction • Soft tissue reconstruction
- Free tissue transfer • Microsurgery • Pedicled perforator flap

KEY POINTS

- MSAP flap is thin and pliable with moderate pedicle length. It is suitable for small to medium-sized defect reconstructions of the lower limb.
- MSAP flap is raised as a pedicled or a free flap for locoregional and distant defect reconstructions and is a workhorse flap capable of reconstructing all anatomic regions of the lower limb.
- CTA, Doppler, indocyanine green, and endoscopic-assisted dissection enhance MSAP flap surgical planning and reduce technical adversities and complications secondary to anatomic variations.
- Tourniquet-assisted dissection, meticulous hemostasis, and high pedicle division above the bifurcation of medial sural artery lessen the risk of arterial spasm and reduce anastomosis challenges.

INTRODUCTION

Meticulous evaluation of tissue defect components in lower extremity reconstruction is the essence of achieving satisfactory functional and aesthetic outcomes. Recent technical refinements of perforator flaps and diverse donor site availabilities permit tailored reconstruction while minimizing donor site morbidity. The medial sural artery perforator (MSAP) flap is a relatively new flap. As first described in 2001, MSAP flap was primarily indicated for lower limb reconstruction.[1,2] The versatility of the MSAP flap accompanies its growing popularity.[3] It is thin and pliable with predictable vascular anatomy. It is raised either as a free flap or a pedicled perforator flap and used predominantly as a fasciocutaneous flap.

Comparing with the anterolateral thigh (ALT) flap, the MSAP flap has shorter pedicle, and perforators are embedded more superficially in medial gastrocnemius muscle. Thus, the intramuscular dissection is less demanding and less traumatic. Like the ALT flap, the MSAP flap can also be harvested as a chimeric flap, providing much-needed volume for the desired reconstruction.

The MSAP flap can be raised with an applied tourniquet, aiding an advantage over the ALT with the bloodless surgical field during dissection. Claimed challenges of this flap consist of anatomic variations, extended intramuscular dissection, and potential donor site morbidity. Preoperative computed tomography angiography (CTA), Doppler-assisted perforator mapping, endoscopic-assisted perforator visualization, and indocyanine green fluorescence imaging enhance MSAP flap surgical planning and reduce technical adversities and complications secondary to anatomic variations. This article describes the versatility of pedicled and free MSAP flaps for lower extremity reconstruction. Surgical indications, specific considerations, and

[a] Department of Plastic and Reconstructive Surgery, Chang Gung Memorial Hospital, Chang Gung Medical College and Chang Gung University, 5, Fu-Hsing Street, Kuei-Shan, Taoyuan, Taiwan; [b] Department of Plastic and Reconstructive Surgery, Epworth Eastern Hospital, 1 Arnold Street, Box Hill, Victoria, Australia; [c] Department of Plastic and Reconstructive Surgery, Chiayi Chang Gung Memorial Hospital, 6, Sec. West, Chia-Pu Road, Putzu City, Chiayi County, Taiwan
* Corresponding author.
E-mail address: lukechlin@gmail.com

Clin Plastic Surg 48 (2021) 249–257
https://doi.org/10.1016/j.cps.2021.01.003
0094-1298/21/© 2021 Elsevier Inc. All rights reserved.

surgical steps of MSAP flap are also examined and explored in detail.

INDICATIONS AND CONTRAINDICATIONS OF MEDIAL SURAL ARTERY PERFORATOR FLAP TRANSFERS

The choice between pedicled and free MSAP flap is based on anatomic regions. Parallel to pedicled medial gastrocnemius flap, pedicled MSAP flap is indicated for knee and the proximal third of the leg reconstructions. In pedicled MSAP flap, the skeletonized vascular pedicle extended the range of flap advancement with a greater arc of rotation. These features enable MSAP flap coverage to the lateral knee and the middle third of the leg, which are traditionally unattainable with pedicled medial gastrocnemius muscle flap. MSAP flap is one of the most effective flaps for small to medium-sized defect reconstructions at all regions of the lower extremity.[4]

The main indication for free MSAP flap in lower extremity reconstruction is resurfacing of the ankle and foot defect with exposed tendon or bone/metalware. These regions generally require a thin and pliable flap to restore the contour so that patients may comfortably wear shoes. In the rare scenario, the chimeric MSAP flap with the inclusion of partial medial gastrocnemius muscle is applied to obliterate dead spaces or augment missing tissue volume, either as a free or a pedicled flap.

The MSAP flap is contraindicated in trauma involving the proximal tibia or medial gastrocnemius muscle because the perforators may be within the zone of injury. Also, hematoma and bruise on the muscle may interfere with the precise identification of the perforator and intramuscular dissection (**Box 1**).

PREOPERATIVE EVALUATION AND SPECIAL CONSIDERATIONS

Preoperative CTA is recommended for preoperative mapping of MSAP flap vascular anatomy.

Box 1
The indication, contraindication, and versatility of MSAP flap.

- MSAP chimeric flap is indicated for bone and metalware coverage, and dead space obliteration.
- Pedicled MSAP flap is an alternative flap for knee and proximal two-thirds of leg defects.
- Free MSAP flap is suitable for foot, ankle, and distal one-third of the leg reconstructions.
- MSAP flap is contraindicated with trauma involving proximal tibia or medial calf.

CTA can identify vascular injuries and variations, and delineate the relationships between perforators and skin paddles. CTA can also map the vascular branching patterns and detect the depth, directions, and intramuscular course of the perforators. This is crucial information for surgical planning and flap design, especially if a chimeric flap is indicated (**Fig. 1**A). In the rare scenario, when medial sural artery anatomy is unfavorable for MSAP flap, CTA also facilitates the design of an alternative flap preoperatively as a backup procedure (**Fig. 1**B).

In our study, the MSAPs were found between 6 and 15 cm from the popliteal crease, and the average number of the perforators is 1.4 (1–3 perforators; n = 1 [34], n = 2 [16], n = 3 [2]). Similar to the study by Hallock,[2] most of the vascular pedicles are located superficially within medial gastrocnemius muscle. The upper limit of the flap size in this series measured 15 × 9 cm[2]. The average pedicle length was 11.0 cm, with a maximum length of 20 cm.

SURGICAL PROCEDURES

Patients were positioned in supine with abducted and externally rotated hip, and 90° flexion of the knee. Tourniquets were routinely used on the thigh. A line was drawn between the midpoint of the popliteal crease and the medial malleolus. Candidate perforators were located by handheld pencil Doppler centered over the drawn line over the midcalf.[5,6] In some of our cases, endoscopy was used to visualize the perforator locations, facilitating the design of the skin paddle (**Fig. 2**A).

Raise of a Fasciocutaneous Flap

The first skin incision was made over the anteromedial border of the designed skin paddle down to the fascia. Everting the anteromedial flap edge with gentle traction facilitates subfascial dissection and perforator identification. Because the Doppler signals of the perforators are loosely correlated with the actual perforator locations, once the perforators were identified, fine design adjustment of the MSAP flap may be needed. The chosen perforators were traced back to the medial sural artery pedicle through retrograde intramuscular dissection. The vascular pedicle was routinely traced proximally to the bifurcation of medial sural artery, because its caliber reduced abruptly after its division.[7] This step permits the inclusion of vessels with greater caliber, reduces the risk of vasospasm, and lessens the technical challenge of the microvascular anastomosis. The posterolateral boundary of the flap was left undivided until sufficient pedicle length was yielded.

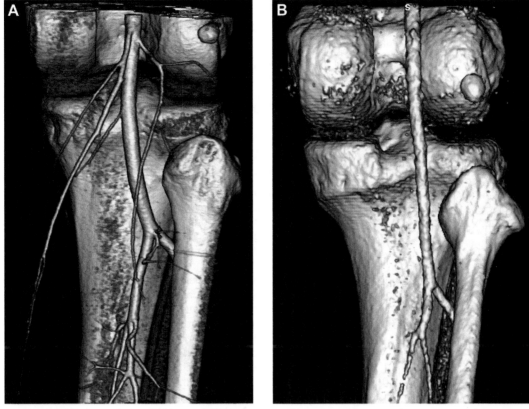

Fig. 1. CTA with three dimensional reconstruction image of posterior knee vascular anatomy. (*A*) Presence of medial and lateral branches of the right medial sural artery, favorable for chimeric flap design. (*B*) Absence of medial and lateral sural arteries, an unfavorable vascular anatomy for MSAP flap.

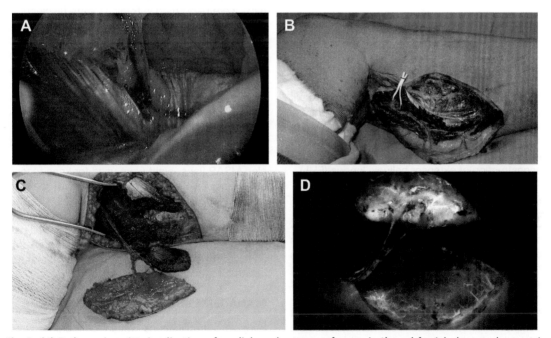

Fig. 2. (*A*) Endoscopic-assist visualization of medial sural artery perforator in the subfascial plane under tourniquet control. (*B*) The posterolateral boundary of the flap was left undivided until sufficient pedicle length was acquired to prevent accidental perforator traction, twisting, or kinking during intramuscular dissection. (*C*) The design of chimeric MSAP flap. The muscle component was based on the distal runoff of the lateral branch. (*D*) Intraoperative indocyanine green fluorescence imaging. The indocyanine green image demonstrated adequate native perfusion of the flap and sufficient residual muscular perfusion of medial gastrocnemius muscle.

This step prevents accidental perforator traction, twisting, or kinking during intramuscular dissection (**Fig. 2**B).

Raise of a Chimeric Flap

The fasciocutaneous flaps were raised mostly based on the lateral branch of the medial sural artery in our patient population. Thus, when designing a chimeric MSAP flap with gastrocnemius muscle, the muscle component was based either on the medial branch or the distal runoff of the lateral branch (**Fig. 2**C).[8] The muscle component of the chimeric flap is designed with 1 to 2 cm of the skeletonized pedicle to enhance the degree of freedom during flap inset.

Raise of a Pedicled Flap

There are four types of pedicled MSAP flap designs to accommodate different defect sizes and locations: (1) propeller flap, (2) peninsular flap, (3) advancement flap, and (4) proximally based island flap. Accurate mapping of the perforators is critical for pedicled MSAP flap design and its subsequent success. Skeletonizing the pedicles from meticulous intramuscular dissection significantly increases the pedicle length, enhances the flap advancement, and inset flexibility. Thus, it strengthens the versatility of the pedicled flap.

Harvest of Adjacent Tissue Components

Anatomically, medial sural artery territory is surrounded by various useful donor tissues and structures. From the same donor site, tendon grafts are harvested from plantaris tenon between the medial gastrocnemius and soleus or from a split Achilles tendon. In addition, saphenous and sural nerve grafts can also be harvested via the same incision site.[6] In our series, three flaps were raised with plantaris tendon grafts for simultaneous reconstruction of extensor hallucis longus (EHL).

Intraoperative Indocyanine Green Fluorescence Imaging

Indocyanine green fluorescence imaging is routinely used in the author's practice. It examines the native perfusion of the flap and its angiosomes and assesses remnant muscular perfusion of medial gastrocnemius muscle (**Fig. 2**D). If generalized reduction in native flap perfusion is present, it prompts a re-examination of vascular pedicle before its division. If regional perfusion insufficiency was detected, the concerned tissue could be discarded to prevent postoperative flap necrosis.

Donor Site Management

The donor site was closed primarily (67.3%; n = 35), skin grafted (15.4%; n = 8), or via delayed primary closure with shoelace technique (17.3%; n = 9). In our experience, a 6-cm flap width is the cutoff for primary closure.

POSTOPERATIVE CARE AND EXPECTED OUTCOME

Patients with free MSAP flap were routinely admitted to the microsurgical intensive care unit for 3 to 5 days of flap monitoring and postoperative care. No routine postoperative anticoagulant was given. Intensive flap monitoring prompts early detection, and timely re-exploration is the key to successful free flap salvage. This is particularly relevant in flaps with venous insufficiency, which is the main cause of re-explorations.[9] In addition, the rehabilitation program starts a few days after surgery to reduce recovery delay. All of the patients were discharged with regular outpatient follow-up. In our series, the incidence of flap re-exploration showed no significant difference in patients with different age, gender, comorbidities, and timing of reconstruction after trauma.

A retrospective study was conducted for examining all patients who received MSAP flaps for lower extremity reconstruction at Chang Gung Memorial Hospital from 2007 to 2019. Fifty-two flaps were performed in total: 47 were fasciocutaneous flaps, and five were chimeric flaps incorporating medial gastrocnemius muscle. The chimeric flap was indicated for bone and metalware coverage and dead space obliteration. Among these 52 MSAP flaps, 17 were pedicled, and 35 were free flaps. In this series, knee and proximal two-thirds of the leg were reconstructed with pedicled flaps, whereas the distal third of leg (n = 3), ankle (n = 3), and foot (n = 29) were reconstructed with free flaps. Reflectively, among those 17 pedicled MSAP flaps, eight were used for knee reconstructions, four for the proximal third of the leg, and five for the middle third of the leg.

Durable soft tissue coverage without tendon/bone/metalware exposure was achieved in all patients receiving MSAP flaps. Early mobilization and physical therapy promoted optimal functional recovery of the injured extremities.

MANAGEMENT OF COMPLICATIONS

Surgical complications within 3 months were recorded. Data points included microvascular complications, compromised wound healing, hematoma, and wound dehiscence. Donor site morbidities were also documented.

In the pedicle flap group, the survival rate was 94.1% (16/17) as opposed to 100% in the free flap group. In this series, there were four free flap re-explorations because of venous congestion, which were all successfully salvaged. There was one complete flap failure in the pedicled group, and the defect was subsequently reconstructed by propeller ALT tensor fascia lata flap. There were two partial necroses in the pedicled group, which were managed with successive debridement and skin graft. No significant donor site morbidity was observed.

REVISION OR SUBSEQUENT PROCEDURES

Most commonly performed revision procedures after lower extremity reconstruction with MSAP flap were single-stage flap debulking surgery (n = 12), scar revision (n = 7), and tenolysis (n = 5). All the debulking procedures were performed for patients with foot reconstruction to enhance the fitting of their shoewear.

CASE DEMONSTRATIONS
Case 1: Pedicled Medial Sural Artery Perforator Flap

A 69-year-old man was referred for necrotic left pretibial wound from a fall into a ditch. Judicious

wound debridements resulted in an 8 × 6 cm² soft tissue defect with the exposed proximal tibia. A pedicled MSAP flap was raised based on a single perforator. The size of the flap was 13 × 7 cm², with an 8-cm pedicle length. The flap was delivered to the defect through a subcutaneous tunnel. Donor site closure with shoelace sutures allowed dynamic wound closure to minimize pedicle compression from postoperative swelling. At 1-month follow-up, a sturdy pretibial wound coverage with aesthetically acceptable outcome was attained (**Fig. 3**).

Case 2: Free Medial Sural Artery Perforator Flap with Plantaris Tendon Graft

A 31-year-old woman was admitted for severe friction injury to the left foot from a motor vehicle accident. She presented with extensive soft tissue defect (15 × 7 cm²) over the dorsal surface of the foot exposing tarsus and metatarsus, and segmental loss of EHL tendon. One-stage soft tissue reconstruction was performed after judicious debridement. A free MSAP flap (15 × 8 cm²) was raised based on one perforator, and plantaris tendon graft was harvested simultaneously for EHL reconstruction. Delayed primary closure of the donor site was achieved by shoelace suture,

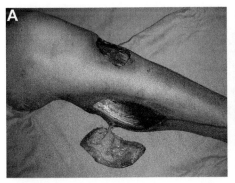 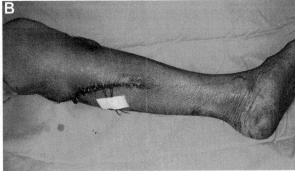

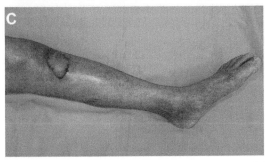 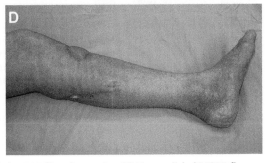

Fig. 3. (*A*) Left pretibial soft tissue defect and the pedicled MSAP flap donor site. (*B*) The pedicled MSAP flap was delivered to the defect through a subcutaneous tunnel. Shoelace sutures were used to minimize tunnel swelling–induced pedicle compression. (*C, D*) Anterior and lateral view of the left leg 1 month after reconstruction.

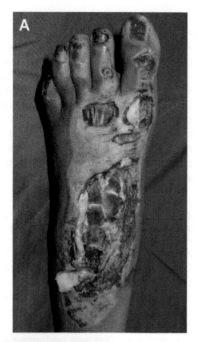
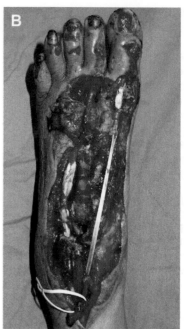
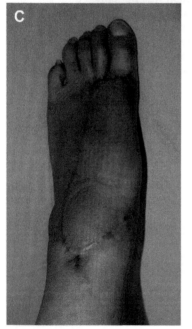
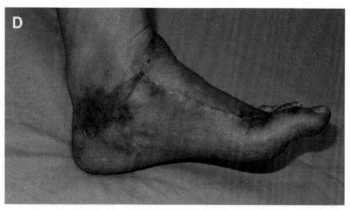

Fig. 4. (*A*) Significant skin loss over the dorsal surface of the left foot with bone exposure and segmental loss of EHL tendon. (*B*) Nonvascularized plantaris graft for EHL tendon reconstruction. (*C*, *D*) Bird's-eye and medial view of the left foot 4 months after revision surgery. The photographs show an acceptable flap contouring to the surrounding tissue of the foot, and thus reduced shoe-wearing difficulties.

the dynamic wound closure technique, and omitted the need for a skin graft. Six months post-reconstruction, the flap was debulked and EHL and extensor digitorum longus to the second toe were tenolyzed for a reduced range of toe flexion. Satisfactory EHL tendon excursion and left foot function restorations were accomplished (**Fig. 4**).

Case 3: Free Chimeric Medial Sural Artery Perforator Flap with a Piece of Medial Gastrocnemius Muscle

A 52-year-old woman was referred for progressive worsening of left medial ankle pain from skin graft–induced scar contracture over the tarsal tunnel. The injury resulted from a motor vehicle accident 3 years ago, causing compound injury involving bimalleolar fracture, proximal phalangeal fracture of left great toe, and degloved skin from the medial malleolus to medial forefoot. Initially, the bimalleolar fracture was managed by external fixation, the proximal phalangeal fracture was stabilized with K-wire, and degloved skin was resurfaced by skin grafts. To reconstruct the medial foot and ankle defect, scar contracture was released, left tarsal tunnel was opened, and the posterior tibial nerve was neurolyzed. Skin graft over the neurovascular bundles was excised, creating a soft tissue defect measuring 15×6 cm^2 with significant dead space over the tarsal tunnel. A free chimeric

MSAP flap (15×9 cm^2) was raised based on two Doppler-detected perforators. End-to-side anastomosis of the medial sural artery to the posterior tibial artery and end-to-end venous anastomosis of vena comitantes were performed. The fasciocutaneous component resurfaced medial ankle and foot, and gastrocnemius muscle obliterated the dead space at the tarsal tunnel. The donor site was managed with primary closure, and the recovery was uncomplicated. The flap was debulked 5 months later to enhance the fitting of shoewear (**Fig. 5**).

DISCUSSION

Clinically, the precise locations of the MSAPs are inconsistent with detected Doppler signals. This discrepancy may result in the flap design change to maximize the inclusion of the detected perforators into the flap. To enhance the accuracy of the flap design, we developed an endoscopic-assisted technique for MSAP flap dissection. Endoscopic-assisted dissection at the subfascial plane aims to visualize and mark the precise locations of the desired perforators, to map and investigate the course of perforators and their "lazy S" tributaries. Endoscopic-assisted dissection technique thus minimizes flap design errors and reduces the risk of iatrogenic perforator injuries caused by the imprecision of handheld Doppler perforator markings.

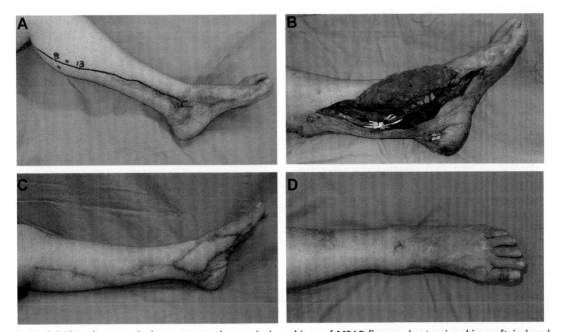

Fig. 5. (*A*) This photograph demonstrates the surgical markings of MSAP flap, and extensive skin graft–induced scarring extending from medial malleolus to medial forefoot. (*B*) The inset of free chimeric MSAP flap. With the extended vascular pedicle to muscle component, the direction of muscle inset was independent of the fasciocutaneous part. (*C, D*) Medial and bird's-eye view of the reconstructed left foot 5 months after debulking surgery.

Although a duplex ultrasound and CTA are used for perforator localization, the endoscope has the advantage of higher magnification and allows complete exploration of the flap vicinity in an atraumatic and radiation-free approach. The endoscopic-assisted approach can aid to avoid raising an MSAP flap that lacks identifiable or favorable perforators and allows early change of surgical plans. Thus, it potentially shortens the operative time and lessens unnecessary donor site dissection and trauma.

The topography of the MSAP has been investigated extensively. All the perforators of the MSAP flap are musculocutaneous and perforators of the region are mostly derived from the medial sural artery. In our intraoperative finding, few of these musculocutaneous perforators at medial gastrocnemius territory originate from the posterior tibial artery. Nevertheless, this anatomic variation does not preclude the use of MSAP flap as long as the perforator is located precisely as mapped. In this situation, the concept of freestyle dissection, proposed by Wei and Mardini,[10] should be applied.

The major concern of using MSAP flap is the donor site morbidity. The most common donor site morbidities are related to the use of skin graft for its secondary defect reconstruction. These reported morbidities include donor site discomfort, hypertrophic and keloid scar, and aesthetically displeasing postoperative appearances. In our practice, the MSAP flap is suitable for small to medium-sized lower extremity defects. We generally confined our flap design to 6 cm in width and used the shoelace suture technique for dynamic donor site closure to avoid skin graft. For large lower extremity defects, thigh-based free flap, such as the ALT flap, is our preferred option.

The medial sural motor nerve injury is a less frequently reported donor site morbidity. The nerve is assumed to be deeper and more proximal to the medial sural artery. However, their proximity is closer in practice; thus, unintentional nerve division can occur. Although the incidence of the nerve severance is predictably high, the resultant medial gastrocnemius dysfunction is rarely significant. If muscle atrophy remains a concern, we recommend repair of the motor nerve, although the significance of functional recovery from the neurorrhaphy, is yet to be determined.

Venous insufficiency is the most common microvascular complication in free MSAP flap reconstruction. The main identifiable reasons for venous congestion include hematoma, kinking and twisting of the vein, and inadequate recipient vein selection. On the contrary, arterial complications in MSAP flaps tend to occur intraoperatively.

Arterial spasm of either the recipient or the donor artery was the major cause. To avoid potential re-explorations, we recommend tourniquet-controlled dissection with meticulous hemostasis, and gentle pedicle dissection and tissue handling. Dividing the artery proximal to the bifurcation of the medial sural artery to its medial and lateral branches ensures adequate vascular caliber is obtained for anastomoses.

SUMMARY

The MSAP flap is a reliable workhorse flap for all small to medium-sized defect reconstructions in the lower extremity. It is harvested as a free or a pedicled flap with options to include multiple tissue components that further expands its versatility.

CLINICS CARE POINTS

- In free MSAP flaps, venous insufficiency occurs more commonly than arterial insufficiency.
- Arterial spasm is the major cause of arterial insufficiency and is more challenging to overcome.
- Intensive flap monitoring prompts early detection, and the timely re-exploration is the key to successful free flap salvage.
- In pedicled MSAP flaps, lengthy dissection has to be performed to provide better mobility of the flap and avoid tension during insetting.

DISCLOSURE

None of the authors has a financial interest in any of the products, devices, or drugs mentioned in this article.

REFERENCES

1. Cavadas PC, Sanz-Gimenez-Rico JR, Gutierrez-de la Camara A, et al. The medial sural artery perforator free flap. Plast Reconstr Surg 2001;108(6):1609–15.
2. Hallock GG. Anatomic basis of the gastrocnemius perforator-based flap. Ann Plast Surg 2001;47(5):517–22.
3. Al Deek NF, Hsiao JC, Do NT, et al. The medial sural artery perforator flap: lessons learned from 200 consecutive cases. Plast Reconstr Surg 2020;146(5):630e–41e.
4. Wong JK, Deek N, Hsu CC, et al. Versatility and "flap efficiency" of pedicled perforator flaps in lower extremity reconstruction. J Plast Reconstr Aesthet Surg 2017;70(1):67–77.
5. Kim HH, Jeong JH, Seul JH, et al. New design and identification of the medial sural perforator flap: an

anatomical study and its clinical applications. Plast Reconstr Surg 2006;117(5):1609–18.

6. Lin CH, Lin CH, Lin YT, et al. The medial sural artery perforator flap: a versatile donor site for hand recon-struction. J Trauma 2011;70(3):736–43.

7. Thione A, Valdatta L, Buoro M, et al. The medial sural artery perforators: anatomic basis for a surgical plan. Ann Plast Surg 2004;53(3):250–5.

8. Lee CH, Chang NT, Hsiao JC, et al. Extended use of chimeric medial sural artery perforator flap for 3-dimensional defect reconstruction. Ann Plast Surg 2019;82(1S):S86–94.

9. Lorenzo AR, Lin CH, Lin CH, et al. Selection of the recipient vein in microvascular flap reconstruction of the lower extremity: analysis of 362 free-tissue transfers. J Plast Reconstr Aesthet Surg 2011; 64(5):649–55.

10. Wei FC, Mardini S. Free-style free flaps. Plast Re-constr Surg 2004;114(4):910–6.

The Optimal Timing of Traumatic Lower Extremity Reconstruction: Current Consensus

Z-Hye Lee, MD[a,1], John T. Stranix, MD[b], Jamie P. Levine, MD[c,*]

KEYWORDS

- Lower extremity trauma • Lower extremity reconstruction • Timing of reconstruction

KEY POINTS

- Although early reconstruction within 72 hours of injury has long been held as the gold standard for treating traumatic lower extremity injuries, recent evidence suggests this ideal window can likely be extended 1 to 2 weeks.
- Advances in local wound care, particularly negative pressure wound therapy, have allowed for successfully temporizing lower extremity wounds.
- Although timing of reconstruction may be less important than previously suggested, expeditious treatment using a multidisciplinary approach remains the ultimate goal.

INTRODUCTION

Lower extremity reconstruction, particularly in the setting of trauma, remains one of the most challenging tasks for the plastic surgeon. Relevant factors to consider include bony restoration, flap choice, and timing. Considerable debate has continued regarding the ideal timing of reconstruction for lower extremity trauma. For nearly 3 decades, early reconstruction within 72 hours of injury has been considered the gold standard. However, with the evolution of microsurgical practices and new advances in wound care, specifically negative pressure wound therapy (NPWT), there has been a paradigm shift in the timing for managing these injuries.

EVIDENCE FOR EARLY TIMING OF RECONSTRUCTION

In 1986, Marko Godina's landmark paper "Early Microsurgical Reconstruction of Complex Trauma of the Extremities" provided evidence for the benefits of free flap coverage within 72 hours from initial injury.[1] His large series of over 500 patients demonstrated lower rates of flap failure and postoperative infection in the early group compared with flaps performed after 72 hours (**Figs. 1–5**). The tenet of early reconstruction in lower extremity trauma came to be accepted as the relative gold standard as subsequent studies provided further corroboration. However, although Godina's original work established some of the guiding principles for free flap reconstruction in lower extremity trauma, there were some limitations. Most notably, his analysis did not control for the learning curve that occurred over time: his first 100 cases had a flap failure rate of 26% compared with only 4% in his last 100 cases, and most of his initial 100 cases were performed in a delayed fashion. Despite this confounding factor, the concept of early coverage within 3 days of injury became the

a Department of Plastic Surgery, The University of Texas MD Anderson Cancer Center, Houston, TX, USA; b Department of Plastic and Maxillofacial Surgery, University of Virginia Health, West Complex 4th Floor, 1300 Jefferson Park Avenue, Charlottesville, VA 22903, USA; c Hansjörg Wyss Department of Plastic Surgery, New York University Langone Health, New York, NY, USA
1 Present address: 2630 Bissonnet Street, Houston, TX 77005.
* Corresponding author. Hansjörg Wyss Department of Plastic Surgery, NewYork University Langone Health, 222 East 41st Street, New York, NY 10016.
E-mail address: Jamie.Levine@nyulangone.org

Clin Plastic Surg 48 (2021) 259–266
https://doi.org/10.1016/j.cps.2021.01.006
0094-1298/21/© 2021 Elsevier Inc. All rights reserved.

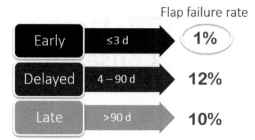

Flap failure rate

Early   ≤3 d   **1%**

Delayed   4 – 90 d   **12%**

Late   >90 d   **10%**

Fig. 1. Results from Godina's landmark paper establishing 72 hours as the ideal window for reconstruction after lower extremity trauma. (*Data from* Godina M. Early microsurgical reconstruction of complex trauma of the extremities. Plast Reconstr Surg 1986;78:285–92.)

standard of care, especially given the rationale of less scarring and fibrosis in the immediate stages after injury. Furthermore, it has been well documented that the onset of significant inflammation in the delayed period after injury can affect all tissue types of the lower extremity, from the skin and muscle to the neurovascular structures, resulting in compromised outcomes after free flap reconstruction.

With the development of regional trauma centers specializing in limb salvage, treatment of severe lower extremity injuries has become standardized with a multidisciplinary approach involving vascular, orthopedic, and plastic surgeons. Open fractures are debrided early and fixated either with temporary external fixators or internal fixation, followed by stable soft tissue coverage, usually in the form of free tissue transfer. However, delays in flap coverage can occur because of delay in referral to a tertiary trauma center, other life-threatening injuries, or attempts at wound closure with skin grafts or local flaps. Given these practical limitations and the arbitrary nature of Godina's original timing groups, several additional studies have investigated the impact of timing on outcomes after free flap reconstruction

of the lower extremity and whether this early safe period of 3 days can be extended (**Table 1**).[2,3]

In particular, several recent studies demonstrated that flaps could be performed in the subacute period within 1 week to as late as several months from injury with comparable rates of flap success.[4] Findings from the authors' institution have demonstrated that flaps performed within 10 days after injury had similar rates of total failures and major complications compared with reconstructions performed within the first 72 hours after injury.[5] A retrospective review by Francel and colleagues[6] of 72 patients with Gustilo IIIB lower extremity fractures demonstrated fewer major complications and decreased time to bony union when performed within 15 days of injury compared with when surgeries were performed 15 to 30 days and more than 30 days from injury. Byrd and colleagues[7] demonstrated the highest rates of infection between 2 and 6 weeks, and Fischer and colleagues[8] similarly showed the lowest infection and fastest bony union with definitive coverage that occurred within the first 10 days after injury.

In contrast, Starnes-Roubaud and colleagues[9] found no difference in flap failure, osteomyelitis, or bony union between lower extremity free flaps performed within 15 days compared to after 15 days from injury. Other studies that expanded the acute period even further demonstrated no significant difference in flap complications. Kolker and colleagues[10] compared reconstructions for below knee lower extremity traumas performed within 21 days versus 22 to 60 days and after 60 days with no significant differences in flap complications. Similarly, Hill and colleagues[11] demonstrated no differences for reconstructions performed within 30 days compared to those performed 31 to 90 days and after 90 days from injury.

WOUND PREPARATION AND MANAGEMENT

Appropriate wound management and debridement are intimately related to the optimal timing of reconstruction in lower extremity trauma. Although wound care has evolved significantly over the past several decades, adequate surgical debridement remains the most critical component for achieving optimal short- and long-term outcomes.[6,12] Failure to eradicate nonviable tissue will ultimately result in infection, which may manifest as osteomyelitis, nonunion, or flap failure. Not all lower extremity wounds are created equal, and severe, heavily contaminated injuries will require serial debridements, while smaller, subacute wounds may require only 1 or 2 trips

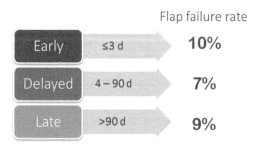

Flap failure rate

Early   ≤3 d   **10%**

Delayed   4 – 90 d   **7%**

Late   >90 d   **9%**

Fig. 2. Current flap failure rates from NYU for early, delayed and late lower extremity reconstruction.

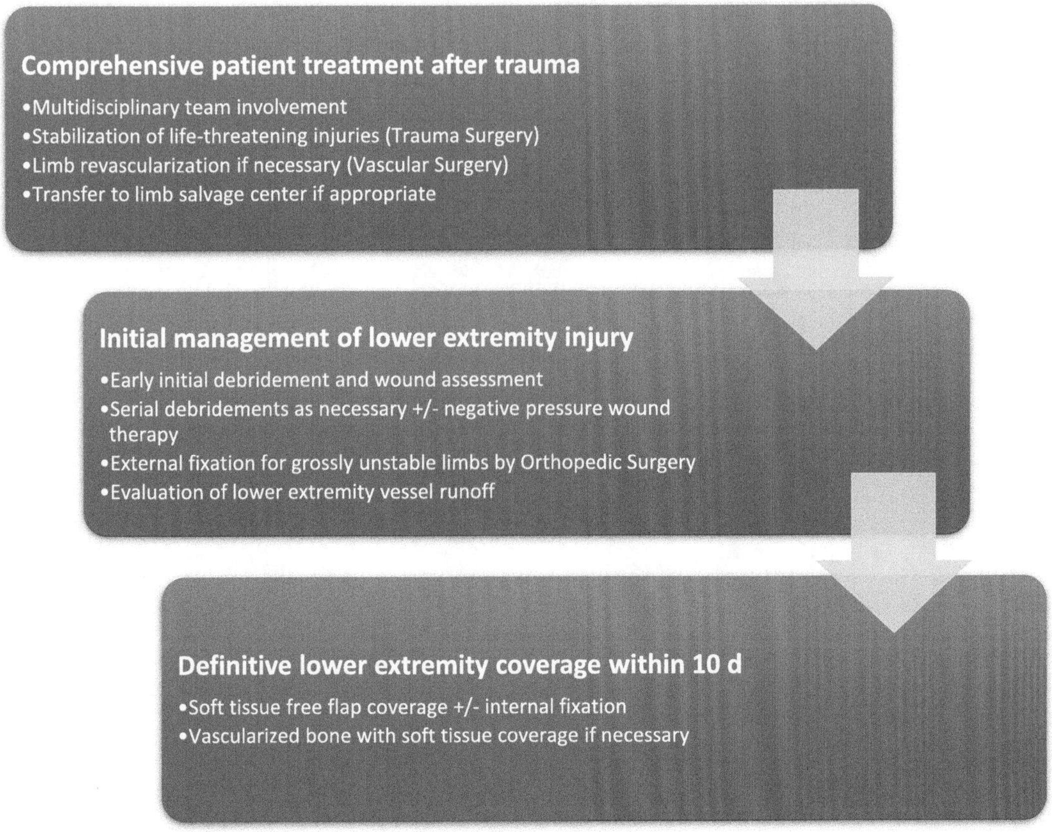

Comprehensive patient treatment after trauma

•Multidisciplinary team involvement
•Stabilization of life-threatening injuries (Trauma Surgery)
•Limb revascularization if necessary (Vascular Surgery)
•Transfer to limb salvage center if appropriate

Initial management of lower extremity injury

•Early initial debridement and wound assessment
•Serial debridements as necessary +/- negative pressure wound therapy
•External fixation for grossly unstable limbs by Orthopedic Surgery
•Evaluation of lower extremity vessel runoff

Definitive lower extremity coverage within 10 d

•Soft tissue free flap coverage +/- internal fixation
•Vascularized bone with soft tissue coverage if necessary

Fig. 3. Workflow for management of lower extremity trauma patients.

to the operating room. Wound cultures should be taken routinely, and there should be a low threshold to maintain patients on tailored antibiotic therapy in preparation for the final reconstruction.

The introduction of NPWT in the late 1990s transformed the management of large traumatic wounds. The placement of an open-cell polymer foam in the wound bed promotes granulation tissue formation on a cellular level and reduces tissue edema. NPWT can be applied after the first debridement and can be used to bridge between serial debridements until the final reconstruction. Although the basic principles of adequate debridement and bony stabilization have remained the cornerstones for successful limb salvage after lower extremity injuries, several studies have highlighted the potentially beneficial role of NPWT in improving the safety of delayed reconstruction, although they have been limited to small subset of patients.[13–16] NPWT remains the preferred approach for temporizing wounds at most institutions because of its effects on edema, improved physiology of healing, logistical ease, and patient comfort.[17] Given the well-delineated benefits of NPWT on wound management, one can potentially attribute its use as a contributing factor for prolonging the safe period of reconstruction from the initial 3-day period proposed by Godina to a more subacute period.[18–20] In addition, this additional time afforded with the use of NPWT may also allow for a better appreciation of the zone of injury prior to microsurgical reconstruction. Establishing inflow and outflow out of the zone of injury to avoid thrombosis is among the most critical elements of free flap success, and with time, the need for arteriovenous loop or vein grafts may become apparent.

However, NPWT is not a substitute for adequate debridement or for prompt definitive soft tissue coverage within the proposed 10-day window. Studies have demonstrated increased bacterial colonization in wounds managed with NPWT as well as a rise in clinically relevant infections for open lower extremity fractures.[21,22] In addition,

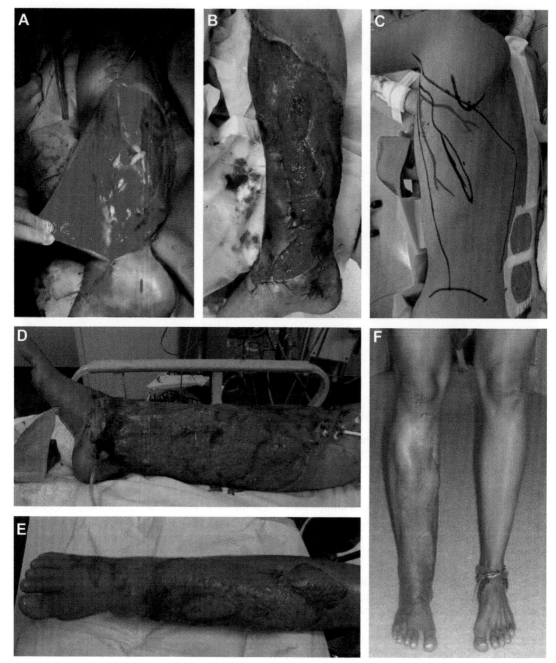

Fig. 4. (*A*) 19-year-old woman with Gustilo 3C right lower extremity open tibia-fibula fracture. (*B*) 8 days after injury after serial debridement and VAC placement. (*C*) Markings for myocutaneous latissimus dorsi free flap. (*D*) Postoperative day 2. (*E*) 4 weeks after reconstruction. (*F*) 18 months after reconstruction.

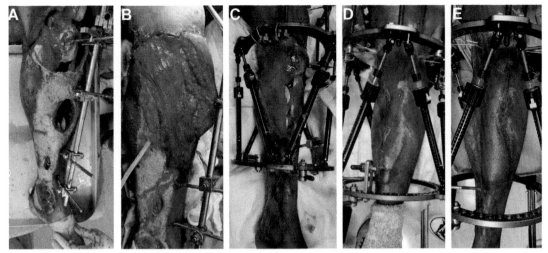

Fig. 5. (*A*) 21-year-old woman with Gustilo 3B right lower extremity open tibia-fibula fracture initially managed with serial debridements and external fixation. (*B*) Soft tissue coverage with myocutaneous latissimus dorsi flap at 3 weeks after injury. (*C*) Appearance of wound after flap failure and debridement followed by serial NPWT dressing changes. (*D*) Significant decrease in wound size after skin graft to most of the wound with persistent exposure of comminuted tibia. (*E*) Fibula free flap for tibial reconstruction and soft tissue coverage with fibula flap skin paddle.

prolonged use of NPWT over bone stripped of periosteum can result in significant osseous desiccation and devitalization. Ultimately, although a revolutionizing adjunct for managing acute wounds, NPWT is only a tool to temporize wounds, and its use should not delay definitive reconstruction.

THE CONSENSUS

Despite the lack of Level 1 evidence and the heterogeneity of studies, the modern paradigm allows for more fluid application of Godina's original principles. Although timely fixation and coverage is always the goal, the guideline for early reconstruction may be less rigidly applied, with the goal of definitive treatment occurring within 7 to 10 days of injury.

There are several benefits to accepting a prolonged initial safe period of reconstruction from a practical standpoint. In a multidisciplinary approach, lengthening the time before safe soft tissue coverage can facilitate a comprehensive treatment plan and ensure the availability of all team members with individual expertise (eg, microsurgical, orthopedic, and vascular). However, increased costs and probability for hospital-related complications caused by extended length of stay must be considered. In addition, a recent study has suggested that sociodemographic variables such as patient's insurance status and treatment at Level 1 trauma center may result in

delay in reconstruction after lower extremity trauma.[23] These variables suggest the use of standardized protocols with a regional referral system to trauma centers with combined orthopedic and reconstructive expertise that would streamline care and minimize unnecessary delays in treatment.

SUMMARY

Based on Marko Godina's original work, microsurgical reconstruction within 3 days of lower extremity trauma has long been advocated as the gold standard. However, with advance in wound care and microsurgical expertise, it appears that this early timing of reconstruction is not as critical and can be extended. In addition, timing of reconstruction is merely 1 variable among many, including patient factors, injury severity, operative technique, and flap type, that likely influence immediate and long-term outcomes. Goals for patients with lower extremity trauma remain unchanged, to provide care in the safest manner and to provide definitive treatment as promptly as possible, ideally within a 10-day window from initial injury.

CLINICS CARE POINTS

- The initial management of a lower extremity trauma patient should entail a multidisciplinary approach involving Orthopedic

Table 1
Articles on timing in lower extremity reconstruction

Author, Year	Study Design (# of Patients)	Outcomes Assessed	Reconstruction Criteria	Timing Windows	Conclusion
Byrd et al,[7] 1985	Prospective (n = 191)	Flap failure Amputation rate Osteomyelitis Time to bony union Length of stay Time to closure	Open tibial fractures (type I-IV)	Acute 1-5 d Subacute 1-6 w Chronic >6 w	Acute best for all outcomes
Godina et al,[1] 1986	Retrospective (n = 532)	Flap failure Infections Time to bony union Length of stay	Lower extremity trauma	Early <72 h Delayed 72 h-3 mo Late >3 mo	Acute best for all outcomes
Francel et al,[6] 1992	Retrospective (n = 72)	Flap failure Reoperations Osteomyelitis SSI Length of stay (LOS) Time to bony union	Gustilo IIIB injuries	<15 d 15–30 d >30 d	<15 d group: Fewer flap failures and reoperations, decreased LOS and time to bony union
Kolker et al,[10] 1997	Retrospective (n = 451)	Flap failure Reoperation	Below knee injuries	Acute <22 d Subacute 22–60 d Chronic >60 d	No difference in outcomes
Karanas et al,[4] 2008	Retrospective (n = 14)	Flap failure Osteomyelitis	Lower extremity trauma	All >72 h	No flap loss in 14 patients
Hill et al,[11] 2012	Retrospective (n = 60)	Flap failure Reoperation SSI	Lower extremity trauma	<30 d 31–90 d >91 d	No significant difference in outcomes Trend toward lower rates of failure among >91 d group
Raju et al,[13] 2014	Retrospective (n = 50)	Flap failure Reoperation Infection	Lower extremity trauma (All received *NPWT* prior to flap)	1 wk 2 wk 3 wk 4 wk 5 wk 6 wk 7 wk	No difference in outcomes
Bellidenty et al,[3] 2014	Retrospective (n = 89)	Flap failure Osteomyelitis	Lower extremity trauma Gustilo 3B injuries (emergency vs delayed cases referred to	Emergency Delayed	Lower failure and infection rates in 'emergency' group, increased in delayed group

(continued on next page)

Table 1
(continued)

Author, Year	Study Design (# of Patients)	Outcomes Assessed	Reconstruction Criteria	Timing Windows	Conclusion
			center for coverage)		
Starnes-Roubaud et al,[9] 2015	Retrospective (n = 51)	Flap failure Osteomyelitis Bony union Ambulation	Lower extremity trauma	<15 d >15 d	No difference in outcomes
Lee et al,[5] 2018	Retrospective (n = 358)	Flap failure Return to OR	Lower extremity trauma	0–3 d 3–9 d 10–90 d >90 d	No difference in outcomes between 0–3 and 3–9 d; higher complications for 10–90 d

Data from Refs.[1,3,4,6,7,9–11,13]

Surgery, Vascular Surgery and Plastic Reconstructive Surgery.

- Patients with complex lower extremity injuries should be ideally be promptly transferred to a tertiary trauma center specializing in limb salvage to avoid delays in treatment
- Definitive treatment with skeletal fixation and soft tissue coverage should happen within 72 hours and no later than 10 days from initial injury.External skeletal fixation with timely soft tissue coverage is the ideal approach for heavily contaminated wounds that are not ready for definitive internal bony fixation.
- While NPWT is a valuable for temporizing and bridging wounds to definitive reconstruction, it does not replace adequate debridement.
- In the setting of critical limb ischemia requiring revascularization, delaying free flap reconstruction is safest given the risk of significant tissue edema and reperfusion injury.

DISCLOSURE

The authors have nothing to disclose.

REFERENCES

1. Godina M. Early microsurgical reconstruction of complex trauma of the extremities. Plast Reconstr Surg 1986;78:285–92.
2. Hertel R, Lambert SM, Müller S, et al. On the timing of soft-tissue reconstruction for open fractures of the lower leg. Arch Orthop Trauma Surg 1999;119(1–2): 7–12.
3. Bellidenty L, Chastel R, Pluvy I, et al. Emergency free flap in reconstruction of the lower limb. Thirty-five years of experience. Ann Chir Plast Esthet 2014;59(1):35-41.
4. Karanas YL, Nigriny J, Chang J. The timing of microsurgical reconstruction in lower extremity trauma. Microsurgery 2008;28(8):632–4.
5. Lee ZH, Stranix JT, Rifkin W, et al. Timing of microsurgical reconstruction in lower extremity trauma: an update of the Godina paradigm. Plast Reconstr Surg 2019;144(3):759–67.
6. Francel TJ, Vander Kolk CA, Hoopes JE, et al. Microvascular soft-tissue transplantation for reconstruction of acute open tibial fractures: timing of coverage and long-term functional results. Plast Reconstr Surg 1992;89(3):478–87.
7. Byrd HS, Spicer TE, Cierney G III. Management of open tibial fractures. Plast Reconstr Surg 1985; 76(05):719–30.
8. Fischer MD, Gustilo RB, Varecka TF. The timing of flap coverage, bone-grafting, and intramedullary nailing in patients who have a fracture of the tibial shaft with extensive soft-tissue injury. J Bone Joint Surg Am 1991;73(09):1316–22.
9. Starnes-Roubaud MJ, Peric M, Chowdry F, et al. Microsurgical lower extremity reconstruction in the subacute period: a safe alternative. Plast Reconstr Surg Glob Open 2015;3(7):e449.
10. Kolker AR, Kasabian AK, Karp NS, et al. Fate of free flap microanastomosis distal to the zone of injury in lower extremity trauma. Plast Reconstr Surg 1997; 99(4):1068–73.
11. Hill JB, Vogel JE, Sexton KW, et al. Re-evaluating the paradigm of early free flap coverage in lower extremity trauma. Microsurgery 2013;33(1):9–13.
12. Yaremchuk MJ, Brumback RJ, Manson PN, et al. Acute and definitive management of traumatic osteocutaneous defects of the lower extremity. Plast Reconstr Surg 1987;80:1–14.

13. Raju A, Ooi A, Ong YS, et al. Traumatic lower limb injury and microsurgical free flap reconstruction with the use of negative pressure wound therapy: is timing crucial? J Reconstr Microsurg 2014;30(6): 427–30.

14. Liu DS, Sofiadellis F, Ashton M, et al. Early soft tissue coverage and negative pressure wound therapy optimises patient outcomes in lower limb trauma. Injury 2012;43(6):772–8.

15. Rinker B, Amspacher JC, Wilson PC, et al. Subatmospheric pressure dressing as a bridge to free tissue transfer in the treatment of open tibia fractures. Plast Reconstr Surg 2008;121:1664–73.

16. Morykwas MJ, Argenta LC. Vacuum-assisted closure: a new method for wound control and treatment: clinical experience. Ann Plast Surg 1997;38: 563–77.

17. Stannard JP, Volgas DA, Stewart R, et al. Negative pressure wound therapy after severe open fractures: a prospective randomized study. J Orthop Trauma 2009;23:552–7. Microsurgery. 2008;28(8):632-4.

18. Hou Z, Irgit K, Strohecker KA, et al. Delayed flap reconstruction with vacuum-assisted closure management of the open IIIB tibial fracture. J Trauma 2011;71(6):1705–8.

19. Steiert AE1, Gohritz A, Schreiber TC, et al. Delayed flap coverage of open extremity fractures after previous vacuum-assisted closure (VAC) therapy - worse or worth? J Plast Reconstr Aesthet Surg 2009;62(5): 675–83.

20. Stannard JP, Singanamala N, Volgas DA. Fix and flap in the era of vacuum suction devices: what do we know in terms of evidence based medicine? Injury 2010;41(8):780–6.

21. Weed T, Ratliff C, Drake DB. Quantifying bacterial bioburden during negative pressure wound therapy: does the wound VAC enhance bacterial clearance? Ann Plast Surg 2004;52(03):276–9. discussion 279–80.

22. Bhattacharyya T, Mehta P, Smith M, et al. Routine use of wound vacuum-assisted closure does not allow coverage delay for open tibia fractures. Plast Reconstr Surg 2008;121(04):1263–6.

23. Shammas RL, Mundy LR, Truong T, et al. Identifying predictors of time to soft-tissue reconstruction following open tibia fractures. Plast Reconstr Surg 2018;142(6):1620–8.

Management of Gustilo Type IIIC Injuries in the Lower Extremity

Heather A. McMahon, MD[a], John T. Stranix, MD[a,*], Z-Hye Lee, MD[b],
Jamie P. Levine, MD[b]

KEYWORDS

- Gustilo IIIC • Open tibia fracture • Limb salvage • Lower extremity free flap
- Lower extremity reconstruction

KEY POINTS

- Gustilo IIIC injuries of the lower extremity are characterized by open tibia fractures with associated vascular injury requiring repair.
- These injuries pose a challenge to the reconstructive surgeon, and controversy remains regarding limb salvage versus primary amputation in these patients.
- Early recognition of vascular injury and subsequent repair is critical, in addition to early and serial debridement with the goal of achieving definitive reconstruction within 7 to 10 days after the injury.
- Reconstructive options for these injuries frequently require free tissue transfer, with the anterolateral thigh flap and the latissimus dorsi myofascial or myocutaneous flaps as the most common flaps used.

INTRODUCTION

Lower extremity fractures are a commonly encountered injury with epidemiologic surveys estimating rates of approximately 17 per 100,000 person years.[1] These fractures occur along a spectrum of severity, with open fractures representing 2.6% of injuries.[2] Most of these open fractures occur in young men as the result of high-energy trauma; however, elderly women involved in lower energy mechanisms also represent a significant proportion of these injuries.[2] Open fractures are classified based on the Gustilo-Anderson Classification, with Gustilo IIIC injuries defined as open fractures with associated arterial injury requiring repair.[3]

Fortunately, Gustilo IIIC injuries are relatively uncommon. Among studies specifically evaluating open tibial fractures, rates of IIIC injuries range from 2.5% to 3.4%.[2,4] Historically, these injuries have the worst prognosis of those patients requiring limb salvage with amputation rates ranging from 20% to as high as 75% to 77% in some studies.[4,5] Numerous investigators have devised a variety of scales and scoring criteria in an attempt to better determine which limbs should proceed to salvage versus primary amputation; however, there is no consensus on their reliability, and they have not been found to be predictive of functional recovery.[6] As a result, the management of these injuries remains controversial.

Proponents of primary amputation cite increased length of stay, increased number and complexity of surgical procedures, high complication rates, and increased cost as the rationale favoring amputation.[7] However, a systematic review of the existing literature on this topic that evaluated complications following limb salvage and amputation in type IIIB and IIIC injuries including osteomyelitis, nonunion, secondary

[a] Department of Plastic and Maxillofacial Surgery, UVA Health, 1215 Lee Street, Box 800376, Charlottesville, VA 22903, USA; [b] Hansjorg Wyss Department of Plastic Surgery, NYU Langone Health, 303 East 33rd Street, New York, NY 10016, USA
* Corresponding author.
E-mail address: jts3v@virginia.edu

Clin Plastic Surg 48 (2021) 267–276
https://doi.org/10.1016/j.cps.2020.12.006

amputation, ischemia, and flap failure did not find significant differences in duration of hospitalization, pain, limb function, or long-term quality of life between the groups.[8]

Equivalent functional outcomes have also been observed when evaluating those patients undergoing reconstruction versus those patients undergoing amputation.[9] In addition, when specifically evaluating cost, several studies have evaluated long-term costs between limb salvage and amputation and have found that patients undergoing amputation incur substantially higher lifetime costs compared with those patients treated with limb salvage.[10]

Lastly, over the course of the nearly 40 years since Gustilo's landmark publication on the topic, significant advancements in initial trauma management, vascular reconstruction, orthopedic fixation, and microvascular techniques have resulted in improved outcomes in this patient population. Single institution data demonstrate a statistically significant decrease in flap failure rates when patients are stratified by timing of reconstruction within their cohort.[11] However, complication rates remain high in these patients due to the significant degree of trauma, with recent studies citing a 9% partial and 15.6% complete flap loss rate, so it is essential to approach these complex patients thoughtfully and in the context of an experienced, multidisciplinary team.[12]

RECONSTRUCTIVE PHILOSOPHY

Various reconstructive options exist for the management of Gustilo IIIC injuries, and determination of the optimal technique is individualized based on the following[13]:

- Mechanism of injury
- Location and severity of the injury
- Degree of soft tissue deficit
- Other concomitant injuries
- Comorbidities

The goals of reconstruction include the following:

- Restoring form and function
- Promoting bony union
- Restoring sensation
- Minimizing donor site morbidity

INITIAL EVALUATION

Gustilo IIIC injuries are often the result of high-energy trauma, so the initial evaluation based on advanced trauma life support (ATLS) is essential to ensure patient stability and address any immediately life-threatening injuries. Once the patient is deemed adequately stable, clinical examination of the affected limb including documentation of the pulse examination is crucial. **Fig. 1** demonstrates those findings seen in a typical Gustilo IIIC injury with significant bony, soft tissue, and vascular injury.

Some debate in the literature exist as to the role of computed tomography (CT) angiograms in this patient population, but many investigators advocate for inclusion of this study in the evaluation if any of the following are present[14]:

- Abnormal pulse or Doppler examination
- Zone of injury over potential free flap recipient vessels
- Zone of injury over any portion of a candidate regional flap and its blood supply

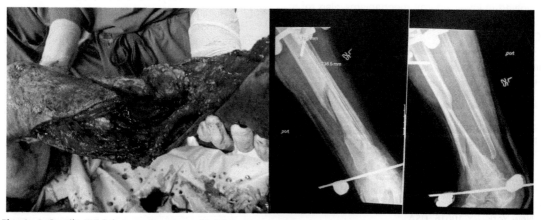

Fig. 1. A Gustilo IIIC injury at the time of initial presentation, demonstrating a large, full-thickness soft tissue defect with devitalized skin, subcutaneous tissue, and muscle (*left*). Radiographic images of this patient following provisional fixation with external fixator demonstrating comminuted, displaced fractures of the tibia and fibula as well as segmental bone loss (*right*).

- Extensive soft-tissue or bony destruction from high-energy mechanism
- Preexisting arterial occlusive disease

In addition, CT angiography represents a less expensive and less invasive option than formal angiography.[14] However, intraoperative angiography remains the gold standard for evaluation of these injuries, and an obviously dysvascular limb should be taken to the operating room emergently following initial ATLS stabilization barring any additional life-threatening injuries requiring intervention.

Antibiotics are another important component in the early management of these patients. Time to receipt of antibiotics after open fracture has been demonstrated to decrease rates of infection, specifically if received within 66 minutes of the injury.[15] Typical regimens include a first-generation cephalosporin, such as cefazolin, as well as gentamycin.[13]

Other immediate interventions that should be initiated in these patients include administration of a tetanus vaccine.[13,16] Many investigators also advocate for administration of low-molecular-weight heparin.[16]

TIMING OF OPERATIVE INTERVENTIONS

Generally, these patients are taken to the operating room within hours of presentation for evaluation, vascular repair, debridement, fasciotomies, and skeletal stabilization. At the time of this initial surgical intervention, the plastic surgeon can provide valuable insight, including the following[14,16]:

- Debridement of devitalized tissues and management of marginal skin flaps
- Incision planning to preserve regional flap options
- Optimal placement of external hardware to allow easier access to potential recipient vessels

We may also be able to aid in the critical determination as to whether primary amputation is indicated. Although decreasing in frequency, the primary amputation rate remains around 17%.[4] Clinical situations that may merit primary amputation include the following[4,16]:

- Warm ischemia time exceeding 4 to 6 hours
- Muscle loss affecting more than 2 lower extremity compartments
- Bone loss exceeding more than one-third the length of the tibia
- Those patients deemed not reconstructable by the multidisciplinary surgical team

The timing of definitive reconstruction depends on the severity of the injury, need for serial debridement, and the patient's other medical needs. Most of the publications evaluating time to coverage outcomes have evaluated IIIa and IIIb injuries, and the application of these results to the more severe IIIC injuries should be considered in the context of each clinical presentation. Some investigators advocate for the "fix and flap" principle with radical debridement, skeletal stabilization, neurovascular repair, and immediate soft tissue reconstruction.[4,16] However, several studies have demonstrated equivalent outcomes when definitive soft tissue coverage is performed within 3 days of injury.[4,17] When it is not possible to complete the reconstruction within 3 days, there is an increase in overall complications; however, recent evidence demonstrates no differences in flap outcomes, including flap failure and major complications, if performed by 10 days.[17] With these data in mind, one should aim to achieve soft tissue reconstruction by 10 days postinjury whenever feasible.

FLAP SELECTION

Because of the extent of soft tissue and vascular injury, most of these fractures require free tissue transfer with a limited, supplemental role for local flaps. For IIIC injuries, most of the publications to date favor muscle over fasciocutaneous flaps. One study evaluated their flap choices and found that 40% were latissimus muscle flaps and 27% were anterolateral thigh flaps (ALT).[18] This preferential use of the latissimus dorsi muscle flap seems to be true for multiple investigators, with others citing a 75% rate of muscle flaps with the latissimus dorsi used in 53% of those cases and was the most commonly used flap overall.[12] Interestingly, studies evaluating the performance of muscle flaps versus fasciocutaneous flaps have found comparable rates of limb salvage and functional recovery between the 2 flap types.[19] We have also found fasciocutaneous flaps easier to elevate for subsequent orthopedic revisions and therefore recommend assessing this factor based on the underlying bone quality and fixation method used at the time of flap coverage. Muscular segments either in combination with a fasciocutaneous flap, as the vastus lateralis with the ALT, or primary muscle flaps can be useful for filling in the more complex 3-dimensional bone loss defects, especially if not being filled in a Masquelet fashion with antibiotic cement.

An additional consideration should include flap size, as increased flap size has been correlated with increased rates of major complications including partial and complete flap loss.[20] Specifically, for flaps greater than 250 cm^2 the rate of major complications is 50% versus 33.6% in less than 250 cm^2 flaps, and the rate of flap failure is 25% versus 11.8%.[20] Increased flap size is an independent predictor of these outcomes, particularly in muscle flaps.[20] Although these findings may be related to flap size serving as a surrogate marker for overall injury severity, they nevertheless provide another variable associated with lower extremity trauma-free flap outcomes. Similar to the timing data reviewed earlier, however, most of the literature is derived from IIIB free flap outcomes and extrapolated to these IIIC injuries.

Primary factors influencing free flap selection:

- Location and size of the defect
- Missing components (skin, muscle, nerve, bone), specifically what needs free tissue coverage and what can be skin grafted
- Vascular bypass conduit type, inflow, and outflow
- Length of vascular pedicle required to perform anastomosis outside of the zone of injury
- Potential recipient vessels (keep in mind that arterial inflow and venous outflow may not be possible in same recipient location)
- Vein graft source for grafting or arteriovenous loop
- Minimizing donor site morbidity

SURGICAL APPROACH

A full understanding of the residual and novel revascularized anatomy is paramount to approaching these complex reconstructions, starting with being available for consultation during the emergent stabilization and revascularization to assist in initial management decisions. A multidisciplinary approach with early and active plastic surgery involvement preserves any residual soft tissue options, optimizes wound management, and provides a more complete evaluation of the defect. Other key steps include the following:

- Serial debridements, including soft tissue and bone, every 48 to 72 hours are often required before definitive coverage and should be part of the reconstructive plan.
- Study the angiogram and plan for multiple recipient vessel options but expect to use vein grafts and determine potential sources preoperatively.
- Have orthopedic surgery available to adjust fixation as needed, to make your dissection approach more straightforward.
- Primary shortening of the limb with a bone gap is an option, if needed.

- Set up the bone for primary repair with immediate coverage or delayed repair after a planned period of healing.

Ideally, a flap is selected that provides adequate soft tissue coverage with ample pedicle length for arterial and venous anastomoses performed beyond the zone of injury in close proximity to each other. In our experience, however, that is unfortunately the exception in these cases and there should be a low threshold to use vein grafts or an arteriovenous loop to complete the microvascular anastomosis.[14] If vein grafting is required, every attempt should be made to reach source vessels as far out of the zone of injury as possible.

When feasible, our prefer to use either the disrupted anterior tibial or posterior tibial vessels proximal to the zone of injury away from the bypass graft and perform end-to-end anastomoses because the distal flow has been disrupted by the injury. Evaluation of our experience, however, has demonstrated higher flap complication rates using injured recipient vessels.[11] We interpret this finding to highlight the insidious nature of the zone of injury—meticulous recipient vessel dissection and inspection are of utmost importance. Although recipient vessels proximal to the zone of injury are typically preferred, our experience does support distal anastomoses from retrograde flow off of the vascular bypass as a viable option without any evidence of increased flap loss.[21] When feasible, the authors' preference is to perform 2 venous anastomoses.

POSTOPERATIVE CARE AND EXPECTED OUTCOME

Despite the often higher level of injury in these patients with IIIC injuries, once free flap coverage has been performed they usually follow standard lower extremity free flap protocols. However, significant heterogeneity exists in the postoperative management of these patients and seems to be largely dictated by surgeon preference.

Flap monitoring protocols typically involve frequent nursing and physician examination including use of a hand-held doppler probe, with some centers also using objective devices such as implantable dopplers or near infrared spectroscopy devices that monitor changes in tissue oxygenation. Regardless of the protocol used, for lower extremity flaps specifically, the data suggest that routine monitoring should be continued for at least 4 days as take-backs occur at an average of 3.7 days postoperatively.[19] We have found suspending limbs from a trapeze via their external fixator frame or a calcaneal pin placed after the free flap to be extremely helpful in maintaining flap elevation during this early period, especially in this cohort with higher complication rates.

Although the evidence suggests equivalent functional recovery and flap failures between muscle flaps and fasciocutaneous flaps, it is important to recognize that fasciocutaneous flaps do have a more frequent take-back rate for suspected vascular compromise.[19] Fortunately, fasciocutaneous flaps have a higher successful salvage rate as compared with muscle flaps, which is posited to be the result of lower metabolic demand in fasciocutaneous flaps and more easily

recognized vascular compromise.[19] It is important to keep these factors in mind when monitoring these flaps postoperatively to maximize the potential for early recognition and flap salvage.

The decision regarding the initiation of flap dependency training is also surgeon and institution dependent, with little high-level evidence to support a specific protocol. Most of the centers begin flap training in the 3 to 7 postoperative day range, and the available data do not show any increased rates of flap compromise with earlier, more aggressive protocols.[22] We typically initiate flap dependency training around the seventh postoperative day but adjust accordingly depending on

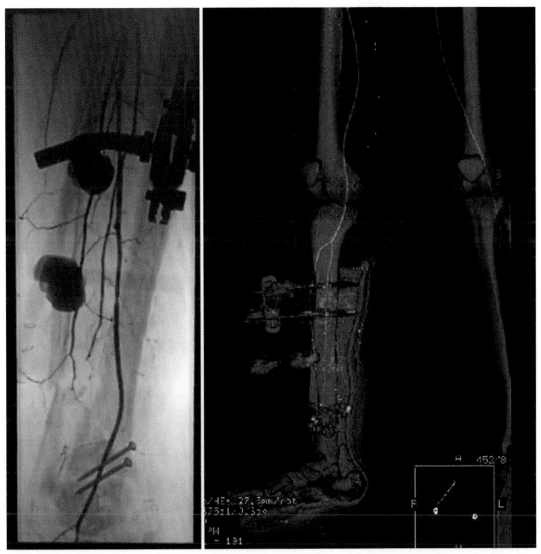

Fig. 2. Still images from formal angiogram (*left*) and CT angiography (*right*) demonstrating single vessel run-off via the anterior tibial artery following emergent bypass reconstruction with reverse saphenous vein graft. CT, computed tomography.

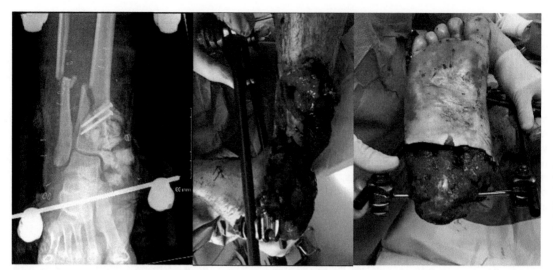

Fig. 3. (*Left*) Radiographs demonstrating fibular shaft fracture and comminuted distal tibial fracture, which has been provisionally fixated with an external fixator and interfragmentary screws. (*Middle*) Intraoperative photograph following 2 prior debridements demonstrating the 30 cm × 15 cm soft tissue defect of the distal lower extremity with exposed underlying bone and hardware. (*Right*) Intraoperative photograph demonstrating the extent of the soft tissue defect extending to the plantar surface of the foot.

the stability of the flap, difficulty of the case, episodes of vascular compromise either during the index procedure or postoperatively, and the overall appearance of the flap including persistence of postoperative edema. Weight-bearing status is typically a joint decision with the orthopedic surgeon managing the patient's bony injury.

Antibiotic duration is also quite variable and controversial, as infection remains one of the most significant complications after open fracture. Recent attempts at systematic review reveal a lack of robust literature on the subject and as a result they concluded that antibiotic prophylaxis is indicated in the immediate management of open tibia

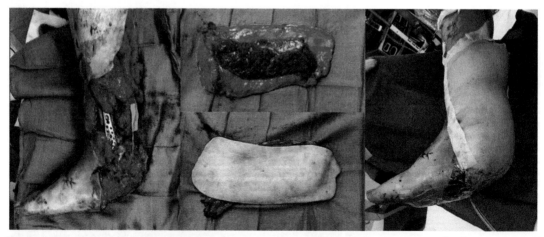

Fig. 4. Intraoperative photograph demonstrating the soft tissue defect following open reduction and internal fixation of the tibia and reconstruction of the tibial nerve with sural nerve cable graft (*left*). A 33 cm × 16 cm free anterolateral thigh flap from the left thigh was harvested with underlying vastus lateralis, iliotibial tract, and tensor fascia lata to facilitate closure of the dead space in the defect and to reconstruct the Achilles tendon, respectively (*middle*). The flap was anastomosed to the posterior tibial vessels and inset into the defect with skin graft placed over the lateral foot due to lack of exposed critical structures not requiring flap coverage (*right*).

fractures but that the ideal duration remains unanswered.[23]

Discharge disposition of these patients is often dictated by their other medical needs and traumatic injuries; however, the majority are able to discharge home after their hospitalization. Regardless of the patient's disposition, specific attention should be paid to the postoperative rehabilitation protocol, as these injuries have the potential to substantially impact functional status and the ability to live independently. Despite the severity of these injuries, recent studies have documented an 83% limb salvage rate in this population.[4,16]

MANAGEMENT OF COMPLICATIONS

Despite appropriate management, patients with IIIC injuries continue to experience substantial major complications including the following:

- Infection
- Thrombosis of arterial reconstruction resulting in limb ischemia
- Partial flap loss
- Complete flap loss
- Nonunion
- Secondary amputation

Infection rates for these injuries are approximately 35% and are best managed when diagnosed early and treated with prompt antibiotic therapy and serial debridements, followed by appropriate wound closure.[3,16] Infection can also include hardware and poorly vascularized retained bony segments, which should be thoughtfully dealt with in combination with your orthopedic colleagues.

Partial and complete flap loss rates have improved; however, they remain substantial in this population with some investigators reporting double the rates of microvascular thrombosis in patients with IIIC injuries as compared with other less severe injury patterns.[12] Recent data found that only 75% of patients underwent reconstruction without flap loss, with a 9.4% partial flap loss rate and 15.6% complete flap loss rate.[12] Other studies corroborate these findings, reporting flap loss rates ranging from 15% to 27%.[16,18]

Rates of secondary amputation are variable and have improved over time, decreasing from 42% in early studies to as low as 5.5% more recently,

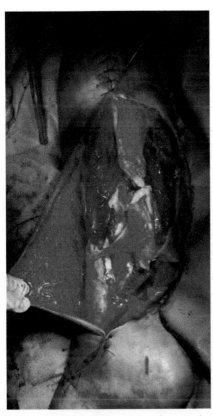

Fig. 5. Intraoperative photograph taken at the time of initial exploration and debridement after right lower extremity Gustilo IIIC injury demonstrating significant soft tissue defect of the medial leg with comminuted tibial fracture.

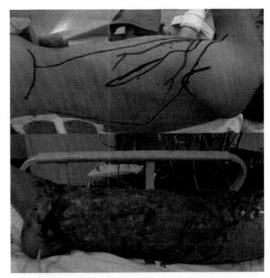

Fig. 6. Operative markings in preparation for the harvest of a free latissimus dorsi myocutaneous flap demonstrating the key anatomic landmarks and the thoracodorsal artery pedicle (top). Immediate postoperative photograph demonstrating reconstruction of the right lower extremity soft tissue defect with free latissimus dorsi myocutaneous flap and split-thickness skin grafts (bottom).

although typical rates seem to range from 16% to 20%.[3,4] Causes of secondary amputation include infection, ischemia, and flap loss resulting in inability to achieve soft tissue coverage.[4] The presence of arterial injury seems to be associated with these elevated amputation rates, with one study reporting a rate of 11.5% in patients with arterial injury compared with 1.5% in those without arterial injury.[18]

REVISION OR SUBSEQUENT PROCEDURES

Secondary revision procedures are common in this patient cohort, with some studies reporting a mean of 2.9 procedures performed.[4] This reinforces the benefit of easier reelevation of fasciocutaneous flaps compared with muscle and should be considered during flap selection. Common secondary procedures include the following[14]:

- Bone grafting
- Tendon reconstruction
- Flap debulking
- Flap liposuction
- Scar revision

CASE DEMONSTRATIONS
Case 1

A 33-year-old man sustained a right lower extremity Gustilo IIIC injury following a motorcycle crash. He initially underwent revascularization of his anterior tibial artery using a reverse saphenous vein graft (**Fig. 2**). He was also noted to have transection of his tibial nerve with a 10 cm gap, comminuted distal tibial and fibular shaft fractures, disruption of the Achilles tendon, and 30 cm by 15 cm soft tissue defect (**Fig. 3**). After 2 debridements, in a joint procedure with orthopedic surgery he underwent open reduction and internal fixation of the right tibia, tibial nerve reconstruction with sural nerve cable grafting, Achilles tendon reconstruction with vascularized tensor fascia lata and iliotibial band, and soft tissue coverage with a left anterolateral thigh flap and split-thickness skin grafts (**Fig. 4**). The anterolateral

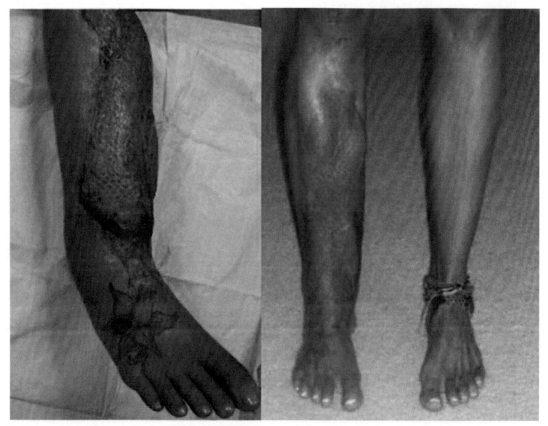

Fig. 7. One-month postoperative photograph following reconstruction with free latissimus dorsi myocutaneous flap and slit-thickness skin graft (*left*). Eighteen-month follow-up photograph demonstrating atrophy of the latissimus flap with improved contour of the right lower extremity (*right*).

thigh flap was anastomosed end to end to the disrupted posterior tibial artery, and 2 venous anastomoses were performed using 3.0 and 2.0 venous couplers, respectively. The left thigh donor site and the lateral foot were then skin grafted to complete the reconstruction.

Case 2

A 19-year-old female pedestrian was struck by a car resulting in a right lower extremity Gustilo IIIC injury (**Fig. 5**). She underwent emergent vascular repair and serial debridements and ultimately required soft tissue coverage with free latissimus myocutaneous flap and split-thickness skin graft (**Fig. 6**). She did not experience any flap loss and at 18 months postoperatively was noted to have excellent improvement in leg contour secondary to atrophy of the latissimus muscle (**Fig. 7**).

DISCUSSION

These cases are the most challenging subgroup within the reconstructive cohort, notorious for persistently high free flap failure and complication rates. After the initial emergent operation with revascularization, a thorough and empathetic discussion with the patient regarding operative expectations, possible options, and potential outcomes is mandatory to guide them through the decision of whether to pursue limb salvage. This decision may also require multiple conversations over time, as the wound itself evolves over the course of serial debridements. If limb salvage is pursued, especially in patients with IIIC injuries, flap selection remains surgeon preference, and we recommend use of the flap you are most comfortable with that provides long pedicle length and adequate coverage, with a low threshold to vein graft. Recipient site vascular flow and positioning may be the most critical factor in the planning of the case and will affect all other decisions thereafter. Backup vascular options are always recommended.

Despite elevated rates of complications including partial and total flap loss, infection, and secondary amputation, equivalent functional outcomes and quality of life are observed between those patients undergoing primary amputation and limb salvage with overall lower lifetime costs for those patients undergoing limb salvage.

SUMMARY

Reconstruction of Gustilo IIIC injuries requires a combined surgical approach in order to achieve limb salvage. Complication rates remain higher than fractures without associated vascular injury;

however, reasonable rates of limb salvage are still able to be achieved with good functional outcomes and result in lower long-term costs to patients and the health care system.

CLINICS CARE POINTS

- The reconstructive team should be involved from the time of initial presentation of these patients to help assess soft-tissue viability and plan incisions to preserve reconstructive options.
- Managing these injuries within an experienced, multidisciplinary team is essential.
- Multiple operative debridements are recommended prior to proceeding with definitive coverage.
- Definitive coverage should ideally be acheieved within 7-10 days of initial injury to minimize complications.
- Flap selection should be based upon surgeon comfort, as well as defect size, pedicle length, recipient vessel availability, need for revision procedures, and minimizing donor site morbidity.
- Have a low threshold to perform vein grafting in these cases.

DISCLOSURE

The authors have nothing to disclose.

REFERENCES

1. Weiss RJ, Montgomery SM, Ehlin A, et al. Decreasing incidence of tibial shaft fractures between 1998 and 2004: information based on 10,627 Swedish inpatients. Acta Orthop 2008; 79(4):526–33.
2. Court-Brown CM, Bugler KE, Clement ND, et al. The epidemiology of open fractures in adults. A 15-year review. Injury 2012;43(6):891–7.
3. Gustilo RB, Mendoza RM, Williams DN. Problems in the management of type III (Severe) open fractures: a new classification of type III open fractures. J Trauma 1984;24(8):742–6.
4. Soni A, Tzafetta K, Knight S, et al. Gustilo IIIC fractures in the lower limb. J Bone Joint Surg Br 2012; 94-B(5):698–703.
5. Flint LM, Richardson JD. Arterial injuries with lower extremity fracture. Surgery 1983;93(1 Pt 1):5–8.
6. Schirò GR, Sessa S, Piccioli A, et al. Primary amputation vs limb salvage in mangled extremity: a systematic review of the current scoring system. BMC Musculoskelet Disord 2015;16(1):372.
7. Hansen STJ. Overview of the severely traumatized lower limb. Reconstruction versus amputation. Clin Orthop Relat Res 1989;243:17–9.

8. Saddawi-Konefka D, Kim HM, Chung KC. A systematic review of outcomes and complications of reconstruction and amputation for type IIIB and IIIC fractures of the tibia. Plast Reconstr Surg 2008;122(6):1796–805.

9. Bosse MJ, MacKenzie EJ, Kellam JF, et al. An analysis of outcomes of reconstruction or amputation after leg-threatening injuries. N Engl J Med 2002; 347(24):1924–31.

10. Chung KC, Saddawi-Konefka D, Haase SC, et al. A cost-utility analysis of amputation versus salvage for gustilo type IIIB and IIIC open tibial fractures. Plast Reconstr Surg 2009;124(6):1965–73.

11. Stranix JT, Lee Z-H, Jacoby A, et al. Not all gustilo type IIIB fractures are created equal. Plast Reconstr Surg 2017;140(5):1033–41.

12. Ricci JA, Abdou SA, Stranix JT, et al. Reconstruction of gustilo type IIIC injuries of the lower extremity. Plast Reconstr Surg 2019;144(4):982–7.

13. Aslan A, Uysal E, Özmeriç A. Clinical study a staged surgical treatment outcome of type 3 open tibial fractures. ISRN Orthop 2014. e-collection 2014(721041).

14. Lachica RD. Evidence-based medicine: management of acute lower extremity trauma. Plast Reconstr Surg 2017;139(1):287e–301e.

15. Lack WD, Karunakar MA, Angerame MR, et al. Type III open tibia fractures: immediate antibiotic prophylaxis minimizes infection. J Orthop Trauma 2015; 29(1):1–6.

16. Arnež ZM, Papa G, Ramella V, et al. Limb and flap salvage in gustilo IIIC injuries treated by vascular repair and emergency free flap transfer. J Reconstr Microsurg 2017;33(S 01):S03–7.

17. Lee ZH, Stranix JT, Rifkin WJ, et al. Timing of microsurgical reconstruction in lower extremity trauma: an update of the godina paradigm. Plast Reconstr Surg 2019;144(3):759–67.

18. Badash I, Burtt KE, Leland HA, et al. Outcomes of soft tissue reconstruction for traumatic lower extremity fractures with compromised vascularity. Am Surg 2017;83(10):1161–5.

19. Stranix JT, Lee ZH, Jacoby A, et al. Forty years of lower extremity take-backs: flap type influences salvage outcomes. Plast Reconstr Surg 2018; 141(5):1282–7.

20. Lee ZH, Abdou SA, Ramly EP, et al. Larger free flap size is associated with increased complications in lower extremity trauma reconstruction. Microsurgery 2020;40(4):473–8.

21. Stranix JT, Borab ZM, Rifkin WJ, et al. Proximal versus distal recipient vessels in lower extremity reconstruction: a retrospective series and systematic review. J Reconstr Microsurg 2018;34(5): 334–40.

22. McGhee JT, Cooper L, Orkar K, et al. Systematic review: early versus late dangling after free flap reconstruction of the lower limb. J Plast Reconstr Aesthet Surg 2017;70(8):1017–27.

23. Isaac SM, Woods A, Danial IN, et al. Antibiotic prophylaxis in adults with open tibial fractures: what is the evidence for duration of administration? A systematic review. J Foot Ankle Surg 2016;55(1): 146–50.

Orthoplastic Approach to Lower Extremity Reconstruction: An Update

Zvi Steinberger, MD[a], Paul J. Therattil, MD[b], L. Scott Levin, MD[c],*

KEYWORDS

- Flap • Free flap • Lower extremity • Orthoplastic • Reconstruction

KEY POINTS

- Complex extremity injuries should be treated with early multidisciplinary collaboration in an orthoplastic approach.
- Using a multidisciplinary orthoplastic approach can help avoid unnecessary extremity amputations.
- There may be improved functional outcomes when implementing a multidisciplinary orthoplastic approach.

INTRODUCTION

The orthoplastic approach to lower extremity reconstruction uses the strength of a multidisciplinary team and the synergy of principles and techniques from orthopedic and plastic surgeons. Although the orthopedic and plastic surgeons are the clinical leaders of the team, there are several critical members that support this approach, including vascular surgeons, infectious disease specialists, musculoskeletal radiologists, physical therapists, prosthetists, pain management physicians, and a specialized nursing staff. This collaboration leads to improved patient outcomes, optimized conditions for bone healing, expediting soft tissue coverage, decreasing length of hospital stay, and avoidance of complications and revision surgeries. The orthoplastic approach not only avoids amputation but also improves patient function and quality of life in the short and long term.[1]

INDICATIONS AND CONTRAINDICATIONS

With the advent of negative pressure wound therapy, the number of lower extremity trauma cases referred for soft tissue reconstruction has decreased, thus resulting in the referral of more complex cases to regional centers. Therefore, many of the patients who may be candidates for extremity salvage and orthoplastic techniques may be transferred from outside institutions, and therefore, it is critical to educate referring centers as to what are potential indications for referral. Open fractures in patients with comorbidities, Gustilo III injuries, dysvascular limbs, concomitant nerve injuries (especially lacking plantar sensation), foot/ankle soft tissue loss, compartment syndrome, crush or blast injuries, or patients with additional social or psychological needs should be considered for transfer and would potentially benefit from a multidisciplinary approach.[1]

Sources of Support: None.
[a] Department of Hand and Microsurgery, Sheba Medical Center, Tel Hashomer, 52621 Ramat Gan, Israel; [b] Department of Plastic and Reconstructive Surgery, Hackensack University Medical Center, 30 Prospect Avenue, Hackensack, NJ 07601, USA; [c] Department of Orthopedic Surgery, University of Pennsylvania, Philadelphia, PA, USA
* Corresponding author. Department of Orthopedic Surgery, Penn Medicine University City, 3737 Market Street, 6th Floor, Philadelphia, PA 19104.
E-mail address: Scott.Levin@pennmedicine.upenn.edu

Clin Plastic Surg 48 (2021) 277–288
https://doi.org/10.1016/j.cps.2020.12.007

PREOPERATIVE EVALUATION AND SPECIAL CONSIDERATIONS

Typically, the orthopedic surgeon stabilizes fractures, whereas the plastic surgeon provides soft tissue coverage. The orthoplastic approach can combine these strengths in a variety of operative circumstances. In the case of lower extremity trauma, the orthopedic surgeon may be providing the initial assessment of the wound as well and determining whether higher rungs of the reconstructive ladder will be necessary to obtain soft tissue coverage with reconstructive plastic surgery assistance. In the case of oncologic defects or diabetic limb salvage, the orthopedic and plastic surgeon can perform preoperative evaluation and planning, intraoperative decision making, and postoperative care in synchrony. Particularly in the trauma setting, the evaluation by both an orthopedic and a plastic surgeon may result in a different result than if only 1 specialist was making the decision between extremity salvage and amputation. This difference may be due to lack of familiarity with more complex reconstructive techniques or fixation options, misconceptions with concomitant nerve injury, differences in length of soft tissue and bony recovery, or complexity of socioeconomic variables.[2] Especially in the latter circumstances, one can see why all members of the orthoplastic team are critical.

SURGICAL PROCEDURES

The orthoplastic approach has been well described, and therefore, in later discussion, the authors touch on the advancements in theory and techniques and discuss the burgeoning areas where rapid change will occur in the coming years.[1]

Pediatric IIIC Injuries

Although Gustilo type IIIC injuries are not exceeding common, and those injuries in children are even less so (2.6% of all open pediatric tibial fractures), the stakes become high at an exponential rate when the case does present itself.[3] Regional tertiary referral centers may be fortunate enough to have a team skilled in pediatric microsurgery dedicated to pediatric vascular injuries, but this is rare.

There are few data regarding Gustilo IIIC injuries in children. Traditionally, based on literature by Gustilo and colleagues and subsequent studies from the 1980s, Gustilo IIIC injuries were rarely considered for extremity salvage because of the high rate of eventual amputation. However, there have been advances since then in all aspects of lower extremity trauma care. We are more facile

with microsurgical techniques and skeletal fixation as well as with trauma and critical care in general. Ricci and colleagues[4] have demonstrated in the adult population that Gustilo IIIC injuries fare no worse than single-vessel Gustilo IIIB injuries with regard to salvage and complication rates and advocated that we are justified in pursuing extremity salvage. We will likely never have the data to demonstrate the same in the pediatric population, but should be compelled to pursue salvage considering the adult outcomes.

In a pediatric IIIC injury, special care must be given to bony healing and growth potential. If there is a significant bony defect, external circular frame fixation may be needed with acute limb shortening and sequential lengthening. A fresh vascular repair may delay the start of limb lengthening. Separately, limb lengthening or bony transport may be complicated by poor soft tissue coverage, which may ultimately necessitate a flap reconstruction in a patient with complex lower extremity vasculature. In these ways, a collaborative approach is critical.

Medial Femoral Condyle to Foot and Ankle

Both persistent nonunion and avascular necrosis (AVN) occur in the setting of vascular compromise. In foot and ankle surgery, the talus and navicular bones are prone to such pathologic condition because of their poor blood supply, which may be further compromised by trauma or surgical manipulation of the surrounding tissues. Long-standing AVN or nonunion may result in painful debilitating arthrosis of the tarsal, subtalar, or ankle joints. Arthrodesis may be the final reconstructive option for such situations. In patients with comorbidities, such as peripheral neuropathies, diabetes, nutritional deficiency, peripheral vascular disease, and tobacco use, the rate of failed primary fusion with nonunion is 28% to 48%.[5]

Various revision options are available for failed foot and ankle fusion, and some include autogenous bone grafting as a way of restoring bone stock to the fusion site for structural support. When the use of conventional procedures, including the use of nonvascularized bone grafts, has failed, more advanced techniques are required, such as vascularized bone grafts.[6]

The medial femoral condyle/trochlea is a versatile graft that can be used as vascularized cortical bone, cancellous bone, cartilage, periosteum, or a chimera of the above. The medial femoral condyle can include skin or muscle to augment the soft tissue with variable size that can help achieve the desired union.[7,8]

Arteriovenous Loop Fibula

Ankle arthrodesis is a solution in select cases of severe pain resulting from ankle arthrosis or may be used as a salvage procedure after failed total ankle arthroplasty. The type of ankle arthrodesis is dictated by the degree of deformity, soft tissue status, and bone quality. In cases with minimal or no deformity, in situ arthrodesis may be performed with minimal arthrotomy or arthroscopically using a percutaneous fixation technique. More severe cases may require open realignment and internal fixation.[9]

When a nonunion potential exists, the role of bone grafting comes in. Potential for union may be compromised by infection, bone defect, osteonecrosis of the talus, and previous nonunion. The source of bone graft is dictated by the amount and type required. The amount of bone graft needed depends on available bone stock, which may be compromised by previous surgery, trauma, or debridement in the setting of infection. The type of bone graft needed may be structural or nonstructural and conventional or vascularized. The distal fibula, distal tibia, and iliac crest are commonly used for nonvascularized bone grafts. The medial femoral condyle, iliac crest, and free fibula are commonly used sources for vascularized bone graft.

In cases whereby a significant bone defect is present, the use of vascularized fibula is most appropriate. In order to avoid contralateral morbidity and distal dissection for recipient vessels, the authors use an ipsilateral "AV loop" vascularized fibula. Surgical technique includes debridement of nonviable bone and soft tissue, ipsilateral free fibula harvest, and lengthening of the pedicle to the fibula. To lengthen the reach of fibula, saphenous vein grafts are anastomosed proximally to the native peroneal vessels, and then the artery and vein of the fibula pedicle are anastomosed to vein grafts[10] (**Fig. 1**).

Lymphatic Bypass

Consideration of persistent posttraumatic lymphedema has not been emphasized when it comes to extremity reconstruction. Although it is recognized that patients that experience significant lower extremity trauma develop some degree of lymphedema, the prevalence and severity are not well described; the cause and lymphatic anatomy have not been described until recently.[11] It is now known that in the lower extremity, the lymphatic vessels originate on either side of the toes, on the foot, and at the lateral thigh. These lymphatics originate just deep to the dermis and travel in the subcutaneous tissue toward the popliteal, femoral, and superficial and deep inguinal nodal basins.[12] In the upper extremity, the superficial lymphatics run with the main subcutaneous veins and do not appear to have major connections with the deep lymphatic system.[13] Based on these anatomic studies, soft tissue injuries in these regions, especially degloving injuries or Morel-Lavallee lesions, may disrupt continuity of lymphatic channels and predispose patients to lymphedema. This finding would make sense in theory, but there are few to no supporting data.

Part of the reason that we have not paid enough attention to lymphedema in our population is because there were not good diagnostic tools or solutions for secondary lymphedema until recently. With the popularization of indocyanine green lymphangiography, the reason certain patients with extremity trauma and reconstruction develop lymphedema and others do not is slowly being elucidated. An interesting observation by Van Zanten and colleagues[11] was that patients who underwent skin grafts, local flaps, or free muscle flaps for extremity reconstruction generally did not have restoration of lymphatic flow. In contrast, Slavin and colleagues[14] found that patients who had fasciocutaneous or musculocutaneous free flaps for extremity reconstruction *did*

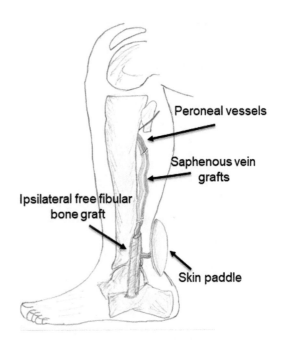

Peroneal vessels

Saphenous vein grafts

Ipsilateral free fibular bone graft

Skin paddle

Fig. 1. An ipsilateral "AV loop" vascularized fibula using the saphenous vein as an "extension cord." The proximal anastomosis was performed to the native peroneal vessels.

have restoration of lymphatic flow. Therefore, the type of tissue transferred (and therefore the type of flap used) and whether it is rich in lymphatics may be critical. In addition, not just the type of flap, but also the orientation and inset of the flap at the extremity may be more important than initially thought because lymphatics have axiality and directionality.[15] Just as inosculation of blood vessels exists, the same is thought to be true for lymphatics. Therefore, if a patient is seen with a circumferential defect of an extremity that was reconstructed with skin grafts and subsequently develops lymphedema, one might consider whether transfer of a free fasciocutaneous flap would provide a bridge of lymphatics to assist in proximal lymphatic transport.[16] More anatomic studies need to be performed on deep lymphatics and the presence of lymphatics (or lack thereof) in muscles.

The development of lymphovenous bypass and vascularized lymph node transfers has given us yet another tool to potentially treat lymphedema. Lymphovenous bypass involves the anastomosis of lymphatics distal to the injury to veins in the area. This technique allows the excess lymphatic fluid at the distal aspect of the extremity to pass through the venous system to the proximal

extremity, thereby bypassing the damaged and nonfunctional lymphatics in between. Lymphovenous bypass is not always an option, especially if there has been severe trauma to the area or long-standing lymphedema, which would result in potentially sclerosed and functionless lymphatics. Vascularized lymph node transfer is an alternative option that involves transfer of lymph nodes as a free flap to an area that is bereft of functional lymphatics. The transplanted lymph node is thought to act as a "sponge" for excess lymph. Although the mechanism is not completely clear, the transfer of functional lymph nodes is thought to cause sprouting of new lymphatics and induce new lymphatic collateral pathways via growth factor signaling. It will also allow for lymphaticovenous drainage, as lymph will flow into the node and can exit via venous outflow.[17] These techniques have primarily been used in iatrogenic lymphatic injuries from oncologic extirpation but have much potential for any cause of secondary lymphedema.

Secondary Aesthetic Refinements

Although limb salvage is the primary goal, salvage rates are quoted at or greater than 90% in tertiary

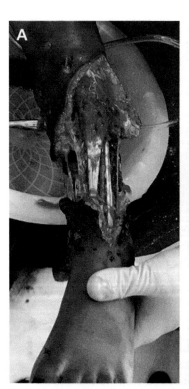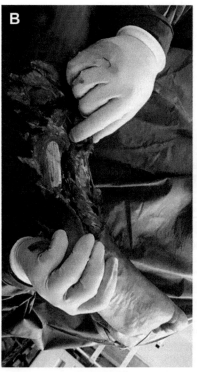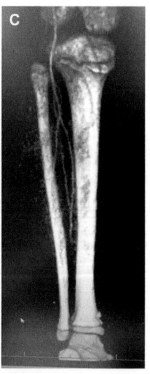

Fig. 2. Presentation of a 7-year-old boy with a severe Gustilo IIIC injury. (*A*) Extensive soft tissue loss of the anterior and lateral aspects of mangled lower extremity. (*B*) Medial aspect of the injured leg. (*C*) CT angiogram demonstrating an abrupt cutoff of all 3 lower leg vessels at the level of the mid tibia.

centers,[18] and therefore, these once secondary aesthetic concerns are now considered much more important to the patient and the surgeon. A secondary surgery rate of near 30% for aesthetic reasons following lower extremity reconstruction using perforator flaps was reported by Hui-Chou and colleagues.[19]

Multiple tools are at the disposal of the reconstructive surgeon to aid in the process: direct excision or debulking, tissue expansion, surgical and nonsurgical scar modification, laser treatment, and suction-assisted lipectomy, the latter of which is the most commonly performed technique.[19] Lower extremity aesthetic considerations should not be of a secondary concern, but should be part of the ultimate reconstructive algorithm for lower extremity limb salvage.

REVISIONS OR SUBSEQUENT PROCEDURES

Some of the more common revisions necessary for patients who have undergone orthoplastic procedures include bone grafting of previous defects and soft tissue flap debulking. A common sequence of events for trauma patients includes (1) multiple debridements to create a healthy wound bed, (2) concurrent bony fixation with placement of an antibiotic spacer or beads as needed, (3) soft tissue coverage with locoregional or free flap, (4) removal of antibiotics spacer with bone grafting (Masquelet technique), and (5) soft tissue debulking as needed.

Bone grafting usually occurs several months after initial reconstruction and requires reelevation of the flap to gain access to the osseous defect. If a

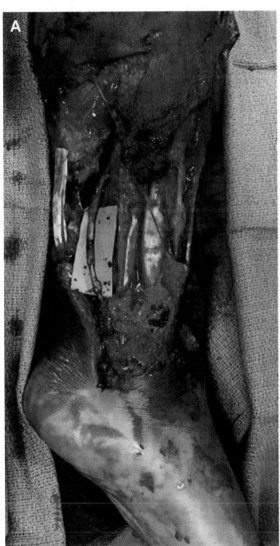
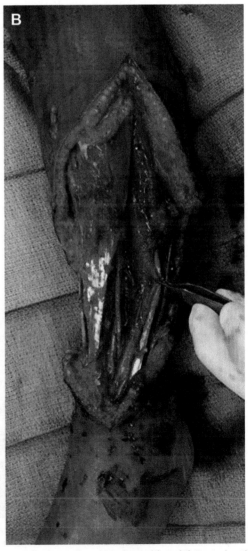

Fig. 3. Revascularization of LLE using greater saphenous vein grafts from the contralateral leg. (A) Posterior tibialis artery bypass. (B) Anterior tibial artery bypass.

free flap was initially performed, care will need to be taken to protect the pedicle as the flap is reelevated. Even if the flap pedicle is injured during the reelevation, there should have been sufficient neovascularization from the periphery to supply the previously transferred tissue, but this is variable and flaps that have been in place for years can be compromised from pedicle injury.[20]

Especially for reconstruction of the foot and ankle, long-term functionality may be compromised by a flap that is too bulky. It is a problem that requires patience on behalf of both the patient and the surgeon. Muscle flaps will undergo a significant amount of atrophy over time, and even fasciocutaneous flaps will decrease in size significantly as edema decreases over the course of months. Therefore, a flap that initially seems too bulky may end up having a near perfect contour. The authors usually assess this potential issue at a visit between 6 and 12 months, depending on the type of flap that was performed. Most often patients complain that they cannot fit into the appropriate footwear, or less often, that the bulk of the flap affects their gait. If the flap is on the plantar surface of the foot, it may prevent normal stance, or may even prevent clearance of the ground during the swing phase. Often these issues are not clear early on, as the patient is nonweight-bearing and is initially not wearing a normal shoe. If debulking is deemed necessary, it can be performed with direct excision or defatting of the undersurface of the flap, by liposuction of a fasciocutaneous flap, or with a combination of both. Again, the pedicle should be protected, especially when performing blind techniques like liposuction. If a perforator flap was performed, location of the perforators should be considered when planning direct excision.

CASE DEMONSTRATION
Case 1

Orthoplastic reconstruction of a Gustilo IIIC injury in a pediatric patient

A 7-year-old boy was airlifted to our pediatric institution after an extensive pit bull dog-bite injury to his left lower extremity (LLE). The patient presented with a severely mangled extremity below the knee with bone exposure, but no fractures. Both dorsalis pedis and posterior tibial pulses were absent, and the foot was cold to touch with no sensation. On computed tomographic (CT) angiography, there was an abrupt cutoff of all 3 lower leg vessels at the level of the mid tibia (**Fig. 2**). The patient was immediately taken to the operating room (OR) where he underwent extensive debridement and, by using his right great saphenous vein, arterial bypass was performed to both the anterior and the posterior tibial arteries to reestablish blood flow to the foot and leg

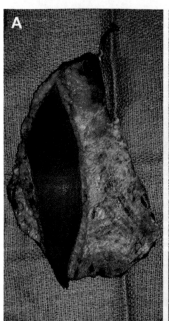
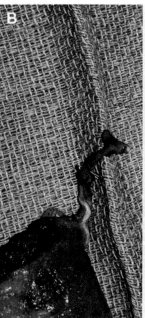
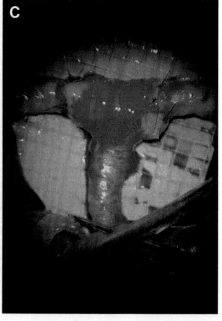

Fig. 4. Soft tissue coverage was performed using a free latissimus myocutaneous flap. (*A*) Free flap after harvest. (*B*) T-junction of the subscapular, circumflex scapular, and thoracodorsal arteries. (*C*) Anastomosis of the flap to the posterior tibial artery using the junction of the subscapular and circumflex scapular arteries as a flow through arterial conduit (as viewed through the operating microscope).

(Fig. 3). Three days later, the patient returned to the OR for soft tissue coverage using a free latissimus dorsi myocutaneous flap. The anastomosis was performed to the posterior tibial artery (above the bypass graft) using the junction of the subscapular and circumflex scapular arteries as a flow through arterial conduit (Fig. 4). The patient eventually had successful skin grafting of the remainder of the flap (Fig. 5). Two years after the injury, the patient's leg remains viable with gross sensation intact and no limb length discrepancy.

Case 2

Free vascularized medial femoral condyle for salvage of tarsometatarsal joint fusion

Our patient was a 47-year-old woman who suffered a Lisfranc fracture-dislocation after falling off a hoverboard. The patient ultimately underwent second tarsometatarsal (TMT) fusion using an anatomically congruent compression plate along with cancellous allograft to the fusion site. Nonunion was diagnosed at 6 months postoperatively. The patient subsequently underwent a revision procedure with removal of hardware, debridement, and fusion with placement of pelvic cancellous bone autograft with compression screw and staples. Seven months later, the patient was diagnosed with a persistent nonunion (Fig. 6). At this point, the patient was referred to the orthoplastic clinic for evaluation, and a free vascularized bone graft was recommended. The patient underwent reconstruction with a free vascularized medial femoral condyle to salvage the second TMT joint fusion (Fig. 7). Evidence of the union was seen at 7 weeks postoperatively (Fig. 8).

Case 3

Ipsilateral Arteriovenous looped free vascularized fibular graft for ankle fusion

Our patient was a 54-year-old woman who was referred to the orthoplastic clinic after being diagnosed with posttraumatic AVN of the talus (Fig. 9). The patient was developing painful ankle osteoarthritis. After evaluation, we planned for an

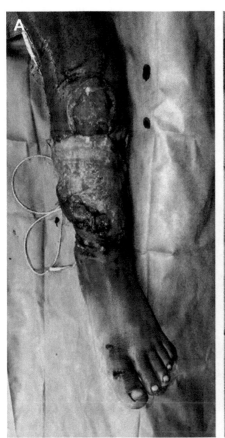
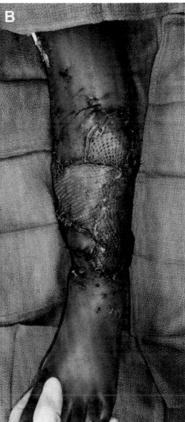
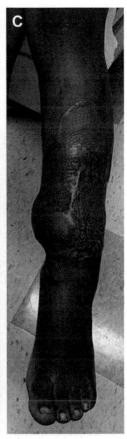

Fig. 5. Status-post orthoplastic limb salvage. (A) Immediate postoperative view of free latissimus myocutaneous flap. Internal Doppler monitoring was used. (B) After final coverage with skin grafting. (C) One year postoperative follow-up visit image; patient demonstrated running and jumping without marked difficulty.

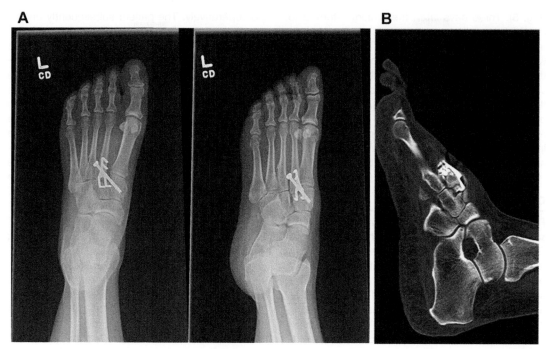

Fig. 6. A 47-year-old woman status-post multiple unsuccessful second TMT fusion attempts. (*A*) Radiograph demonstrating nonunion of the second TMT with a compression screw and plate overlying the joint. (*B*) CT scan of the foot, demonstrating nonunion at the attempted fusion site.

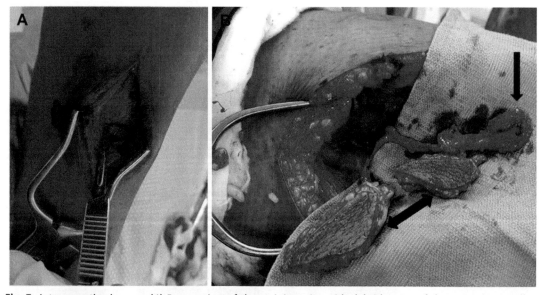

Fig. 7. Intraoperative images. (*A*) Preparation of the recipient site with debridement of the nonunion to allow room for proper insetting of the free flap. The scalpel is located at the prepared bed for the bone graft. (*B*) Free vascularized bone graft (*single-headed arrow*) with medial femoral condyle. This flap can be harvested with an accompanying skin island (*double-headed arrow*) to allow easy external monitoring. In this case, the authors decided, because of the superficial flap's location, not to use skin paddles for monitoring.

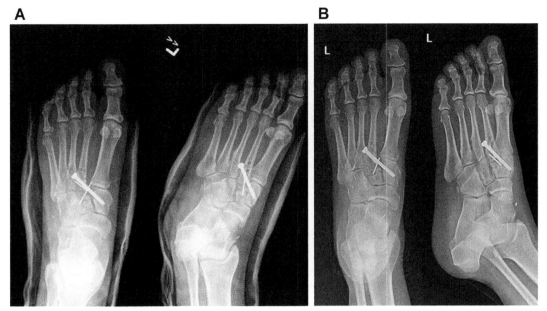

Fig. 8. Postoperative radiographs. Patient underwent free vascularized bone graft to the second TMT joint from the medial femoral condyle. (*A*) Immediate postoperative view with medial femoral condyle segment bridging the nonunion. (*B*) Seven-week postoperative images demonstrating union of the second TMT joint.

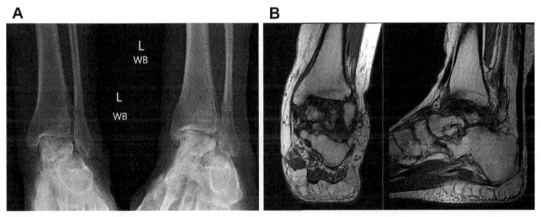

Fig. 9. Posttraumatic AVN of the left talus in a 53-year-old patient. (*A*) Preoperative radiograph demonstrating AVN of the talus with associated tibiotalar osteoarthritis. (*B*) MRI demonstrating AVN and fragmentation of the talus.

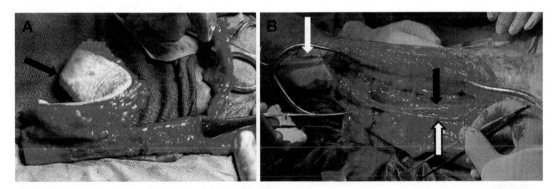

Fig. 10. Intraoperative images. (*A*) An ipsilateral free fibula flap after harvest with skin island (*arrow*) for postoperative monitoring. (*B*) After insetting of the flap with the use of the saphenous vein as an AV loop. Color, temperature, and capillary refill of the skin island can assist in monitoring the patency of the vascular bypass. The saphenous vein graft used as venous outflow (*black arrow*), saphenous vein as arterial inflow (*black outlined arrow*), and insetting of the skin island (*white arrow*).

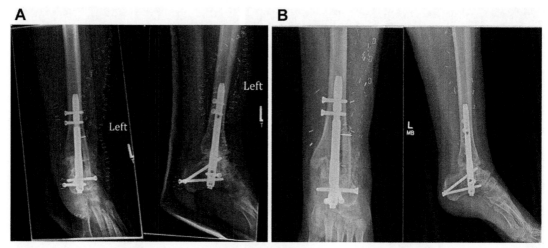

Fig. 11. Postoperative radiographs. (*A*) Immediate postoperative shot with fibular graft positioned as bridging live tissue between the tibia and talus to assist in bone healing and union. (*B*) Three-month postoperative images demonstrating the first signs of callus formation and integration of the vascularized bone graft.

ipsilateral AV loop free vascularized fibular graft along with stable intramedullary nail fixation of the ankle and subtalar joints. After fixation was accomplished, we harvested the ipsilateral fibula as a free bone graft along with a skin island and inset it to bridge the gap between the distal tibia and calcaneus. To extend the reach of the pedicle for inset of the flap at the ankle, an AV loop was formed using the origin of the peroneal vessels and a saphenous vein graft (**Fig. 10**). Evidence of callus formation was visible at 2-month follow-up (**Fig. 11**).

DISCUSSION
Pearls for Developing the Orthoplastic Approach: Teamwork, Awareness, and Education

Teamwork
In order to build an orthoplastic surgery team, some basic principles must be followed. The orthoplastic approach is based on the ability to attack complex problems of varied causes (trauma, tumors, congenital anomalies, complex infections) by diagnosing and treating the various aspects of the problem. In order to deliver such care to patients, a multidisciplinary team should be assembled consisting of orthopedic and plastic surgeons with microsurgical capabilities that hold mutual respect of each other's knowledge and expertise. The team members must understand that "turf battles" or propriety ownership of cases is counterproductive and will preclude success.

Awareness
As orthoplastic surgery is a relatively new field, this puts the burden of proof on our shoulders.

Thus, when building an orthoplastic surgery team, the critical members must be available 24 hours a day, 7 days a week, 365 days a year for consultation and deployment. In addition, potential referring and collaborating specialties, such as primary care physicians, endocrinologists, vascular surgeons, oncologic surgeons, and other surgical specialists, should be aware of the existence of such a team and educated on the value and capabilities of the orthoplastic approach.

Education
Developing a new field can be achieved through a combination of efforts. First, we must learn from the experience of others and share our own experiences through multidisciplinary conferences. Second, we must push the field forward through clinical and basic science research. Finally, we must have a vehicle to spread current knowledge and future achievements that can also be used as a reference in the form of a journal (*Orthoplastic Surgery* by Elsevier).

SUMMARY

The focus of the orthoplastic approach thus far has been to broaden the scope and increase the rate of functional limb salvage via multidisciplinary evaluation, operative planning, and execution. Here, the authors discuss adjunctive techniques that will optimize the final functional result or aid the surgeon in difficult situations when complications arise in these complex reconstructive cases.

CLINICS CARE POINTS

General

- Complex extremity injuries should be treated with early multidisciplinary collaboration using an orthoplastic approach.
- Utilizing a multidisciplinary orthoplastic approach can help avoid unnecessary extremity amputations.

Pediatric IIIC injuries

- With pediatric IIIC injuries, special thought must be given to bony healing and growth potential. For example, limb lengthening may be delayed by a fresh vascular repair.
- Limb lengthening may result in poor soft tissue coverage, which may ultimately necessitate a flap reconstruction in a patient with complex lower extremity vasculature.

Medial Femoral Condyle to Foot & Ankle

- When revising various failed foot and ankle fusions, decision-making should take into account soft tissue coverage, bone stock, and the size of the defect.
- The medial femoral condyle/trochlea is a versatile flap that can be used as vascularized cortical bone, cancellous bone, cartilage, periosteum, or a chimera of the above.
- The medial femoral condyle can include skin or muscle to augment the soft tissue coverage to help achieve the desired union.

AV Loop Fibula

- When significant bone defects are present, one should consider the use of a vascularized free fibula bone graft.
- In order to avoid contralateral comorbidity, we have adopted the use of an ipsilateral AV loop free fibula with the use of saphenous vein graft to bridge the gap formed.
- For monitoring purposes, a skin island can be included.

Lymphatic Bypass

- In the lower extremity, the lymphatic vessels originate on either side of the toes, the foot, and at the lateral thigh, just deep to the dermis and travel in the subcutaneous tissue proximally.
- Since lymphatics have axiality and directionality, type, orientation and inset of the flap at the extremity may affect lymphatic transport.
- Lymphovenous bypass, when possible, allows the excess lymphatic fluid to bypass the damaged and nonfunctional lymphatics in the zone of injury.

Secondary Aesthetic Refinements

- Aesthetics of the lower extremity should be considered as part of the reconstructive algorithm for limb salvage.
- When deciding to revise a free flap reconstruction, the operating surgeon must consider location of the pedicle and keep it protected.
- Patience is critical when considering flap revisions, as muscle and fasciocutaneous flaps will decrease in size significantly over the course of months. Therefore, wait 6-12 months until considering revisions for bulk or skin excess.

DISCLOSURES

The authors have no conflicts of interests or sources of funding to disclose.

REFERENCES

1. Azoury SC, Stranix JT, Kovach SJ, et al. Principles of orthoplastic surgery for lower extremity reconstruction: why is this important? J Reconstr Microsurg 2019; 1(212). https://doi.org/10.1055/s-0039-1695753.
2. Swiontkowski MF, MacKenzie EJ, Bosse MJ, et al. Factors influencing the decision to amputate or reconstruct after high-energy lower extremity trauma. J Trauma 2002. https://doi.org/10.1097/00005373-200204000-00005.
3. Laine JC, Cherkashin A, Samchukov M, et al. The management of soft tissue and bone loss in type IIIB and IIIC pediatric open tibia fractures. J Pediatr Orthop 2016. https://doi.org/10.1097/BPO.0000000000000492.
4. Ricci JA, Abdou SA, Stranix JT, et al. Reconstruction of Gustilo type IIIc injuries of the lower extremity. Plast Reconstr Surg 2019. https://doi.org/10.1097/PRS.0000000000006063.
5. Backus JD, Ocel DL. Ankle arthrodesis for talar avascular necrosis and arthrodesis nonunion. Foot Ankle Clin 2019;24(1):131–42.
6. Haddock NT, Alosh H, Easley ME, et al. Applications of the medial femoral condyle free flap for foot and ankle reconstruction. Foot Ankle Int 2013;34(10): 1395–402.
7. Haddock NT, Wapner K, Levin LS. Vascular bone transfer options in the foot and ankle: a retrospective review and update on strategies. Plast Reconstr Surg 2013;132(3):685–93.
8. Kazmers NH, Thibaudeau S, Gerety P, et al. Versatility of the medial femoral condyle flap for extremity reconstruction and identification of risk factors for

nonunion, delayed time to union, and complications. Ann Plast Surg 2018;80(4):364–72.

9. Nihal A, Gellman RE, Embil JM, et al. Ankle arthrodesis. Foot Ankle Surg 2008;14(1):1–10.

10. Piccolo PP, Ben-Amotz O, Ashley B, et al. Ankle arthrodesis with free vascularized fibula autograft using saphenous vein grafts: a case series. Plast Reconstr Surg 2018;142(3):806–9.

11. Van Zanten MC, Mistry RM, Suami H, et al. The lymphatic response to injury with soft-tissue reconstruction in high-energy open tibial fractures of the lower extremity. Plast Reconstr Surg 2017. https://doi.org/10.1097/PRS.0000000000003024.

12. Pan WR, Wang DG, Levy SM, et al. Superficial lymphatic drainage of the lower extremity: anatomical study and clinical implications. Plast Reconstr Surg 2013. https://doi.org/10.1097/PRS.0b013e31829ad12e.

13. Suami H, Taylor GI, Pan WR. The lymphatic territories of the upper limb: anatomical study and clinical implications. Plast Reconstr Surg 2007. https://doi.org/10.1097/01.prs.0000246516.64780.61.

14. Slavin SA, Upton J, Kaplan WD, et al. An investigation of lymphatic function following free-tissue transfer. Plast Reconstr Surg 1997. https://doi.org/10.1097/00006534-199703000-00020.

15. Yamamoto T, Iida T, Yoshimatsu H, et al. Lymph flow restoration after tissue replantation and transfer: importance of lymph axiality and possibility of lymph flow reconstruction without lymph node transfer or lymphatic anastomosis. Plast Reconstr Surg 2018. https://doi.org/10.1097/PRS.0000000000004694.

16. Pereira N, Cámbara Á, Kufeke M, et al. Post-traumatic lymphedema treatment with superficial circumflex iliac artery perforator lymphatic free flap: a case report. Microsurgery 2019. https://doi.org/10.1002/micr.30437.

17. Schaverien MV, Badash I, Patel KM, et al. Vascularized lymph node transfer for lymphedema. Semin Plast Surg 2018. https://doi.org/10.1055/s-0038-1632401.

18. Fischer JP, Wink JD, Nelson JA, et al. A retrospective review of outcomes and flap selection in free tissue transfers for complex lower extremity reconstruction. J Reconstr Microsurg 2013;29(6):407–16.

19. Hui-Chou HG, Sulek J, Bluebond-Langner R, et al. Secondary refinements of free perforator flaps for lower extremity reconstruction. Plast Reconstr Surg 2011;127(1):248–57.

20. Yoon AP, Jones NF. Critical time for neovascularization/angiogenesis to allow free flap survival after delayed postoperative anastomotic compromise without surgical intervention: a review of the literature. Microsurgery 2016. https://doi.org/10.1002/micr.30082.

Functional Restoration in Lower Extremity Reconstruction

Chih-Hung Lin, MD

KEYWORDS

- Vascularized bone flap • Medial plantar flap • Microsurgical functional reconstruction
- Knee contracture • Foot equinovarus contracture

KEY POINTS

- All reconstruction should have functional goals using either local flap or free flap to restore the lost function.
- If local flap or tendon transfer cannot provide the basic function, microsurgical reconstruction is indicated for bony, soft tissue, and sensation restoration.
- Major functional unit rebuilding is the goal for jeopardized function in lower limbs.
- Free tissue transfer can have the advantage of composite tissue inclusion and spatial arrangement using the fascial component for tendon or muscle defect reconstruction.

INTRODUCTION

Various trauma or tumor surgery on lower limbs can result in not only soft tissue envelope defects but also variable functional deficits. Numerous resurfacing procedures are available to repair the defects. Improvements in sterile technique, the use of antibiotics, bony fixation, and microvascular reconstruction have shifted the management paradigm of mutilating limb and limb salvage to functional restoration. The ultimate goal of reconstructing a lower extremity is to achieve painless, stable weight-bearing walking, which requires adequate bone union, a pliable stable joint, and a sensate sole.

In the scenario of open wounds, all the vital structural defects can be well recognized and assessed, and the required recipient neurovasculature is exposed entirely.[1] It is best to plan either a 1-stage or staged reconstructive strategy. Severely contaminated or mutilated limbs make the viability of the traumatized tissue questionable, so the lesion may require repeated debridement before the coverage reconstruction. If the wound infection or contamination is under control,

functional reconstruction can be combined with the resurfacing procedure to provide a simultaneous soft tissue and functional restoration.

The authors believe that functional reconstruction should incorporate conventional or microsurgical methods for the restoration of functional loss. Methods such as vascularized bone transfer, bone grafting or distraction, tendon transfer, free functioning muscle transfer, and sensate glabrous skin for plantar defect resurfacing are all designed for functional considerations.

The restoration of a stable, strong femur or tibial bony structure is essential for weight bearing. Conventional bone graft or bone substitute can be used for small-segment bony defects.

Improvements in microsurgical free tissue outcomes contribute to the functional result and quality of life. Establishment of comprehensive wound repair, bony union, and motor unit transplant is the standard for adequate lower extremity functional restoration.

Despite the psychological advantages of limb salvage, the return to premorbid status is equivalent to limb amputation. Thus the reconstructive procedures should be designed to accomplish

Plastic and Reconstructive Surgery, Chang Gung Memorial Hospital and University, 5, Fu-Hsing street, Kweishan District, Taoyuan city 333, Taiwan
E-mail address: chihhung@cgmh.org.tw

Clin Plastic Surg 48 (2021) 289–297
https://doi.org/10.1016/j.cps.2021.01.009
0094-1298/21/© 2021 Elsevier Inc. All rights reserved.

comprehensive coverage and functional management to shorten the disability and return to work times.

INDICATIONS AND CONTRAINDICATIONS OF PREFERRED RECONSTRUCTIONS, INCLUDING RATIONALE AND TIMING

The Lower Extremity Assessment Project (LEAP), the first and only prospective, multi-institutional cohort study of several scoring systems on severe lower extremity trauma, found no association between loss of plantar sensation and the need for late amputation, dispelling one of the classic absolute indications for amputation.[2] A comparison of functional outcomes between the amputated and salvaged cohorts found no significant differences.

The scores are not definitely compatible with the functional outcomes. Even low scores tend to have higher lower limb salvage rate. Many patients with high scores have successful salvage or functional outcomes. Recontracture surgery is not appropriate for reconstructable limbs.[2,3] Thus, reconstructable limbs are related to the facility of the hospital or collaborative team. Appropriate referral of the traumatized patients to a competent team at the right time is essential.

However, before the definite reconstruction, all patient should have justified damaged control for the polytrauma insult. Particularly in patients presenting with impending lethal triad, the overwhelming pathophysiologic effect of severe inflammatory response syndrome or complementary antiinflammatory response syndrome can be life threatening.[4–7]

In recent decades, free tissue transfers, local flaps, or pedicle perforator flaps have been widely used for posttraumatic lower limb defect reconstruction. Resurfacing surgeries aim at wound repair, either skin, muscle, or osteocutaneous flaps.[8–11] To go a step further, functional restoration can enhance the benefit for functional deficits of lower limbs. Simultaneous or secondary tendon transfer, or arthrodesis, is applied for functional purposes. Composite free tissue can comprise different components to improve the functional unit loss in various reconstructions.[8]

Established Principles and Surgical Approaches

Beyond the resurfacing procedure, there are several functional deficits that benefit from free tissue transfer or microsurgery, including (1) bony structure rebuilding to allow weight bearing; (2) contracture release of knee, ankle, or toe joints; (3) muscle or tendon defects; (4) denervation; and (5) durable weight-bearing soles.

1. Bony structure rebuilding to allow weight bearing

   Conventional bone grafting is feasible for small bone defects in well-vascularized recipient sites. Vascularized bone flap transfer is indicated for unfavorable situations and Illizarov bone transportation is another alternative. Vascularized bone flap is preferable for (1) segmental bone defects >6 cm with/without soft tissue defect, (2) chronic osteomyelitis, (3) pseudoarthrosis, (4) multiple failure in conventional bone grafting, and (5) poor vascularity of recipient site. There are many donor bone flaps that fit the mentioned indications, such as fibula, iliac crest, and rib flap. Fibular flap possesses more cortical bone strength, constant blood supply, and less donor site morbidity. Stress fracture is common after bone flap transfer, thus protective brace and crutch walking should be applied for both internal fixation or temporary external fixator removal until there is adequate bony hypertrophy. The double-barrel fibular flap can also provide more area and volume in cross section for long bone defects. Therefore, fibular flap is the first option for long bone reconstruction.

   The functional purpose is to have bony union, adequate bone hypertrophy, and full weight bearing within 2 years with the least chronic osteomyelitis and stress fracture (**Fig. 1**). Comparing the donor site and recipient morbidity, and the functional outcomes among the fibular flap, iliac flap, and rib flap,[12–14] the fibular flap was the best for lower extremity bony reconstruction, which can be performed as a double barrel for the volume augmentation to increase the strength for weight loading and less stress fracture(**Fig. 2**). Iliac flap can have good bony union, but less hypertrophy, and limited bony length is available. The serratus anterior combined rib flap is a membranous bone that is thin and requires a lengthy time for bone hypertrophy and consolidation, but, with the accompanying latissimus dorsi muscle based on the thoracodorsal pedicle, this composite flap can reconstruct extensive defects. In bilateral tibiofibular open IIIB fractures, the serratus anterior-rib flap can be an alternative method to rebuild the bilateral lower limb composite defect (**Fig. 3**).

   The segmental tibial defect in an open IIIB fracture can be reconstructed in 1-stage

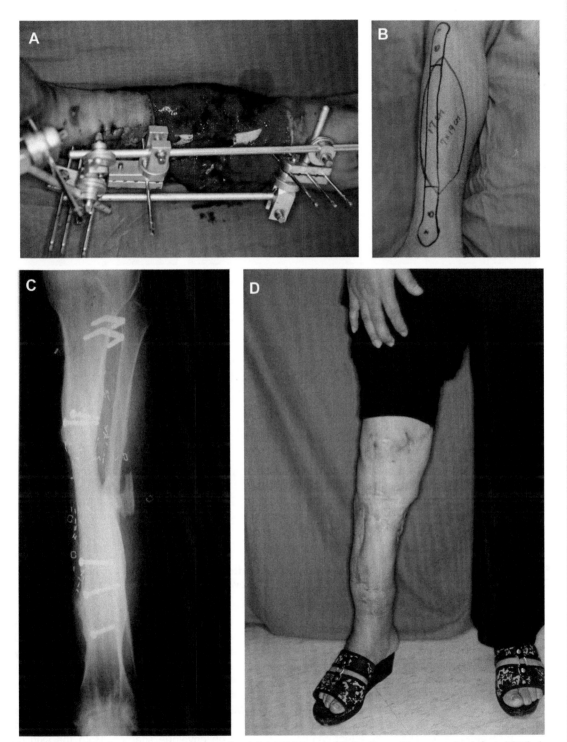

Fig. 1. (*A*) This female patient in her 40s sustained right tibial open IIIB fracture with composite defect. (*B*) Fibular osteocutaneous flap. (*C*) Advanced bony hypertrophy. (*D*) Eight-year follow-up.

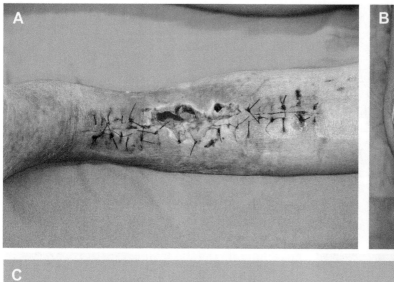
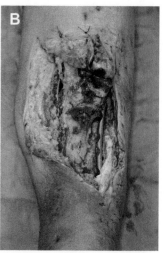
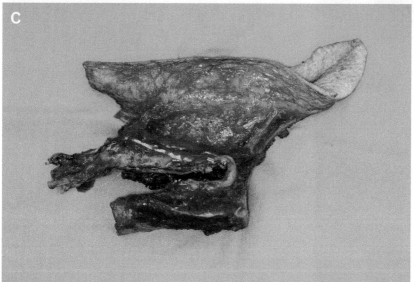
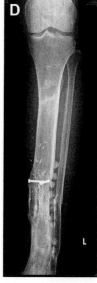

Fig. 2. (*A*) Left tibial chronic osteomyelitis soft tissue defect after sequestrectomy. (*B*) Composite defect. (*C*) Double-barrel fibular flap. (*D*) Bony hypertrophy at 10-year follow-up.

surgery or a 2-stage procedure. Some surgeons prefer soft tissue coverage as the first choice, followed by second-stage vascularized bone transfer. This technique can be indicated in a more extensive defect or severely contaminated wound, and can achieve viable soft tissue coverage with a healthy pedicle for a free soft tissue flap for wound repair. The bony defect can be implanted with an antibiotic spacer for infection control. A vascularized bone transfer is performed after the traumatized lesion is well treated. If the defect is not too bad, as mentioned, a 1-stage vascularized osteocutaneous flap is justified for composite tibia and soft tissue defect

reconstruction. Even in stable tibia or femur chronic osteomyelitis, a vascularized bone flap can achieve intercalary segmental bone defect repair after comprehensive sequestrectomy.

2. Contracture release of knee and ankle

Mutilating lower extremity trauma may have muscle contracture after damage, and skin envelope scarring. Both the skin or muscle fibrosis nearing the knee or ankle joints tend to result in knee stiffness, flexion contracture, or ankle equinovarus contracture. Both knee and ankle contracture cause incommodious, limping gait. Releasing the contracture is needed for balanced, harmonious walking. Diligent

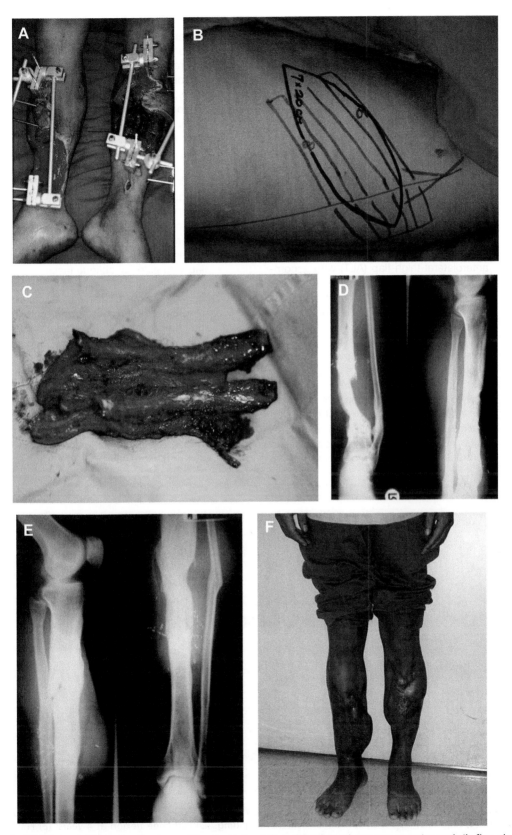

Fig. 3. (*A*) Bilateral tibia open fracture with composite defect. (*B*) Bilateral serratus anterior and rib flap elevation. (*C*) Composite serratus-rib flap. (*D*) Right tibia union and bone hypertrophy at 3 years. (*E*) Left tibia union. (*F*) Full weight bearing at 3-year follow-up.

rehabilitation can improve the flexion contracture to achieve knee full extension. In stiff knees caused by direct quadriceps trauma and skin envelope, or extensive quadriceps adhesion to the fractured femur, release of the muscle from the surrounding tissue may be adequate to achieve passive full knee flexion. If quadriceps lysis is not enough, a patellar tendon lengthening or quadricepsplasty will be required. Furthermore, the anterior knee skin is much too tight because of the shortness of the pliable envelope for knee flexion, so a free skin flap is indicated. In patellar tendon contracture that is not suitable for lengthening, a tendon allograft or vascularized fascia lata is indicated.[15] An anterolateral thigh flap (ALT) with accompanying vascularized fascia lata cord is justified for composite skin and patellar tendon defect reconstruction, or the vascularized fascia lata can be used as a gliding tissue for separation of quadriceps from the fracture site to prevent adhesion (**Fig. 4**).

Ankle equinovarus contracture is common after lower leg trauma because of either bed-ridden positioning or gastrocnemius muscle contracture. This contracture results from the muscle or soft tissue contracture. The posterior compartment is volumetric strong muscle group than the anterior and lateral compartment for ankle dorsiflexion. In the early stage, the contracture can be corrected by rehabilitation or adjustable external fixator progressively, but, in the chronic stage, Achilles tendon or gastrocnemius muscle lengthening is needed. In cases of inadequate skin coverage on the Achilles tendon area, a local soft tissue flap or free skin flap is indicated for the heel soft tissue repair after the Achilles tendon lengthening. If the Achilles tendon is unhealthy, disrupted, or badly contracted, a free composite fascia rod and skin flap will be needed, such as an ALT flap with accompanying vascularized fascia late or groin flap with external oblique fascia.

3. Muscle or tendon defect

After high-energy damage or compartment syndrome, the muscle and soft tissue may be crushed or devascularized. When there is adequate soft tissue coverage, various tendon transfers can accomplish functional reconstruction. For example, the posterior tibialis or the peroneus longus can be used for anterior tibialis loss. In the distal lower leg and ankle area with a paucity of soft tissue envelope, segmental tendon loss thus occurs because of extensive crush or avulsion injury. Thus, a free

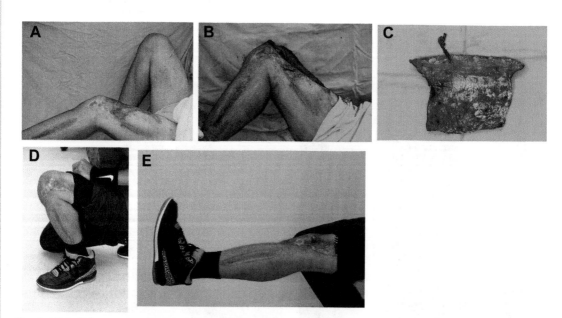

Fig. 4. (*A*) Left femur open fracture with stiff knee. (*B*) Left knee split-thickness skin graft scar excision, quadriceps lysis. (*C*) Right ALT flap with vascularized fascia for gliding. (*D*) Full knee flexion at 4 years. (*E*) Full knee extension.

skin flap with simultaneous tendon transfer or accompanying fascial rod for tendon replacement is needed.

When there is composite soft tissue and muscle loss, free functioning muscle transfer is indicated. Either gracilis or rectus femoris functioning muscle can be used for anterior tibialis and extensor halluces longus.[16] However, for weight-bearing purposes, a strong donor muscle is required, hence a rectus femoris functioning muscle is preferred for composite gastrocnemius, or quadriceps defects in 1-stage reconstruction (**Fig. 5**).

4. Denervation of major nerve

Nerve dysfunction can be caused by compression or disruption. Different from the upper limb, the outcome of decompression is worse because of more distal nerve regeneration from the lumbar spinal cord. However, nerve repair is indicated for essential functional deficit. Femoral nerve is fundamental for the quadriceps, which is important for knee extension. Sciatic nerve provides the motor nerve to the biceps, semitendinosus, and semimembranosus for knee flexion; to the lower leg posterior tibial nerve innervating gastrocnemius and soleus weight bearing; and sensory nerve for plantar sensation. The common peroneal nerve has a deep peroneal nerve for the anterior tibialis for ankle dorsiflexion, peroneus longus/brevis for ankle valgus, and extensor halluces longus/extensor digitorum longus for toe extensions.

Nerve repair or nerve grafting may be performed for the reinnervation or denervated targets to restore essential function. Nerve decompression of the compressed common peroneal nerve or tarsal tunnel have been performed often. If nerve repair is not feasible for denervated muscle, tendon transfer or muscle transfer will be indicated.

5. Durable weight-bearing sole

Painless stable walking is crucial for every patient, and balanced bilateral lower limbs may cause much less walking stress to the planter weight-bearing soles. Bilateral feet bony structure, curvature, and position are important. All efforts are designed to achieve precise bony, ligament, and tendon repair followed by comprehensive rehabilitation.

The weight-bearing sole requires adequate stability, durability, and sensitivity. Free skin flaps or skin grafted muscle flaps have been used for extensive healing of soft tissue defects. The skin flap possesses thick, durable skin, and partial innervated skin, but the excessive

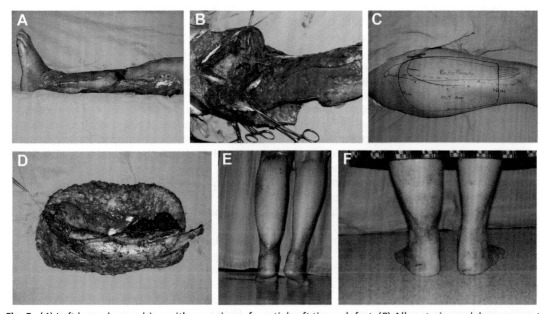

Fig. 5. (*A*) Left lower leg avulsion with near-circumferential soft tissue defect. (*B*) All posterior and deep compartment lost. (*C*) Right ALT with functioning rectus femoris flap donor site planning. (*D*) Flap elevated. (*E*) Standing on toes. (*F*) Full weight bearing.

subcutaneous fat tends to have more shearing force and cause unstable walking. The skin grafted muscle flap may have sensory nerves, such as innervation by the posterior tibial nerve to the latissimus dorsi thoracodorsal mixed nerve, but the muscle cannot achieve adequate protective sensation. Postoperative protection is crucial to prevent the occurrence of trophic ulcers. The bulky skin or muscle flaps make the soft tissue unstable and cause excessive shearing force for ordinary walking. Sensation can be overemphasized; it is common after a free flap for a heel defect for an intractable trophic ulcer to develop on the undamaged glabrous plantar skin. This situation can be assessed from the excessive shearing stress across the free flap but accretion on the weight-bearing plantar skin.

If trophic ulcers develop, skin flaps may make skin flap partial elevation possible as rotational flap mobilization for ulcer repair, but skin grafted muscle may not be available for flap mobilization, whereas another free flap or innervated medial plantar flap is another option.

Medial plantar flap is performed on the non–weight-bearing instep area where the character of the entire forefoot and hindfoot glabrous skin flap is similar. The medial plantar flap can be elevated to provide sensation based on the branch of the medial plantar nerve; possesses durable, innately hyperkeratinized skin; and has adequate stability for walking because of its dense fibroseptum.

If the posterior tibial neurovascular bundle is healthy, this medial plantar flap can be transferred as an innervated pedicle flap for hindfoot coverage, most commonly hindfoot melanoma ablation. However, in most cases of trauma, the ipsilateral instep area was involved or a forefoot defect has occurred, so free contralateral instep flap is indicated. In addition, in forefoot defects with healthy insteps, the instep flap can be elevated as a free flap to the ipsilateral forefoot defect with intercalary arterial and nerve defects bridged with vein or nerve grafts.[17,18]

DISCUSSION

With the development of extremity microsurgery in the last several decades, the reconstruction ladder algorithm has evolved from simple wound coverage with either skin graft or local flap to free tissue transfer. In aesthetic considerations, it is common that a free flap can provide better, healthy tissue to create an aesthetic appearance and less secondary recipient site violation. Considering functional restoration, the choice of surgical procedure concerns much more than the wound repair; it also includes how to provide the best possible reliable functional outcome to the patient. Major functional unit rebuilding is the goal for functional jeopardized lower limbs. The sensory or motor nerve can provide predictable functional recovery, but less so for the lower limb, and the nerve repair or grafting should be compared with the available tendon transfer for reconstructing functional deficit. Local flaps usually are useful for neighboring and small defects, but, for extensive and composite defects, free tissue transfer is required.

Free flap for wound repair with accompanying tendon transfer can be a predictable procedure. However, the lower limb may not have suitable donor tendon for transfer, so a composite tissue reconstruction may be preferred. Free tissue transfer can have the advantage of composite tissue inclusion and spatial arrangement, especially in the situation of functional reconstruction to provide the fascial component for tendon or muscle defect reconstruction.

SUMMARY

The ultimate goal of reconstructing a lower extremity is to achieve painless, stable, weight-bearing walking, which requires adequate bone union, pliable stable joints, and sensate sole. All reconstructive procedures should be designed to accomplish comprehensive coverage and functional management to shorten the disability time and return to work. Simultaneous or secondary tendon transfer, or arthrodesis, can be applied for functional purposes. Composite free tissue can comprise different components to improve the functional unit loss in the various reconstructions.

CLINICS CARE POINTS

- Definite functional restoration will be evaluated and decided during the surgery.
- Tendon or muscle reconstruction require adequate tension and postoperative immobilization for at least 6 weeks.
- Free tissue transfers will be monitored in a microsurgical ICU by experienced nursery.
- Rehabilitation program will be initiated one week after surgery when the wound heals well.

DISCLOSURE

The author has nothing to disclose.

REFERENCES

1. Godina M. Early microsurgical reconstruction of complex trauma of the extremities. Plast Reconstr Surg 1986;78:285.
2. Bosse MJ, McCarthy ML, Jones AL, et al. The insensate foot following severe lower extremity trauma: an indication for amputation? J Bone Joint Surg Am 2005;87:2601–8.
3. Bosse MJ, MacKenzie EJ, Kellam JF, et al. An analysis of outcomes of reconstruction or amputation after leg-threatening injuries. N Engl J Med 2002;347:1924–31.
4. Seekamp A, Regel G, Frank H, et al. Parameters of multiple organ dysfunction fail to predict secondary amputation following limb salvage in multiply traumatized patients. Injury 1999;30:199–207.
5. Keel M, Trentz O. Pathophysiology of polytrauma. Injury 2005;36:691–709.
6. Holcomb JB. Damage control resuscitation. J.Trauma 2007;62:S36–7.
7. Engel H, Lin C-H, Wei F-C. Role of microsurgery in lower extremity reconstruction. Plast Reconstr Surg 2011;127:228–39.
8. Lin C-H, Wei F-C, Lin Y-T, et al. Lateral circumflex femoral artery system: warehouse for functional composite free-tissue reconstruction of the lower leg. J Trauma 2006;60(5):1032–6.
9. Koshima I. A new classification of free combined or connected tissue transfers: introduction to the concept of bridge, Siamese, chimeric, mosaic, and chain-circle flaps. Acta Med Okayama 2001;55:329–32.
10. Khouri RK, Shaw WW. Reconstruction of the lower extremity with microvascular free flaps: a 10 year experience with 304 consecutive cases. J Trauma 1989;29:1086.
11. Lin C-H, Wei F-C, Levin SL, et al. The functional outcome of lower- extremity fractures with vascular injury. J Trauma 1997;43(3):480–5.
12. Lin C-H, Wei F-C, Chen H-C, et al. Outcome comparison in traumatic lower extremity reconstruction by using various composite vascularized bone transplantation. Plast Reconstr Surg 1999;104(4):984–92.
13. Lin C-H, Sukru Y. Revisiting the serratus anterior rib flap for composite tibial defects. Plast Reconstr Surg 2004;114(7):1871–7.
14. Yazar S, Lin C-H, Wei F-C. One-stage reconstruction of composite bone and soft-tissue defects in traumatic lower extremities. Plast Reconstr Surg 2004;114(6):1457–66.
15. Ulsal AE, Ulsal BG, Lin Y-T, et al. The advantage of free tissue transfer in the treatment of posttraumatic stiff knee. Plast Reconstr Surg 2007;119:203.
16. Lin C-H, Lin Y-T, Yeh J-T, et al. Free functioning muscle transfer for lower extremity posttraumatic composite structure and functional defect. Plast Reconstr Surg 2007;119(6):2118–26.
17. Zelken JA, Lin C-H. An Algorithm for forefoot reconstruction with the innervated free medial plantar flap. Ann Plast Surg 2016;76(2):221–6.
18. Löfstrand JG, Lin CH. Reconstruction of defects in the weight-bearing plantar area using the innervated free medial plantar (instep) flap. Ann Plast Surg 2018;80(3):245–51.

Supermicrosurgery in Lower Extremity Reconstruction

Joon Pio Hong, MD, PhD, MMM*, Changsik John Pak, MD, PhD,
Hyunsuk Peter Suh, MD, PhD

KEYWORDS

• Microsurgery • Supermicrosurgery • Lower extremity reconstruction • Perforator to perforator

KEY POINTS

- Supermicrosurgery is defined as manipulation of vessels less than 0.8 mm, often requiring different thinking and tools.
- Perforators can be used as a recipient source (perforator-to-perforator supermicrosurgery), minimizing the need for extensive dissection to find recipient vessels.
- Perforators also allow reconstruction, where axial arteries are not available due to trauma, atherosclerosis, or other causes.
- Like a perforator flap based on a single perforator, the limits of a single perforator as a recipient should be understood.

INTRODUCTION

Microsurgery is a general term for surgery requiring the use of an operating microscope; in the field of reconstructive surgery, various procedures are performed, such as replantation, flap transfer, autotransplantation or allotransplantation, revascularization, neurorrhaphy, lymphatic surgery, and others. The core principles of microsurgery encompass (1) proper working environment, including microscopes and loupes; (2) preoperative evaluation and planning; (3) microsurgical technique from elevation, pedicle dissection, recipient preparation, microanastomosis, to flap insetting; and (4) postoperative care.[1] The reconstructive microsurgery usually involves the anastomosis of vessels of approximately 1 mm to 2 mm in vessel diameter. In some instances of larger vessels, anastomosis can be done under loupe magnification. The overall success rates for reconstructive microsurgery in the lower extremity using these principles are approximately 93% to 100%.[2] Although lower extremity reconstructive microsurgery remains the highest rung of the reconstruction ladder, the goal of microsurgery is stretched to achieve not only soft tissue coverage but also function and acceptable aesthetics through a more efficient reconstructive elevator approach, simplifying the stages of reconstruction.

The wide zone of injury, however, usually associated with trauma frequently leaves the extremity with injured vessels; the increase in chronic diseases among the general population leaves the axial arteries calcified; the axial arteries often are difficult to approach, especially when reconstructing the upper leg including the knee; and, when using a single axial artery, there is a fear of steal phenomenon, making lower extremity reconstruction challenging. These situations frequently result in limited availability of good pulsatile axial arteries as choices for recipient vessels. Even when using these limited axial arteries as recipient sources, the possibilities of having steal phenomenon and injuring the functioning artery may deter surgeons from using these axial arteries. Thus, utilizing the

Department of Plastic Surgery, Asan Medical Center, University of Ulsan, 88 Olympicro 43 gil, Songpagu, Seoul 05505, Korea
* Corresponding author.
E-mail address: joonphong@amc.seoul.kr

Clin Plastic Surg 48 (2021) 299–306
https://doi.org/10.1016/j.cps.2020.12.009

recipient from the contralateral leg spared from injury in a cross-leg fashion can be a reliable source. Although this approach deserves to be recognized and should be considered an alternative solution, the process is painstaking not only for surgeons but also for patients. Knowing that the first key to having a successful outcome for microsurgical reconstruction is having a reliable recipient source, it must be asked how to overcome these difficulties in finding a reliable recipient.

In the era of perforator flaps, which are cutaneous or fasciocutaneous flaps based on a single perforator, it is remarkable to see a flap with a large skin dimension have a successful outcome reflecting the influence of a single perforator. The authors hypothesized that if a single perforator is capable of supplying the skin vascularity, it could be used as a recipient source.[3,4] In the past, it was believed that there was a significant risk for failure in using vessels with diameter less than 1 mm.[5] Since the early days of microsurgery, there has been substantial improvement of microscopes, technique, instruments, training, knowledge, and imaging, allowing microsurgeons to perform anastomosis of vessels less than 1 mm without worrying about the outcome. Hence, the term, *supermicrosurgery technique*, is defined as microsurgical anastomosis of vessels with a diameter less than 0.8 mm facilitated by using smaller and finer instruments.[6,7] This technique frequently is applied to lymphaticovenous anastomosis (LVA) to treat lymphedema, fingertip replantation, finger/toe reconstruction, and nerve flaps and in soft tissue reconstruction. The use of a perforator as a recipient vessel in the lower extremity falls into this domain because a majority of the perforators used are less than 0.8 mm, and numerous articles have validated the efficacy of the approach.[3,4,8–10] In this article, principles, indications, preoperative evaluation, surgical procedures, postoperative care, and management of complications after perforator-to-perforator supermicrosurgery are presented and reviewed.

INDICATIONS AND CONTRAINDICATIONS

Any perforators that are pulsating can be indicated for use as a recipient source. These perforators can be found within the defect while débriding or adjacent to this zone. Unlike burns and radiation wounds, the zone of injury, especially in trauma, is difficult to define and the definition remains unclear.[11] Nevertheless, the zone of injury concept should be considered and using a vessel within the zone avoided if a good alternative exits nearby, because perivascular changes within the zone

may occur and lead to increased friability of vessels and perivascular scarring of recipient vessels, resulting in higher incidence of thrombosis after anastomosis. If choosing to use a recipient vessel within the zone, clinical presentation of vessel wall pliability and quality of blood from transected vessel need to be feasible to have a successful outcome.[12] This idea was validated further by using a perforator as a recipient adjacent to or within zone of injury.[4] When large vessels are readily available or superficially located, however, then these vessels should be chosen as it will be technically easier. In cases of large axial vessels anatomically located deep to the muscles, injured or calcified, patients benefit the most from using a perforator as a recipient.

A large perforator with adequate flow is able to supply a large territory of skin. When using a perforator as a recipient, the limit of perfusion from the perforator needs to be understood. It would not be feasible to use a perforator to supply a large muscle or a chimeric flap that requires abundance of flow. Thus, an adequate indication to use the perforator as a recipient vessel would be a skin or fasciocutaneous flap that is sufficiently supplied by vascularized by 1, 2, or 3 angiosomes. Although multiple variables may determine the success of the flap after perforator-to-perforator approach, a simple and safe way to determine the adequacy of flap size is to see the viability of the flap during the elevation before cutting the pedicle based on a single perforator.

PREOPERATIVE EVALUATION AND SPECIAL CONSIDERATIONS

When microsurgical reconstruction is planned, evaluating the vascular status of the lower extremity is essential not only to understand the vasculature of the major axial arteries but also to identify potential recipient arteries as well as potential donor sites. The use of preoperative arteriography for lower extremity reconstruction is considered when physical/Doppler examination reveals inconclusive vascular status or chronic vascular disease is suspected. According to the authors' experience, 75% to 80% of lower extremity reconstructions that involve trauma, chronic wounds, and oncologic reconstruction undergo detailed vascular evaluation. The computed tomographic angiography (CTA) is minimally invasive and can be obtained easily, revealing adequate information facilitating the planning and the surgical procedure.[13,14] The invasive angiogram is reserved for patients who need intervention to revascularize the extremity or if the presence of foreign bodies makes CTA difficult to read. From both modalities, when looking at defect region, perforators often are identifiable, allowing consideration as a recipient vessel. Then, using a handheld Doppler, the location of the target perforator can be pinpointed. The use of duplex ultrasound, however, is becoming the main modality in identifying perforators. It has multiple advantages over CTA and handheld Doppler. It is able not only to provide real-time reading of the exact anatomic location and pathway in respect to the skin surface but also to provide physiologic information, such as flow velocity and volume.[15] Perforator velocity greater than 15 cm/s to 20 cm/s as a recipient in ischemic diabetic foot reconstruction is shown to be reliable with acceptable success.[16] Despite the use of these preoperative diagnostics, the key remains to be identifying a good pulsatile perforator during the operation.

SURGICAL PROCEDURE

While excising or débriding, perforators that are pulsating within the zone of injury/defect may be seen and may be selected for use as recipient. Working in the zone of injury/defect, however, can be difficult and tedious. Thus, moving away from this zone and based on the prior markings for potential recipient perforators can make the process for locating recipient perforators easier. When exploring for the perforators, they can be found in the same manner as elevating the flap above the fascia if located under the skin or can be searched subfascially depending on surgeon preference.[11,12] Initially, the recipient perforators are searched under loupe magnification and, upon location, further dissection is carried out under microscope. If the target perforator is within the zone of defect, dissection is recommended under the microscope to minimize injury to the vessel, which can be surrounded by scarring. A strong visible pulse of the perforator is the main indicator for use.[3,4,6] When the perforator diameter is too small or with spasm, then dissection can proceed more proximal to the source vessel, which has larger diameter and is less sensitive to manipulation. **Fig. 1** shows the approach to securing the recipient perforator. After determining the perforator feasible to use as a recipient vessel, the required pedicle length of the flap is measured. Also, definitive débridement is performed, preparing the recipient site ready for flap coverage. The flap for coverage then is elevated with a corresponding pedicle length and dimension of skin for coverage. Usually, a short pedicle suffices, saving operating time for pedicle dissection. Swelling must be anticipated, however, and it must be ensured that swelling does not increase tension to the anastomosis site

and thus harvest an extra centimeter or 2. Prior to transecting the pedicle from the donor site, status of the recipient perforator is checked again. A strong pulse or a pulsatile flow after opening the vessels is the indicator to proceed for anastomosis. This allows the surgeon to fix the problem before it becomes a major problem.

Once the flap is harvested and ready for anastomosis, the perforator vessels should be dilated to increase the vessel diameter. Special instrument, such as fine dilators, forceps, and microscissors, designed for supermicrosurgery help to make the process smoother. Although these fine instruments for supermicrosurgery may not be essential, the authors feel that the dilator is critical because it can dilate the vessels to a comfortable diameter to anastomose. The diameter easily can dilate up to 0.8 mm to 1 mm without injuring the vessels. After dilation, for diameters less than 0.8 mm but greater than 0.5 mm, an 11-0 or 12-0 nylon suture with a 50-μm to 30-μm needle can be used. If smaller than 0.5 mm, a 12-0 nylon suture with 50-μm to 30-μm needle is used. The anastomosis is the same as any microsurgery anastomosis. The authors' experience shows that minimum of 6 stitches but an average of 9 stitches can be performed.[3,4,6] After anastomosis, brisk bleeding from the margin of the flap is confirmed and the flap is set over the defect. If in doubt, imaging using indocyanine green (ICG) helps determine if the flap is being well perfused.

POSTOPERATIVE CARE AND EXPECTED OUTCOME

The classic subjective signs to monitor flaps can be different when using the perforator as a recipient vessel. The ideal inflow from 1 perforator to the other does not induce overflow, which makes the capillary refill evident. Thus, typical subjective monitoring can be difficult other than monitoring temperature and using pinprick to determine the viability. Using ICG imaging may help determine viability but cannot be repeated frequently because the dye may take a long time to wash out. The preferred objective monitoring method is using duplex ultrasound to measure the velocity of the pedicle and comparing with intraoperative baseline to determine the patency of the anastomosis. Drop in more than 30% of the velocity may be a sign to take back for a second look.

Hydration is important in supermicrosurgery, especially when using a perforator as a recipient vessel because dehydration may lower the blood pressure and peripheral circulation shuts down first, including the perforators to the extremity skin. A urine output of 0.75 mL/kg/h to 1 mL/kg/

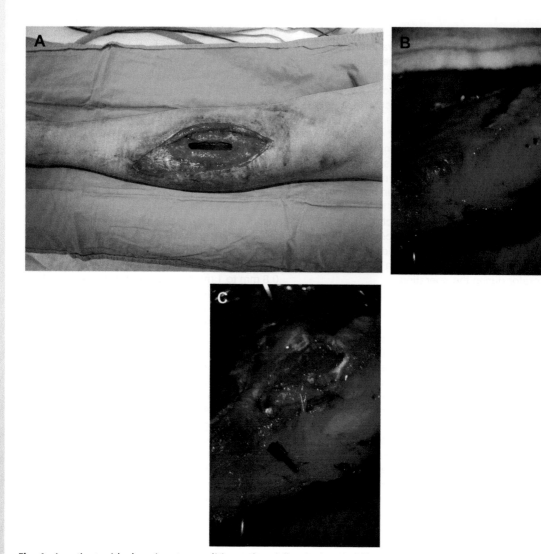

Fig. 1. A patient with chronic osteomyelitis on the midleg is shown. Prior to surgery, a handheld Doppler was used to mark a potential perforator outside the defect as a recipient (*A*). Prior to final débridement and elevation of the flap, the recipient should be secured first, confirmed by firm pulse. Exploration for the recipient was done suprafascially and a perforator was noted on the marked region (*B*). While exploring the recipient, superficial veins also should be saved as a lifeboat for veins. Further dissection of the recipient perforator artery and vein is done under the microscope, confirming a firm pulse and preparing the vessels for microanastomosis (*C*).

h denotes good hydration. Occasionally, when, in spite of adequate fluid replacement, the blood pressure remains low, an infusion of low-dose dopamine (3–5 µg/kg/min) can be used.[4,6,16,17] The immediate postoperative patient position also may make a difference. In order to maximize the flow to the leg, keeping patients on a sitting position is recommended because the flow to the leg increases. This is opposite to using high-flow axial arteries as recipient vessel, where elevation of the leg is recommended to reduce the flow and to allow better venous drainage of the flap.

The debate continues whether or not to use antithrombotic therapy, such as low-molecular-weight heparin, heparin, and dextran.[18,19] Even use of aspirin remains to be controversial regarding flap survival despite evidence showing impairment of thrombin generation. Use of anticoagulation for cases of small vessels, significant size mismatch, vein graft, vessels of poor quality, intraoperative thrombosis–forming patients, or hypercoagulable patients, however, should be considered.[18,19] Further study on the effect of anticoagulation therapy after supermicrosurgery is warranted.

Early compression of flaps from day 4 or 5 begins using bandages providing pressure of 30 mm Hg to 40 mm Hg is another part of the management, with benefits, such as reducing swelling, collapsing dead spaces, minimizing hematoma collection, and preventing shearing while not affecting the hemodynamics of the flap.[20] With compression, depending on bone status, ambulation begins on postoperative day 4 or day 5, and the patient usually is discharged from the hospital within 7 days to 10 days if no other problems were noted.

When the authors reviewed the recent experience from 2011 to 2017, 429 free flaps for te lower extremity (excluding all diabetes-related reconstruction) were performed. The defects were caused by various cases from trauma (42.8%), tumor (35.4%), and others. Most of the flaps were elevated on the superficial fascia plane to be elevated as superthin flaps, where a majority of the flaps were superficial circumflex iliac perforator (SCIP) flaps (50.8%) and anterolateral thigh flaps (40.2%). The overall limb salvage rate was 98.8% and total flap failure rate was 6.1%. When evaluated further between supermicrosurgery technique (108 cases [26.5%]) and classic microsurgery (299 cases [73.5%]) there was no significant difference in outcome of the flap, showing the efficacy and validity of the supermicrosurgery approach. A higher portion of classical approach is used in daily practice, however, reserving supermicrosurgery for cases when the axial artery is not readily available as a recipient.

MANAGEMENT OF COMPLICATIONS

Complications are inevitable in a percentage of patients in supermicrosurgery. The incidence of venous complications, however, is less than classical microsurgery and incidence of arterial insufficiency is higher. This tendency is most likely from the hemodynamics of the perforator artery being sensitive to perfusion.[3,4,6,16,21] As discussed previously, this is why hydration is important. It is good postoperative care and monitoring that determine the success or failure of the reconstruction and also permit early intervention, leading to salvage of a failing free flap.

REVISION OR SUBSEQUENT PROCEDURES

As with any flap, when a flap is in distress due to either venous or arterial cause after perforator-to-perforator supermicrosurgery, immediate exploration is performed. When the cause is arterial, dehydration can be a common reason whereas spasms from pedicle tension can occur from hematoma or swelling. When spasm occurs, repositioning the pedicle during exploration to minimize tension and stripping the adventitia layer of the artery at the point of obstruction may help restore the perfusion. Venous complications may be more difficult to overcome as the thrombosis develops in the small caliber of the perforator and its branches making it difficult to remove; thus, early intervention may be critical.

The most subsequent procedure after reconstruction is contouring of the bulky flap. When superthin flaps are used, this is less of a problem but nevertheless in obese patients secondary debulking procedure still may be needed.

CASE DEMONSTRATIONS
Case 1

A 58-year-old woman presents with a chronic osteomyelitis of the right upper tibia with unstable scar. The patient had burn injury 30 years ago, which was treated with secondary intension. The histology report showed no malignant transformation. The patient underwent skin resection with cortical bone débridement. During the débridement, a perforator, presumably from the medial geniculate system, was noted with a pulsatile artery (0.4 cm) and an accompanying vein (0.6 cm) under the microscope. After confirming the perforator as the recipient, a 16-cm × 7-cm SCIP flap was elevated to cover the defect. Perforator-to-perforator anastomosis was performed after dilatation of the vessels to a comfortable working diameter (artery of 0.8 cm and vein of 1.5 cm) using a dilator after resection of the vessels. Pulsatile flow was confirmed visually and the flap refill was noted followed by insetting of the flap. The patient at 3 years shows good contour (**Fig. 2**).

Case 2

A 42-year-old man presents with a sarcoma of the left leg with positive margin from the biopsy. A wide skin along with partial muscle resection was performed leaving a 16-cm × 9-cm defect of the medial upper leg. A pulsatile perforator was noted during resection, most likely originating from the posterior tibial artery. After confirming the recipient vessel, a 7-cm × 15-cm flap was elevated. Perforator-to-perforator anastomosis was performed to the artery and the accompanying vein; then, an additional superficial vein was anastomosed to a superficial vein from the recipient site. The radiation therapy began after 3 weeks of surgery. The patient at 5 years shows good contour of the leg (**Fig. 3**).

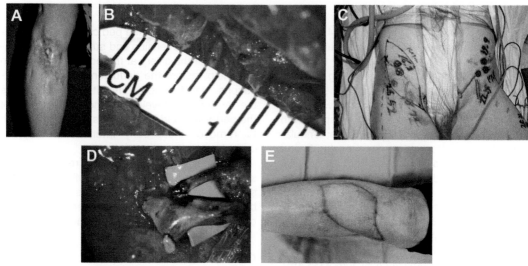

Fig. 2. A 58-year-old woman presents with a chronic osteomyelitis of the right upper tibia with unstable scar (*A*). The patient underwent skin resection with cortical bone débridement, during which a strong pulsatile perforator, presumably from the medial geniculate system, was found (artery, 0.4 cm, and an accompanying vein, 0.6 cm) under the microscope (*B*). After confirming the perforator as the recipient, a 16-cm × 7-cm SCIP flap was elevated to cover the defect (*C*). Perforator-to-perforator anastomosis was performed after dilatation of the vessels to a comfortable working diameter (artery of 0.8 cm and vein of 1.5 cm), using a dilator after resection of the vessels (*D*). Pulsatile flow was confirmed visually and the flap refill was noted followed by insetting of the flap. The patient at 3 years shows good contour (*E*).

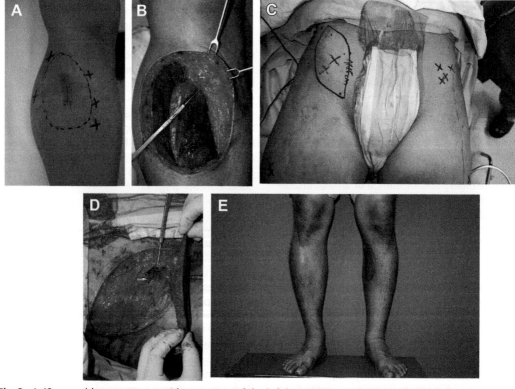

Fig. 3. A 42-year-old man presents with a sarcoma of the left leg with positive margin from the biopsy (*A*). A wide skin along with partial muscle resection was performed leaving a 16-cm × 9-cm defect of the medial upper leg, during which a pulsatile perforator was noted, most likely originating from the posterior tibial artery (*B*). After confirming the recipient vessel, a 7-cm × 15-cm flap was elevated (*C*). The SCIP perforator and the vein str shown (*D*). Perforator-to-perforator anastomosis was performed to the artery and the accompanying vein; then, an additional superficial vein was anastomosed. The radiation therapy began after 3 weeks of surgery. The patient at 5 years shows good contour of the leg (*E*).

DISCUSSION

Supermicrosurgery, although perceived as a new concept, is an inevitable and natural evolution of microsurgery. Like the concept of perforator flaps, which evolved from random pattern flaps, fasciocutaneous flaps, and musculocutaneous flaps, by identifying detailed anatomy and physiology, thus leading to better understanding and application of perforators, supermicrosurgery is an evolution of microsurgery applied to smaller vascular structures. Like most evolution, the fundamental principles remain similar but the details in approach differ considerably, which may lead to improving the outcome after supermicrosurgery.

1. A better working environment with enhanced microscopes makes supermicrosurgery doable. Recent technological advances in microscopes have allowed a higher magnification and brighter light source, increasing the clarity of the surgical field during the procedure. The addition of various imaging tools mounted on the microscope, especially the built-in ICG imaging, allows viewing the flap perfusion on the table and predicting potential flap area with low perfusion.[6]
2. Preoperative evaluation using not only handheld Doppler but also preoperative CTAs and the use of color duplex imaging enhance the details of the perforator level, allowing adequate planning for supermicrosurgery.[4,6,14,15,22,23] These preoperative imaging allow the surgeon to have more choices, less limitation, and greater degree of freedom, especially when choosing recipient vessels.
3. Supermicrosurgical technique requires more finesse and a longer learning curve. This is true for any surgery because accumulation of experience dictates all outcomes. A beginner, however, when performing LVA supermicrosurgery, still may have a reasonable result as long as abiding by the principle of supermicrosurgery. As experience accumulates, better proficiency can be expected by decreasing anastomosis and dissection time.[6,24]
4. Postoperative care is different for the supermicrosurgery approach, based on understanding the physiology as well as anatomy, as discussed previously.

Supermicrosurgery has been the latest contribution to reconstructive surgery.[25] As the saying goes, "practice makes perfect"; supermicrosurgery is no exception.[6] Practice in various training models provides technical skills and confidence and allows reducing trial errors in real clinical application. From using synthetic models to small rat vessels, training allows practicing a wide variety of techniques and helps achieve the proficiency needed for successful outcomes. This technique now is applied frequently in LVA to treat lymphedema, distal fingertip replantation, finger/toe reconstruction, and nerve flaps and in soft tissue reconstruction using perforators, providing solutions to problems once thought difficult.[6,7,25,26] The use of supermicrosurgery is one of the latest innovations in reconstructive surgery; and application to the lower extremity, by understanding the principles and applying them to various reconstruction scenarios, will enable surgeons to meet further challenges, continuing the long tradition of innovations in plastic and reconstructive surgery.

SUMMARY

The application of supermicrosurgery has added new advantages that conventional microsurgery could not provide. Using these small perforators as recipients can be minimally invasive which does not require searching and dissecting for major arteries and veins that are located deep under the skin and enables to save time. Furthermore, these perforators can provide many more choices in selecting recipient vessels and eliminates the need for a long pedicled flap which reduces elevation time. The application of supermicrosurgery truly opens the era for freestyle reconstruction and redefines the limits for reconstruction.[6]

CLINICS CARE POINTS

- Preoperative imaging provides detailed anatomical and physiological information on perforators.
- Identify and confirm the status of the recipient first to estimate the dimension of the flap and pedicle.
- Postoperative hydration is essential as the perforators are sensitive to dehydration.

CONFLICT OF INTEREST

All the authors of this article do not have any conflict of interest to declare in relation to the content of this article.

REFERENCE

1. Tamai S. History of microsurgery–from the beginning until the end of the 1970s. Microsurgery 1993;14(1): 6–13.
2. Xiong L, Gazyakan E, Kremer T, et al. Free flaps for reconstruction of soft tissue defects in lower extremity: a meta-analysis on microsurgical outcome and safety. Microsurgery 2016;36(6):511–24.

3. Hong JP, Koshima I. Using perforators as recipient vessels (supermicrosurgery) for free flap reconstruction of the knee region. Ann Plast Surg 2010; 64(3):291–3.

4. Hong JP. The use of supermicrosurgery in lower extremity reconstruction: the next step in evolution. Plast Reconstr Surg 2009;123(1):230–5.

5. Khouri RK, Shaw WW. Reconstruction of the lower extremity with microvascular free flaps: a 10-year experience with 304 consecutive cases. J Trauma 1989;29(8):1086–94.

6. Hong JPJ, Song S, Suh HSP. Supermicrosurgery: principles and applications. J Surg Oncol 2018; 118(5):832–9.

7. Masia J, Olivares L, Koshima I, et al. Barcelona consensus on supermicrosurgery. J Reconstr Microsurg 2014;30(1):53–8.

8. Tashiro K, Harima M, Yamamoto T, et al. Locating recipient perforators for perforator-to-perforator anastomosis using color Doppler ultrasonography. J Plast Reconstr Aesthet Surg 2014;67(12):1680–3.

9. Mureau MA, Hofer SO. Perforator-to-perforator musculocutaneous anterolateral thigh flap for reconstruction of a lumbosacral defect using the lumbar artery perforator as recipient vessel. J Reconstr Microsurg 2008;24(4):295–9.

10. Koshima I, Inagawa K, Yamamoto M, et al. New microsurgical breast reconstruction using free paraumbilical perforator adiposal flaps. Plast Reconstr Surg 2000;106(1):61–5.

11. Loos MS, Freeman BG, Lorenzetti A. Zone of injury: a critical review of the literature. Ann Plast Surg 2010;65(6):573–7.

12. Isenberg JS, Sherman R. Zone of injury: a valid concept in microvascular reconstruction of the traumatized lower limb? Ann Plast Surg 1996;36(3): 270–2.

13. Duymaz A, Karabekmez FE, Vrtiska TJ, et al. Free tissue transfer for lower extremity reconstruction: a study of the role of computed angiography in the planning of free tissue transfer in the posttraumatic setting. Plast Reconstr Surg 2009;124(2):523–9.

14. Suh HP, Kim Y, Suh Y, et al. Multidetector computed tomography (CT) analysis of 168 cases in diabetic patients with total superficial femoral artery occlusion: is it safe to use an anterolateral thigh flap without CT angiography in diabetic patients? J Reconstr Microsurg 2018;34(1):65–70.

15. Dorfman D, Pu LL. The value of color duplex imaging for planning and performing a free anterolateral thigh perforator flap. Ann Plast Surg 2014;72(Suppl 1):S6–8.

16. Suh HS, Oh TS, Lee HS, et al. A new approach for reconstruction of diabetic foot wounds using the angiosome and supermicrosurgery concept. Plast Reconstr Surg 2016;138(4):702e–9e.

17. Suominen S, Svartling N, Silvasti M, et al. The effect of intravenous dopamine and dobutamine on blood circulation during a microvascular TRAM flap operation. Ann Plast Surg 2004;53(5):425–31.

18. Senchenkov A, Lemaine V, Tran NV. Management of perioperative microvascular thrombotic complications - the use of multiagent anticoagulation algorithm in 395 consecutive free flaps. J Plast Reconstr Aesthet Surg 2015;68(9):1293–303.

19. DeFazio MV, Hung RW, Han KD, et al. Lower extremity flap salvage in thrombophilic patients: managing expectations in the setting of microvascular thrombosis. J Reconstr Microsurg 2016;32(6):431–44.

20. Suh HP, Jeong HH, Hong JPJ. Is early compression therapy after perforator flap safe and reliable? J Reconstr Microsurg 2019;35(5):354–61.

21. Suh HS, Oh TS, Hong JP. Innovations in diabetic foot reconstruction using supermicrosurgery. Diabetes Metab Res Rev 2016;32(Suppl 1):275–80.

22. Choi DH, Goh T, Cho JY, et al. Thin superficial circumflex iliac artery perforator flap and supermicrosurgery technique for face reconstruction. J Craniofac Surg 2014;25(6):2130–3.

23. Suh HS, Jeong HH, Choi DH, et al. Study of the medial superficial perforator of the superficial circumflex iliac artery perforator flap using computed tomographic angiography and surgical anatomy in 142 patients. Plast Reconstr Surg 2017; 139(3):738–48.

24. Pereira N, Lee YH, Suh Y, et al. Cumulative experience in lymphovenous anastomosis for lymphedema treatment: the learning curve effect on the overall outcome. J Reconstr Microsurg 2018;34(9): 735–41.

25. Badash I, Gould DJ, Patel KM. Supermicrosurgery: history, applications, training and the future. Front Surg 2018;5:23.

26. Koshima I, Yamamoto T, Narushima M, et al. Perforator flaps and supermicrosurgery. Clin Plast Surg 2010;37(4):683–9. vii-iii.

Lower Extremity Reconstruction After Soft Tissue Sarcoma Resection

Rajiv P. Parikh, MD, MPHS[a], Justin M. Sacks, MD, MBA[b],*

KEYWORDS

- Lower extremity reconstruction • Soft tissue sarcoma • Free flap • Microsurgery • Clinical oncology
- Reconstructive surgery

KEY POINTS

- Localized extremity soft tissue sarcomas (ESTS) frequently arise in the lower extremity and account for 1% of all adult tumors.
- Oncological treatment of ESTS involves wide surgical resection, often combined with perioperative radiation therapy. After tumor resection, many patients will have complex soft tissue defects that require reconstructive surgery to achieve functional limb restoration.
- The role of amputation in the treatment of ESTS has steadily declined. Advancements in adjuvant therapy and reconstructive surgical techniques, including microsurgical free-tissue transfer, functional muscle transfer, and vascularized bone transfer, have made functional limb salvage attainable in greater than 90% of patients.
- A multidisciplinary team of oncological surgeons, radiation oncologists, medical oncologists, plastic surgeons, and physical therapists is essential to optimizing oncological and functional outcomes in patients with ESTS.

INTRODUCTION

Soft tissue sarcomas (STS) are a heterogenous group of tumors with mesenchymal origin that account for 1% of all cancers.[1] Anatomically, greater than 30% of STS arise in the lower extremities.[1] Surgical resection with wide margins is the primary treatment option for localized extremity soft tissue sarcoma (ESTS). Surgical treatment must balance oncological considerations with functional considerations. Historically, the extent of resection to attain local control resulted in substantial morbidity and, often, amputation.[2] Over the last 40 years, the role of amputation in ESTS has steadily declined due to radiation therapy (RT) and the publication of landmark studies demonstrating no improvement in overall survival (OS) for patients undergoing amputation versus limb-sparing surgery combined with adjuvant therapy.[2,3] Today, tumor resection with an emphasis on limb preservation is attainable in greater than 90% of patients with ESTS.[4–6]

Because limb preservation has become standard, maintaining or restoring functionality of the limb is imperative. Unfortunately, the combination of wide resection and RT in the lower extremity often results in functional compromise and complex wounds. In these scenarios, reconstructive surgery plays an integral role. The goals of reconstructive surgery following surgical resection are functional limb restoration and wound closure that minimizes complications and delays in adjuvant treatment. Inclusion of plastic surgeons improves the rates of limb salvage and enhances

[a] Plastic and Reconstructive Surgical Service, Center for Advanced Reconstruction, Memorial Sloan Kettering Cancer Center, 1275 York Avenue, New York, NY 10065, USA; [b] Division of Plastic and Reconstructive Surgery, Department of Surgery, Washington University School of Medicine in St. Louis, 660 South Euclid Avenue, Suite 1150 NWT, St Louis, MO 63110, USA
* Corresponding author.
E-mail address: jmsacks@wustl.edu

Clin Plastic Surg 48 (2021) 307–319
https://doi.org/10.1016/j.cps.2021.01.007
0094-1298/21/© 2021 Elsevier Inc. All rights reserved.

functional and aesthetic results following ESTS resection.[7]

In this article, the authors outline important considerations in the multidisciplinary care of patients with ESTS and propose an anatomic and defect-centered approach to lower extremity reconstruction that emphasizes functional limb restoration. In cases where limb preservation is not possible, the authors advocate for amputation with contemporary reconstructive surgical techniques to maximize residual limb function with a prosthesis and minimize neuropathic pain.

PREOPERATIVE EVALUATION: MULTIDISCIPLINARY CARE, IMAGING, AND STAGING

Patients should be evaluated in comprehensive cancer centers by a multidisciplinary team, including oncological surgeons, orthopedic surgeons, plastic and reconstructive surgeons, medical oncologists, and radiation oncologists. Patients with ESTS treated at high volume cancer centers have significantly better survival rates and functional outcomes.[8] In addition, this may avert unplanned excisions of ESTS, which are associated with increased rates of local recurrence and can contribute failed limb salvage.[9]

MRI remains the standard for evaluating soft tissue masses.[5] MRI provides detailed visualization of tissue planes and compartments, facilitating staging and surgical planning (**Fig. 1**). With imaging, the reconstructive surgery team can anticipate the defect and plan accordingly.

Diagnosis of ESTS is confirmed with histologic assessment. Tissue specimens are most frequently obtained with core needle biopsy, but a carefully planned excisional biopsy is also suitable for small tumors. ESTS are staged according to the American Joint Committee on Cancer (AJCC) 8th edition system.[10] Histologic grade, tumor size, and depth are drivers of prognosis in ESTS. Additional adverse prognostic factors are older age, proximal tumor location, and local recurrence.[4]

ONCOLOGICAL TREATMENT: ROLE OF SURGICAL RESECTION, RADIOTHERAPY, AND CHEMOTHERAPY

The National Comprehensive Cancer Network (NCCN) guidelines recommend wide surgical resection with oncologically appropriate margins for localized ESTS.[5] Resection of the tumor pseudocapsule and a margin without microscopic disease (>1 cm) significantly reduce local recurrence.[11] The NCCN guidelines also support RT and chemotherapy as adjuvant options.

RT can reduce the risk of local recurrence in ESTS with high-risk features (high-grade tumors, large tumors, deep tumors, tumors abutting neurovascular structures, and tumors with select histologic subtypes).[3,12,13] Preoperative and postoperative RT are demonstrated to facilitate

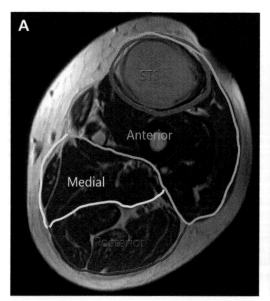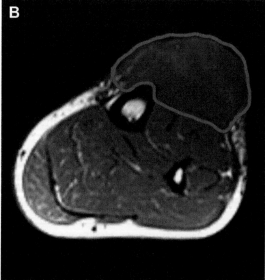

Fig. 1. MRI allows visualization of the tumor in relation to soft tissue compartments and neurovascular structures. (*A*) ESTS of the anterior thigh with involvement of the rectus femoris muscle. (*B*) ESTS of the anterior lower leg in the pretibial location.

limb preservation. When indicated, our preference is preoperative RT. Preoperative RT involves lower doses and irradiates a smaller tissue volume, resulting in lower rates of fracture, joint stiffness, tissue fibrosis, and functional compromise compared with postoperative RT.[13] A recent study of more than 27,000 patients with ESTS demonstrated preoperative RT independently predicts R0 (margin-free) resections and may improve OS.[12] Furthermore, prior publications have confirmed preoperative RT does not increase wound complications in patients undergoing reconstructive surgery after sarcoma resection and may be associated with fewer complications compared with postoperative RT.[14] In situations where oncologically appropriate margins are not obtained, reresection with negative margins and/or adjuvant RT are indicated.[5]

The role of chemotherapy should be determined on a case-by-case basis. Across the heterogenous group of STS, a meta-analysis of randomized controlled trials revealed chemotherapy has only had marginal efficacy on reducing local recurrence and improving OS.[15] The NCCN guidelines support chemotherapy as a Category 2A recommendation (uniform consensus that the intervention is appropriate based on lower-level evidence).[5] Ultimately, the potential benefits of chemotherapy should be balanced with the associated systemic toxicities.

LIMB SALVAGE: INDICATIONS AND CONTRAINDICATIONS

The decision to proceed with limb salvage is influenced by oncological and functional considerations. Limb preservation with adjuvant therapy is oncologically equivalent to amputation in regard to disease-free survival and OS.[2–4] Traditionally, if resection involved neurovascular structures or compromised residual limb function, then amputation was performed.[2] In the current paradigm, these factors are no longer contraindications to limb salvage. Preoperative RT can improve local control and reduce the aggressiveness of resection. Even when tumors involve neurovascular structures, studies have demonstrated limb salvage is feasible if these structures can be reconstructed.[16,17] Furthermore, if large resections of muscle compartments are necessary for local control, function can be restored with techniques such as functional muscle transfers. With multidisciplinary collaboration and careful planning, functional limb preservation and restoration can be accomplished in most patients.

However, limb salvage is not always warranted. If function is expected to be poor even after reconstructive surgery, then amputation is a better option. Often, this occurs in recurrent tumors that are large, multifocal, or proximally located.[2] Other common indications for amputation are in fungating tumors or when tissue contamination is present.[2,18] In patients with metastatic disease and a painful tumor, amputation may provide an equivalent palliative benefit with a shorter recovery period. When amputation is indicated, contemporary reconstructive surgical techniques, as discussed later, should be used to optimize outcomes.

Timing of Reconstruction

Immediate reconstruction has several advantages and is our preferred approach. Foremost, it obviates an open wound that may potentially delay adjuvant therapy. In addition, it facilitates earlier rehabilitation. Surgically, it enables a more straightforward operation, as tissue edema, fibrosis, and scar formation are minimal. Immediate reconstruction is also associated with less morbidity and a lower risk of wound infection and dehiscence compared with delayed reconstruction.[19] The main indication for delayed reconstruction is resection with uncertain margin status. In these cases, the authors advocate for placement of a vacuum-assisted closure device followed by definitive reconstruction when margins are clear.

RECONSTRUCTIVE SURGICAL PROCEDURES: ANATOMIC AND DEFECT-SPECIFIC APPROACH

The approach to reconstruction is dictated by defect size, location, expected functional loss, involvement of underlying structures, and receipt of RT. Primary wound closure can be achieved following resection of most small tumors. In wounds with vascular tissue at the base, skin grafting can be attempted; however, in our experience, skin grafting to a radiated field has unfavorable outcomes. Factors known to cause major wound healing complications requiring more involved reconstructive approaches are RT, tobacco use, diabetes, tumor size (>10 cm), proximity to the skin surface (<3 mm), and exposure of major neurovascular structures.[20,21] When reconstructive surgery is indicated, we advocate for an anatomic and defect-specific approach that emphasizes functional restoration. We present our algorithm for reconstruction of defects located in the thigh and lower leg in **Figs. 2** and **3**, respectively.

Thigh

Proximal and middle thigh
Locoregional soft tissue reconstruction Wide resection of ESTS in the proximal or mid-thigh

Reconstruction of Thigh Defects after Soft-Tissue Sarcoma Resection

Primary Closure Not Possible or High-Risk Wounds

| Proximal and Middle Thigh | Distal Thigh/Knee |

Reconstructive Requirements based on Defect Characteristics

| Locoregional Soft-Tissue Coverage | Free Flap Soft-Tissue Coverage | Free Functional Muscle Transfer | Free Flap Soft-Tissue Coverage | Locoregional Soft-Tissue Coverage |

Goal: Coverage ± deadspace obliteration | Goal: Restoration of Quadriceps | Goal: Coverage ± deadspace obliteration

Rectus abdominis	Rectus abdominis	Latissimus dorsi FFMT	Rectus abdominis	Reverse ALT
ALT	Contralateral ALT	Contralateral Rectus	ALT	Gastrocnemius
Sartorius	Latissimus dorsi	femoris FFMT	Latissimus dorsi	Keystone/Propeller
Gracilis	Chimeric flaps from		Gracilis	
Rectus femoris	subscapular/LFCA		Parascapular	
Keystone/Propeller	systems		SCIP	
Gluteus maximus			Lateral Arm	
Biceps femoris			Radial Forearm	

Fig. 2. Algorithm for reconstruction of thigh defects after sarcoma resection.

results in defects that can frequently be reconstructed with locoregional flaps. Local fasciocutaneous flaps and pedicled muscle or myocutaneous flaps are both reasonable options. The pedicled rectus abdominis flap with a vertically (vertical rectus abdominis musculocutaneous), obliquely, or transversely (TRAM) oriented skin paddle can reconstruct a variety of defects in the anterior, medial, or lateral proximal thigh. Additional muscle flaps commonly used in this region are the gracilis, rectus femoris, sartorius, and vastus lateralis. The anterolateral thigh (ALT) flap is our preferred fasciocutaneous option for coverage of defects in the anterior or medial proximal thigh. In the posterior proximal thigh, soft tissue reconstruction with gluteus muscle or biceps femoris muscle flaps are frequently used.

In the mid-thigh, muscle flap options for anterior, medial, and lateral defects still include the rectus femoris, vastus lateralis, sartorius, and gracilis, with the addition of the vastus medialis and adductor longus muscles.[22] The ALT flap is the primary fasciocutaneous option for the mid-thigh; keystone flaps and free-style propeller flaps can also be designed to reconstruct a variety of mid-thigh defects. Posteriorly, the biceps femoris and semimembranosus are the best local options for reconstruction.

Free flap soft-tissue reconstruction Recurrent tumors, large tumors, and radiation often result in defects requiring free tissue transfer for reconstruction after resection. In a prior series of ESTS cases over 20 years published by the senior author, free-flap reconstruction was necessary in

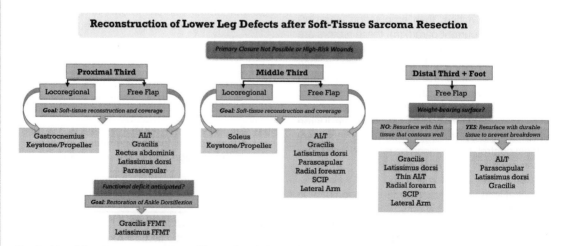

Reconstruction of Lower Leg Defects after Soft-Tissue Sarcoma Resection

Primary Closure Not Possible or High-Risk Wounds

| Proximal Third | Middle Third | Distal Third + Foot |

| Locoregional | Free Flap | Locoregional | Free Flap | Free Flap |

Goal: Soft-tissue reconstruction and coverage | Goal: Soft-tissue reconstruction and coverage | Weight-bearing surface?

Gastrocnemius	ALT	Soleus	ALT	NO: Resurface with thin tissue that contours well	YES: Resurface with durable tissue to prevent breakdown
Keystone/Propeller	Gracilis	Keystone/Propeller	Gracilis		
	Rectus abdominis		Latissimus dorsi	Gracilis	ALT
	Latissimus dorsi		Parascapular	Latissimus dorsi	Parascapular
	Parascapular		Radial forearm	Thin ALT	Latissimus dorsi
			SCIP	Radial forearm	Gracilis
			Lateral Arm	SCIP	
				Lateral Arm	

Functional deficit anticipated?

Goal: Restoration of Ankle Dorsiflexion

Gracilis FFMT
Latissimus FFMT

Fig. 3. Algorithm for reconstruction of lower leg defects after sarcoma resection.

~ 30% of proximal and mid-thigh wounds.[6] A variety of options exist. Most studies have not demonstrated significant differences in outcomes based on free flap choice.[6,14,23] Donor- and recipient-site considerations should guide flap selection. These include the required pedicle length for anastomoses, donor morbidity, and the defect depth/size.

For large defects, the lastissimus dorsi (LD) and rectus abdominis are the commonly used free muscle flaps. Both can be harvested with a skin paddle. The contralateral ALT and parascapular flap are reliable free fasciocutaneous flaps. Both can be harvested to include muscle if deadspace obliteration is required. In addition, the subscapular and lateral femoral circumflex arterial systems (LFCA) enable harvesting of large chimeric flaps for composite tissue replacement, when indicated. Whenever possible, our preference is to avoid flaps from the contralateral lower extremity that have any functional morbidity to avoid downgrading the healthy limb.

Distal thigh, knee, and popliteal regions
Locoregional soft-tissue reconstruction In the distal thigh, locoregional flap choices are limited. The workhorse local flaps are the reverse ALT and gastrocnemius muscle flap. The reverse ALT flap can cover a variety of defects in the distal thigh and peripatellar region (**Fig. 4**). During flap harvest, it is important to confirm retrograde flow through the communicating branches of the distal descending LFCA and the lateral superior genicular artery. If inadequate, the flap can be converted to a standard free ALT; if venous congestion occurs, the flap can be reinset and delayed. Inclusion of tensor fascia lata can provide vascularized tissue for patellar tendon reconstruction, when indicated. The lateral or medial gastrocnemius can be used; in general, the medial gastrocnemius provides better coverage of larger and/or more proximal defects. The arc of rotation and proximal reach of the gastrocnemius flap can be improved by using a posterior midline approach and dissecting off the pes anserinus and/or medial condyle.[24]

Free flap soft-tissue reconstruction In distal thigh defects, the ALT, TRAM, and latissimus dorsi free flaps are good options for large defects. For smaller defects, options include the free gracilis, radial forearm, parascapular, lateral arm, and superficial circumflex iliac artery perforator (SCIP) flaps (**Fig. 5**). One of the challenges to reconstruction in the distal thigh/knee is the potential lack of adequate recipient vessels for microvascular anastomosis near the zone of reconstruction. In these situations, an arteriovenous (AV) loop can be created proximally in the thigh using the femoral system, and flap vessels can be anastomosed safely to the AV loop (**Fig. 6**).

Thigh—skeletal reconstruction
Local invasion to the femur may occur in primary or recurrent ESTS. After resection, segmental bone defects may be present. Restoration of skeletal integrity can be accomplished with several techniques, including segmental bone transport, endoprostheses, massive allografts, vascularized

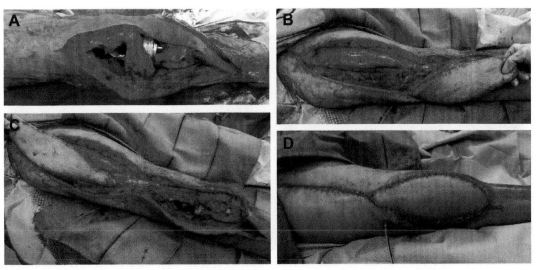

Fig. 4. Reverse ALT flap for coverage of a distal thigh/knee defect after ESTS resection and skeletal reconstruction with an endoprosthetic joint replacement. (*A*) Exposed endoprosthesis. (*B*) Flap harvest. (*C*) Flap transfer on retrograde perfusion. (*D*) Flap inset and defect closure.

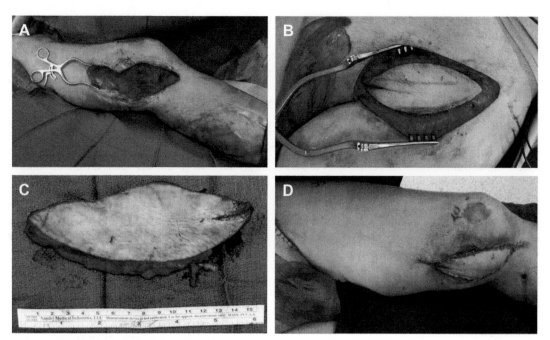

Fig. 5. SCIP flap for reconstruction after RT and resection of a recurrent ESTS at the distal thigh/medial knee. (*A*) Defect at medial knee. (*B*) SCIP flap from left groin. (*C*) SCIP flap after harvest. (*D*) Flap inset and defect closure.

bone grafts, and combined vascularized bone grafts with massive allografts.[25,26] In coordination with Orthopedic Oncology, the optimal method for skeletal reconstruction can be selected. In femoral shaft defects, both endoprostheses and massive allografts are imperfect options with high complication and long-term failure rates.[25] In comparison, vascularized free fibula bone grafts, either alone or in combination with massive

allografts, can reliably restore skeletal integrity and provide good functional outcomes.[27,28]

Our preference for femoral shaft reconstruction is the Capanna technique with a vascularized fibula graft placed within the intramedullary canal of an allograft (**Fig. 7**).[26] This provides strong structural support that tolerates load-bearing forces following hypertrophy and remodeling of the fibula. When there is periarticular involvement, a

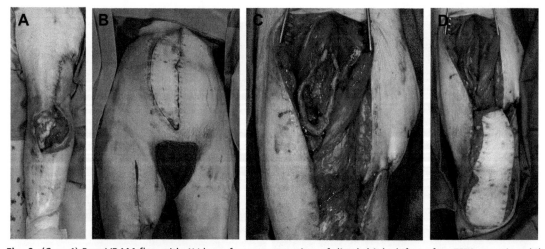

Fig. 6. (Case 1) Free VRAM flap with AV loop for reconstruction of distal thigh defect after ESTS resection. (*A*) Distal thigh/knee defect after radiation and ESTS. No suitable recipient vessels were found in zone. (*B*) VRAM flap delay and (*C*) AV loop creation for planned microvascular flap transfer at second stage. (*D*) Free VRAM flap with anastomoses to AV loop. VRAM, vertical rectus abdominis musculocutaneous.

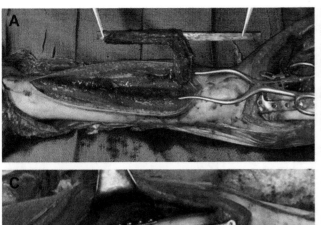
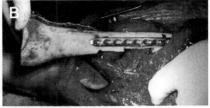
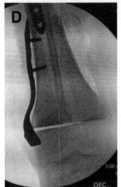
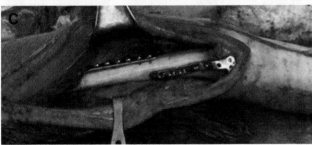

Fig. 7. Pedicled vascularized fibula bone transfer with allograft for reconstruction after ESTS resection with involvement of the distal femur. (*A*) Fibula flap isolated on peroneal vessels. (*B*) Fibula placed inside massive allograft to create an autograft-allograft construct for skeletal reconstruction. (*C*) Construct secured in place with hardware. (*D*) Radiographic imaging demonstrating fibula autograft-cadaveric allograft reconstruction of skeletal defect.

megaprosthesis is usually indicated to restore hip or knee joint function in adults. In contrast, skeletally immature patients with periarticular involvement present a unique challenge, as maintenance of growth potential is crucial. In this population, a vascularized fibula graft can be harvested with inclusion of the proximal epiphysis to optimize limb growth potential (**Fig. 8**).[29]

Thigh—composite functional defects: reconstruction with free functional muscle transfer

If the majority or entirety of an anatomic compartment is resected for local control, functional loss is certain to occur. In the thigh, loss of knee extension and joint stabilization is potentially debilitating. We advocate for free functional muscle transfer (FFMT) to restore quadriceps function. Key principles in FFMT include patient willingness to rehabilitate; an available donor motor nerve with adequate axons to power the transfer; full passive range of motion; a donor muscle with contractile strength, excursion, and force generation similar to the native muscle being replaced; and inset at the appropriate muscle resting length to achieve optimal contraction. Maximal length of the tendinous insertion and origin should be included to facilitate inset. The neurotized LD, based on the thoracodorsal neurovascular pedicle, is the

optimal donor to restore knee extension.[30,31] The contralateral rectus femoris is another potential donor option for FFMT.[32] The motor branch to the rectus femoris is the most lateral of the femoral nerve branches in the thigh and enters the muscle in the proximal aspect. The downside to the rectus femoris FFMT is a decrease in quadriceps extension of the donor limb.

The proximal femoral nerve motor branches corresponding to the resected muscle should be preferentially used to innervate the FFMT. Primary tension-free coaptation is often possible; when not possible, sural nerve cable grafting can be performed to bridge the nerve gap. The FFMT is secured to the new origin in the thigh proximally with bone tunnels or suture anchors; if part of the native rectus femoris origin remains, this can also be used to secure the FFMT. The resting length of the muscle should be restored during inset. The distal tendinous aspect of the muscle is then secured to the native patella tendon to recreate the neo-quadriceps. Patients undergoing FFMT should be counseled on the importance of rehabilitation and that functional recovery will occur over a few years.

Lower leg

Locoregional soft-tissue reconstruction In the lower leg, the role of locoregional coverage is

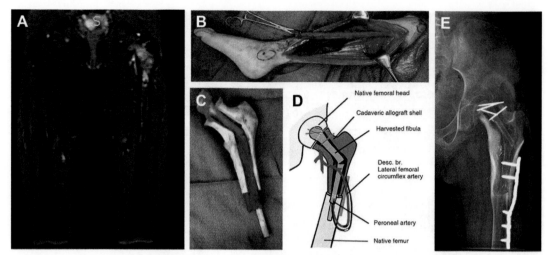

Fig. 8. (Case 2) Free vascularized fibula bone transfer with allograft for reconstruction after resection of a femoral neck sarcoma in a pediatric patient. Vascularized fibular epiphyseal transfer was chosen to maximize growth potential in this skeletally immature patient. (*A*) MR imaging of sarcoma. (*B*) Free fibula harvest in leg. (*C*) Fibula vascularized autograft placed inside cadaveric femur allograft. The fibula was fractured to recreate the native anatomy. (*D*) Schematic demonstrating operative procedure. (*E*) Radiographic imaging of skeletal reconstruction with autograft-allograft construct. (*From* Seu MY, Haley A, Cho BH, et al. Proximal femur reconstruction using a vascularized fibular epiphysis within a cadaveric femoral allograft in a child with Ewing sarcoma: a case report. *Plast Aesthet Res* 2017;4:209-214; with permission.)

limited to small- and medium-sized defects. The gastrocnemius is ideal for proximal leg defects. The soleus muscle can be used for coverage of pretibial defects in the middle third; however, harvest of the soleus has donor-site morbidity and can downgrade remaining limb function. Local perforator-based flaps, including propeller flaps, have been described as an alternative option for small defects in the lower leg.[33]

Free-flap soft-tissue reconstruction Free tissue transfer is necessary in more than 60% of patients after sarcoma resection in the lower leg.[6] In comparison to the thigh, there is less need for dead-space obliteration, and thus bulky flaps, in the leg. For medium to large defects, our preferred flap options are the latissimus dorsi, gracilis, and ALT. To minimize donor-site morbidity, the latissimus muscle can split and harvested on the descending branch of the thoracodorsal vessel. For smaller defects, the SCIP, lateral arm, gracilis, and radial forearm are reliable options (**Fig. 9**).

Skeletal reconstruction In cases where bony resection of the tibia is required, reconstruction of segmental bone gaps can be accomplished with segmental bone transport, endoprostheses, osteoarticular allografts, vascularized bone grafts, and combined vascularized bone grafts with allografts.[25] For proximal tibia reconstructions, the most commonly used techniques are

endoprosthetic joint replacement and osteoarticular allografts. Unfortunately, the failure rates at 10 years for both techniques can be higher than 40%.[34] In skeletally immature patients, fibular epiphyseal transfer can reconstruct proximal tibial defects and enable longitudinal limb growth.[35] For mid-shaft tibial defects, the vascularized fibula is an excellent option in both adults and children. Unlike femur reconstruction, we do not find it critical to use allograft with vascularized fibula for tibia reconstruction. Prior work from Memorial Sloan Kettering Cancer Center demonstrated good functional and bony union outcomes with fibula-only reconstruction of tibia defects.[28] By avoiding an allograft, there is also less theoretic risk for infection.[25,34]

Composite functional defects: reconstruction with functional muscle transfer Sarcoma resection in the lower leg may result in major functional deficits. Resections involving the anterior and lateral compartments lead to instability and compromised dorsiflexion at the ankle (foot drop). In these situations, functional muscle transfers are a potential solution. Both FFMTs and pedicled, functional muscle transfers have been described. The gastrocnemius neuromusculotendinous transfer, as described by Ninkovich, is an excellent local option.[36] In this procedure, the gastrocnemius is transferred anteriorly and part of the superficial Achilles tendon is secured distally to the remaining

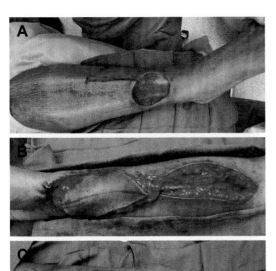

Fig. 9. Free radial forearm flap for reconstruction of a distal third leg defect after ESTS resection. (*A*) Defect. (*B*) Flap harvest. (*C*) Flap after inset.

tendons of the anterior compartment. Orthotopic reinnervation is performed by dividing the tibial motor nerve to the gastrocnemius and coapting it to the proximal stump of the peroneal nerve.[36] This technique avoids the disadvantages, including the need for extensive motor reeducation, of other local antagonistic muscle/tendon transfers. The gracilis FFMT is our other preferred choice to restore dorsiflexion. Harvest of the gracilis to include the entire fascial covering and length on the distal tendinous insertion is essential.[32,37] The obturator motor branch to the gracilis enters the muscle on the medial, deep surface just proximal to the vascular pedicle. Coaptation is performed to the proximal stump of the peroneal nerve in the leg.

Foot and ankle Reconstruction of foot and ankle defects after sarcoma resection most commonly involves free tissue transfer due to the paucity of local options. The goal of reconstruction is functional restoration to enable ambulation and stable weight bearing. Although considerable debate remains on the optimal flap composition, prior studies and systematic reviews have demonstrated equivalent outcomes for fasciocutaneous versus muscle flaps in foot and ankle reconstruction.[6,38] The defect location (weight bearing vs

non–weight-bearing surface) and size should guide reconstructive decision-making.

Our preference is to use thin fasciocutaneous flaps or muscle flaps to resurface ankle and dorsal foot defects. These flaps will contour and allow patients to ambulate in shoes without secondary debulking procedures. The gracilis is a versatile option for foot and ankle defects (**Fig. 10**).[37] For the weight-bearing surface, our preference is to use the ALT flap (**Fig. 11**). This flap provides robust coverage that can withstand repetitive pressure without wound breakdown. A few other commonly used flaps for the weight-bearing surface are the latissimus, gracilis, lateral arm, and parascapular. If local control requires extensive resection of structures critical to gait biomechanics and postural stability, then amputation may provide equivalent quality of life outcomes with an accelerated rehabilitation period compared with limb salvage.[18]

Contemporary approach to amputation
When limb preservation is not feasible, we advocate for a contemporary approach to amputation that incorporates reconstructive surgery principles with recent technical advancements including targeted muscle reinnervation (TMR), regenerative peripheral nerve interfaces, and/or agonist-antagonist myoneural interfaces. A comprehensive discussion of these techniques is beyond the scope of this article, but excellently detailed by Herr and colleagues recently.[39] All of these techniques potentially enable neural control of advanced prostheses and mitigate postamputation neuropathic pain. Our preference is to perform TMR when amputations are necessary for ESTS. In our experience, minimizing neuropathic pain is the foremost consideration in limb amputation, as it significantly enhances quality of life; TMR effectively accomplishes this goal. Unfortunately, advanced prostheses remain cost-prohibitive for most patients.[39] Furthermore, the 5-year survival for patients with high-risk ESTS continues to be suboptimal at ~ 50%, precluding many patients from receiving an advanced prosthetic device.[4]

Reconstructive surgery techniques are also valuable in cases where soft-tissue coverage is required to maintain optimal length. Maintaining length is important because more proximal amputations result in higher metabolic demand and are associated with worse survival.[2] In these cases, fillet flaps or free tissue transfer are both options. Fillet flaps involve isolating vascularized soft tissue from the amputated extremity and then transferring it for stump coverage.[40] If fillet flaps cannot be performed, then free flaps can reliably maintain residual limb length to facilitate function in a standard prosthesis.

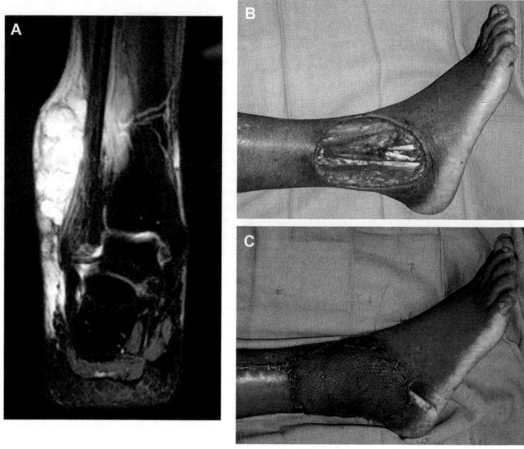

Fig. 10. Free gracilis muscle with STSG for reconstruction of an ankle defect after ESTS resection. (*A*) MRI of tumor. (*B*) Defect of lateral ankle with exposed structures. (*C*) Gracilis muscle flap with STSG after inset.

POSTOPERATIVE CARE

Physical therapists are an integral part of our team and work closely with patients to develop a personalized rehabilitation program based on the reconstructive procedure performed and patients' functional goals. Early postoperative rehabilitation is important to prevent physical deconditioning from prolonged inactivity and to optimize functional recovery. For soft-tissue reconstructions, ambulation can be initiated when

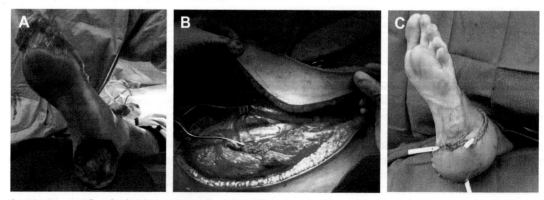

Fig. 11. Free ALT flap for heel reconstruction after ESTS resection. (*A*) Defect with exposed calcaneus. (*B*) ALT flap isolated on pedicle before transfer. (*C*) Reconstruction of heel defect after ALT flap inset.

wounds are healing appropriately. For bony reconstructions, weight bearing is progressively allowed following signs of clinical and radiographic union. Individualized protocols are implemented for rehabilitation of functional muscle transfers and in patients undergoing amputations.

MANAGEMENT OF COMPLICATIONS

Wound complications can occur in up to 50% of patients after reconstruction of sarcoma defects.[6,19,20] Most wound complications can be managed with local wound care. If adjuvant therapy is required, then reoperation for wound closure is indicated to avoid delays. Close oncological monitoring is critical to detect recurrence or spread. Local recurrence occurs in ~ 20% of patients with ESTS. When local recurrence occurs, reresection with adjuvant therapy can be attempted. Depending on the defect, flap readvancement or additional flap coverage may be necessary; however, if local control and maintaining function is not possible with reresection, then amputation is indicated.

CASE DEMONSTRATIONS
Case 1: Reverse Anterolateral Thigh for Distal Thigh/Knee Coverage

An adult woman presented with an ESTS that involved the distal right thigh soft tissue with invasion into bone (see **Fig. 4**). She was treated with preoperative RT and planned curative resection of soft tissue and bone. Skeletal reconstruction was performed with an endoprosthetic joint arthroplasty (see **Fig. 4**A). A reverse pedicled ALT flap was performed for soft tissue reconstruction (see **Fig. 4**B, C, D).

Case 2: Vascularized Free Fibula Within Allograft for Pediatric Hip Joint Reconstruction

An 8-year-old woman presented with an extremity sarcoma involving the left femoral neck (see **Fig. 8**).[29] The oncological plan was for curative resection of the proximal femur. After discussion, we planned for reconstruction of the acetabulofemoral joint using a vascularized free fibula autograft placed inside a cadaveric femoral head allograft. The fibular epiphyseal transfer maintains the patient's growth potential; the allograft shell provides a scaffold for fibular growth and structural integrity. During resection, the native femoral head cap was preserved. The descending branch of the LFCA was dissected to serve as the recipient vessels. The free fibula was then harvested

using standard technique and fractured to recreate the native anatomy of the femoral neck. A cadaveric femoral allograft was reamed out to facilitate placement of the fibular autograft within the allograft. This composite autograft-allograft was then fixated to recreate the joint. Following fixation, the microvascular anastomoses were performed (peroneal vessels to descending branch of the lateral femoral circumflex artery).

Case 3: Free Anterolateral Thigh Flap for Heel Coverage

A 37-year-old man presented with an ESTS involving the left heel (see **Fig. 11**). The oncological plan was for curative resection without adjuvant therapy. Immediate reconstruction with a free ALT flap was planned. The ALT flap was chosen because it provides durable soft tissue coverage that can withstand repetitive pressure without wound breakdown. A 2-perforator flap was raised using a subfascial approach. An end-to-side anastomosis was performed to the anterior tibial artery at the ankle level.

SUMMARY

Adjuvant therapy and advancements in reconstructive surgical techniques, including microsurgical free tissue transfer, functional muscle transfer, and vascularized bone transfer, have made limb salvage the standard of care for most patients with ESTS. After tumor resection, many patients will require reconstructive surgery with locoregional or free tissue transfer for functional limb restoration. A defect- and anatomic-centered approach to reconstruction, as described in this article, will facilitate decision-making and ensure appropriate flap selection. A multidisciplinary approach that includes plastic surgeons is essential to optimizing functional outcomes in patients with ESTS.

CLINICS CARE POINTS

- Extremity soft tissue sarcomas require a multi-disciplinary treatment team to optimize oncological and functional outcomes.

- An anatomic and defect-specific approach that emphasizes functional restoration is integral to reconstruction after oncological resection/treatment.

- Free tissue transfer is often necessary to restore structural stability and/or provide adequate soft-tissue coverage.

- With involvement of reconstructive plastic surgeons, functional limb salvage is attainable for a majority of patients with extremity soft tissue sarcomas.

DISCLOSURE

J.M. Sacks is the Co-Founder of LifeSprout.

REFERENCES

1. Howlader N, Noone AM, Krapcho M, et al. SEER Cancer Statistics Review, 1975-2017. Bethesda (MD): National Cancer Institute; 2020.
2. Clark MA, Thomas JM. Amputation for soft-tissue sarcoma. Lancet Oncol 2003;4(6):335–42.
3. Rosenberg SA, Tepper J, Glatstein E, et al. The treatment of soft-tissue sarcomas of the extremities: prospective randomized evaluations of (1) limb-sparing surgery plus radiation therapy compared with amputation and (2) the role of adjuvant chemotherapy. Ann Surg 1982;196(3):305–15.
4. Weitz J, Antonescu CR, Brennan MF. Localized extremity soft tissue sarcoma: improved knowledge with unchanged survival over time. J Clin Oncol 2003;21(14):2719–25.
5. von Mehren M, Randall RL, Benjamin RS, et al. Soft Tissue Sarcoma, Version 2.2018, NCCN clinical practice guidelines in oncology. J Natl Compr Canc Netw 2018;16(5):536–63.
6. Bridgham KM, El Abiad JM, Lu ZA, et al. Reconstructive limb-salvage surgery after lower extremity soft tissue sarcoma resection: a 20-year experience. J Surg Oncol 2019;119(6):708–16.
7. Agrawal N, Wan D, Bryan Z, et al. Outcomes analysis of the role of plastic surgery in extremity sarcoma treatment. J Reconstr Microsurg 2013;29(2):107–11.
8. Gutierrez JC, Perez EA, Moffat FL, et al. Should soft tissue sarcomas be treated at high-volume centers? An analysis of 4205 patients. Ann Surg 2007;245(6):952–8.
9. Pretell-Mazzini J, Barton MD Jr, Conway SA, et al. Unplanned excision of soft-tissue sarcomas: current concepts for management and prognosis. J Bone Joint Surg Am 2015;97(7):597–603.
10. Amin M, Edge S, Greene F. AJCC cancer staging manual. 8th edition. Switzerland: Springer International Publishing; 2017.
11. Biau DJ, Ferguson PC, Chung P, et al. Local recurrence of localized soft tissue sarcoma: a new look at old predictors. Cancer 2012;118(23):5867–77.
12. Gingrich AA, Bateni SB, Monjazeb AM, et al. Neoadjuvant radiotherapy is associated with r0 resection and improved survival for patients with extremity soft tissue sarcoma undergoing surgery: a national cancer database analysis. Ann Surg Oncol 2017;24(11):3252–63.
13. Haas RL, Gronchi A, van de Sande MAJ, et al. Perioperative management of extremity soft tissue sarcomas. J Clin Oncol 2018;36(2):118–24.
14. Chao AH, Chang DW, Shuaib SW, et al. The effect of neoadjuvant versus adjuvant irradiation on microvascular free flap reconstruction in sarcoma patients. Plast Reconstr Surg 2012;129(3):675–82.
15. Pervaiz N, Colterjohn N, Farrokhyar F, et al. A systematic meta-analysis of randomized controlled trials of adjuvant chemotherapy for localized resectable soft-tissue sarcoma. Cancer 2008;113(3):573–81.
16. Martin E, Dullaart MJ, Verhoef C, et al. A systematic review of functional outcomes after nerve reconstruction in extremity soft tissue sarcomas: a need for general implementation in the armamentarium. J Plast Reconstr Aesthet Surg 2020;73(4):621–32.
17. Nishinari K, Krutman M, Aguiar Junior S, et al. Surgical outcomes of vascular reconstruction in soft tissue sarcomas of the lower extremities. J Vasc Surg 2015;62(1):143–9.
18. Erstad DJ, Ready J, Abraham J, et al. Amputation for extremity sarcoma: contemporary indications and outcomes. Ann Surg Oncol 2018;25(2):394–403.
19. Sanniec KJ, Velazco CS, Bryant LA, et al. Immediate versus delayed sarcoma reconstruction: impact on outcomes. Sarcoma 2016;2016:7972318.
20. Baldini EH, Lapidus MR, Wang Q, et al. Predictors for major wound complications following preoperative radiotherapy and surgery for soft-tissue sarcoma of the extremities and trunk: importance of tumor proximity to skin surface. Ann Surg Oncol 2013;20(5):1494–9.
21. Schwartz A, Rebecca A, Smith A, et al. Risk factors for significant wound complications following wide resection of extremity soft tissue sarcomas. Clin Orthop Relat Res 2013;471(11):3612–7.
22. Kleiber G, Parikh RP. Comprehensive lower extremity anatomy. In: Song DH, Neligan PC, editors. Plastic surgery: trunk and lower extremity, vol. 4, 4th edition. London: Elsevier Health Sciences; 2017. p. 1–50.
23. MacArthur IR, McInnes CW, Dalke KR, et al. Patient reported outcomes following lower extremity soft tissue sarcoma resection with microsurgical preservation of ambulation. J Reconstr Microsurg 2019;35(3):168–75.
24. Veber M, Vaz G, Braye F, et al. Anatomical study of the medial gastrocnemius muscle flap: a quantitative assessment of the arc of rotation. Plast Reconstr Surg 2011;128(1):181–7.
25. Panagopoulos GN, Mavrogenis AF, Mauffrey C, et al. Intercalary reconstructions after bone tumor resections: a review of treatments. Eur J Orthop Surg Traumatol 2017;27(6):737–46.

26. Capanna R, Bufalini C, Campanacci M. A new technique for reconstructions of large metadiaphyseal bone defects. Orthop Traumatol 1993;2(3): 159–77.
27. Chang DW, Weber KL. Use of a vascularized fibula bone flap and intercalary allograft for diaphyseal reconstruction after resection of primary extremity bone sarcomas. Plast Reconstr Surg 2005;116(7): 1918–25.
28. Chen CM, Disa JJ, Lee HY, et al. Reconstruction of extremity long bone defects after sarcoma resection with vascularized fibula flaps: a 10-year review. Plast Reconstr Surg 2007;119(3):915–24 [discussion: 925–6].
29. Seu MY, Haley A, Cho BH, et al. Proximal femur reconstruction using a vascularized fibular epiphysis within a cadaveric femoral allograft in a child with Ewing sarcoma: a case report. Plast Aesthet Res 2017;4:209–14.
30. Innocenti M, Abed YY, Beltrami G, et al. Quadriceps muscle reconstruction with free functioning latissimus dorsi muscle flap after oncological resection. Microsurgery 2009;29(3):189–98.
31. Muramatsu K, Ihara K, Miyoshi T, et al. Transfer of latissimus dorsi muscle for the functional reconstruction of quadriceps femoris muscle following oncological resection of sarcoma in the thigh. J Plast Reconstr Aesthet Surg 2011;64(8): 1068–74.
32. Lin CH, Lin YT, Yeh JT, et al. Free functioning muscle transfer for lower extremity posttraumatic composite structure and functional defect. Plast Reconstr Surg 2007;119(7):2118–26.
33. AlMugaren FM, Pak CJ, Suh HP, et al. Best local flaps for lower extremity reconstruction. Plast Reconstr Surg Glob Open 2020;8(4):e2774.
34. Aponte-Tinao LA, Ayerza MA, Albergo JI, et al. Do massive allograft reconstructions for tumors of the femur and tibia survive 10 or more years after implantation? Clin Orthop Relat Res 2020;478(3):517–24.
35. Innocenti M, Delcroix L, Romano GF, et al. Vascularized epiphyseal transplant. Orthop Clin North Am 2007;38(1):95–101, vii.
36. Ninković M, Ninković M. Neuromusculotendinous transfer: an original surgical concept for the treatment of drop foot with long-term follow-up. Plast Reconstr Surg 2013;132(3):438e–45e.
37. Franco MJ, Nicoson MC, Parikh RP, et al. Lower extremity reconstruction with free gracilis flaps. J Reconstr Microsurg 2017;33(3):218–24.
38. Fox CM, Beem HM, Wiper J, et al. Muscle versus fasciocutaneous free flaps in heel reconstruction: systematic review and meta-analysis. J Reconstr Microsurg 2015;31(1):59–66.
39. Herr HM, Clites TR, Srinivasan S, et al. Reinventing extremity amputation in the era of functional limb restoration. Ann Surg 2020;273(2):269–79.
40. Ver Halen JP, Yu P, Skoracki RJ, et al. Reconstruction of massive oncologic defects using free fillet flaps. Plast Reconstr Surg 2010; 125(3):913–22.

Free Tissue Transfer for Patients with Chronic Lower Extremity Wounds

Jenna C. Bekeny, BA, Elizabeth G. Zolper, BS, John S. Steinberg, DPM,
Christopher E. Attinger, MD, Kenneth L. Fan, MD, Karen K. Evans, MD*

KEYWORDS

- Chronic wound • Wound healing • Surgical flaps • Free flap • Free tissue transfer • Limb salvage
- Foot ulcer • Diabetic foot

KEY POINTS

- Patient optimization with multidisciplinary care, including vascular surgeons to address local ischemia and podiatric or orthopedic surgeons to address bony stability and biomechanics, is critical for long-term, durable flap success.
- Successful surgical management of chronic lower extremity wounds relies on aggressive surgical débridement to achieve a healthy wound bed.
- Wound closure with free tissue transfer preserves limb length, promotes ambulation, and reduces mortality in a highly comorbid population.

INTRODUCTION

Chronic wounds of the lower extremity can be defined as wounds that fail to regain normal functional and anatomic characteristics within 3 months. Recent data indicate that chronic wounds affect as many as 1% to 2% of the population in developed nations, with rates increasing as the population ages and becomes more comorbid.[1,2] Steady increase in this pathology makes the economic impact wide and far-reaching. Among Medicare beneficiaries, 15% of patients are diagnosed with chronic wounds, which is estimated to cost Medicare $28.1 billion to $96.8 billion per year for infection control, surgical procedures, and continued wound care.[2]

The effect of lower extremity wounds is devastating to patient quality of life, pain measures, and, ultimately, survival. Patients with chronic wounds consistently score lower on patient-reported outcomes for physical functioning and pain.[3] When wounds are persistent and progressive, risk for major lower extremity amputation (LEA) increases. For diabetics, chronic lower extremity wounds have a mortality rate of 43% to 55% within 5 years.[4] After major LEA for any chronic wound, however, mortality rates increases to nearly 80% at 5 years, likely due to decline in functional ability, increased cardiovascular exertion, and exacerbation of existing comorbidities.[4] Accordingly, diabetic foot ulcers have surpassed diabetic coma as the primary driver of mortality in this population. Although a young healthy adult may recover from an amputation, a comorbid patient with a lower baseline ability to perform activities of daily living may not. Preservation of limb length not only has functional benefits but also survival benefits.[5]

Providers should strive for early, definitive wound management with a multidisciplinary approach to soft tissue coverage. Up to 80% of major LEAs can be avoided when local flaps or free tissue transfer (FTT) is used for chronic wound closure.[6,7] Efficacious treatment relies on thorough medical and

Department of Plastic Surgery, MedStar Georgetown University Hospital, 3800 Reservoir Road Northwest, First Floor PHC Plastic Surgery, Washington, DC 20007, USA
* Corresponding author.
E-mail address: Karen.K.Evans@gunet.georgetown.edu
Twitter: JBekeny (J.C.B.); ezolper (E.G.Z.); KenFanMD (K.L.F.)

Clin Plastic Surg 48 (2021) 321–329
https://doi.org/10.1016/j.cps.2021.01.004
0094-1298/21/© 2021 Elsevier Inc. All rights reserved.

wound histories, complete physical examination, patient optimization, and appropriate selection of treatment modality. Management must be tailored to the individual patient, underlying disease process, and wound characteristics. Often, this requires careful coordination of both medical and surgical therapies for permanent wound closure. This article aims to outline the authors' tertiary wound care center's multidisciplinary approach to management of chronic lower extremity wounds with a specific emphasis on the value and success rate of FTT.

INDICATIONS AND CONTRAINDICATIONS

Traditional contraindications to microvascular surgery include the presence of hypercoagulable disease, peripheral vascular disease, and severe uncontrolled comorbidities. A large majority of the chronic wound population, however, are afflicted by these pathologies, and many chronic wound patients can have successful reconstruction and salvage. The authors' group begins with a comprehensive approach to patient evaluation and treatment selection. Absolute contraindications include intolerance of prolonged anesthesia, infections recalcitrant to débridement, complete absence of local vascular flow from a major artery, noncompliance, and pyoderma gangrenosum.

Historically, the guiding principles for lower extremity wound coverage came from the traditional reconstructive ladder, which originally was described by Mathes and Nahai.[8] Simple techniques often are sufficient for small or superficial ulcers on a non–weight-bearing surface. These include primary closure and closure with skin grafts. Attempting primary closure in areas of high tension with limited soft tissue mobility often is unsuccessful. Any wound with severe infection requires wide, radical débridement of biofilm. Wide regions of débridement and removal of nonviable bone and tendon obviates consideration of simple closure techniques.

Local flaps from intrinsic muscles of the foot offer limited tissue bulk for coverage and are limited to wounds that measure approximately 3 cm × 6 cm in size. The medial plantar flap is a common choice for local coverage of the foot. Unfortunately, significant mobility is difficult to achieve, limiting the utility of this flap, especially for posterior heel ulcers. Options for the distal third of the leg are especially limited in the vasculopath. The distally based superficial peroneal flap often has insufficient blood flow through the peroneal artery to vascularize the distal tip, which generally is the most needed area. Options for middle leg include the gastrocnemius, soleus, and tibialis

anterior turnover flaps. In the proximal leg, the gastrocnemius has proved to be the workhorse flap. Fasciocutaneous flaps, however, may be ideal in highly active patients to limit donor site morbidity.[9] Local coverage options are reserved for the unique case where the amount of devitalized tissue is limited.

Due to the limitations of primary closure, graft placement, and local flaps for chronic lower extremity wound treatment, a better modus operandi is the reconstructive elevator, first suggested by Dr Gottlieb in 1985.[10] By proceeding to FTT, this approach to wound treatment restores durable form and function resistant to high levels of shear forces in the ambulatory patient. In the patient with a lower extremity wound, the lower rungs of the reconstructive ladder may succumb to friction with shoe wear or ambulation, resulting in surgical wound breakdown.

PERIOPERATIVE EVALUATION AND SPECIAL CONSIDERATIONS

The authors' management algorithm (**Fig. 1**), requires multidisciplinary collaboration, radical surgical débridement to achieve a culture negative wound bed, angiography to define vasculature anatomy, vein studies to identify reflux, hypercoagulable studies to determine propensity for perioperative thrombosis, and a biomechanical examination to identify and address mechanical factors that propagate lower extremity wounds. **Table 1** outlines characteristics of patients presenting to the authors' wound clinic for limb salvage with FTT. Clinics serving a similar population may adapt the authors' strategy to patient evaluation to suit their needs.

History and Physical Examination

Because comorbid conditions are known to inhibit wound healing and prevent FTT success, these pathologies must be identified through a thorough patient history and any preexisting conditions must be optimized before surgery. **Table 2** outlines the main conditions posing concern.

Special attention needs to be paid to a patient's vascular status and biomechanical examination to determine best treatment options and likely outcomes. A complete vascular work-up entails ankle-brachial index, angiogram, and venous duplex ultrasound. Within the authors' practice, as many as 67.8% of patients have arterial pathology identified on preoperative angiography, and as many as 27.5% patients require some form of vascular intervention.[11] Lower extremity duplex ultrasound assists in selection of recipient veins for FTT by ruling out vessels with significant reflux or

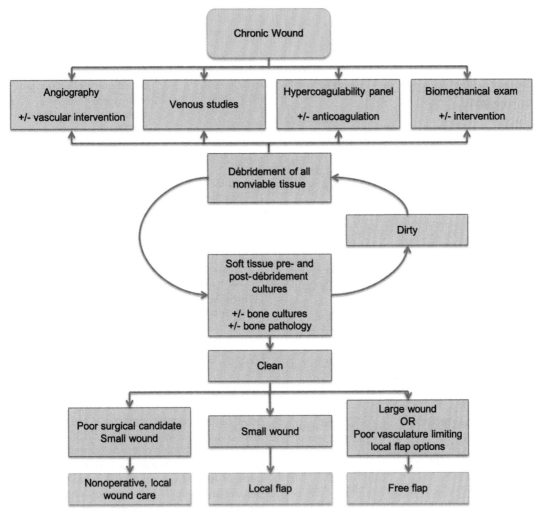

Fig. 1. Management algorithm. The authors' management strategy for chronic lower extremity wounds depends on multidisciplinary management of all factors contributing to wound development and persistence. All patients undergo vascular evaluation and intervention if necessary (angiography and venous duplex ultrasound), hypercoagulability laboratory assessment, biomechanical examination, and intensive surgical débridement to a clean wound bed.

other venous anomalies.[12] In the authors' series, venous insufficiency (defined as <0.5 s of reflux) was detected in 39.0% of patients: 27.2% in the deep thigh, 10.2% in the superficial calf, and 6.78% in the deep calf. Deep vein thrombosis was found in 6.78% of patients, requiring anticoagulation.[12] Identification of these issues reduces complications, yielding a high flap success rate; in this series, flap success reached 98.3%.

All patients must receive a biomechanical examination to evaluate mechanical issues contributing to wound formation, because recurrence may occur if unaddressed. Patients with conditions leading to chronic wounds, especially diabetes mellitus, have alterations in plantar pressure and gait phase timing.[13] Assessment of gait, foot

position, and range of motion to determine need for Achilles tendon lengthening or gastrocnemius recession is critical.

Infection Control

The gold standard for eradicating wound bed infection includes serial débridement supplemented with culture-guided antibiotics until negative cultures are obtained. Débridement yields a wound bed free from granulation tissue and removes hyperkeratotic tissue that hinders epidermal cell migration. Serial débridement clears bacteria, which contribute to biofilm formation, chronic infection, and treatment failure. Wide excision to a healthy wound bed is necessary.

Table 1 Average characteristics for patients with wounds undergoing free tissue transfer	
Characteristic	Average (SD) or N (%)
Demographics	
Age	55.5 (14.7)
Gender	
Female	61 (29.0%)
Male	149 (71.0%)
Body mass index	29.21 (6.25)
Smoking	
Yes	97 (46.2%)
No	113 (53.8%)
Comorbid conditions	
Diabetes	114 (54.3%)
Peripheral vascular disease	48 (22.9%)
Congestive heart failure	11 (5.2%)
Chronic obstructive pulmonary disease	4 (1.9%)
Cerebrovascular accident/transient ischemic attack	13 (6.2%)
Vascular Status	
Deep venous thrombosis	6 (2.9%)
Venous reflux	70 (33.3%)
Arterial vessel supply to the foot	
One vessel	27 (12.9%)
Two vessels	53 (25.2%)
Three vessels	130 (61.9%)

These demographics and comorbid conditions are representative of 210 patients with wounds who underwent FTT at the authors' institution. Patients managed with less intensive surgical and nonsurgical means often are older, more comorbid, and more challenging to treat.

Table 2 Perioperative patient evaluation	
Medical history	Diabetes: hemoglobin A_{1c} <6.5%, perioperative blood glucose <200 mg/dL Smoking: encourage to quit, must abstain for at least 6 wk Nutrition: prealbumin should be tracked in the perioperative period
Vascular examination	Ankle-brachial index Angiogram Venous duplex ultrasound
Biomechanical examination	Gait Foot position Range of motion
Infection control	Serial débridement Culture-guided antibiotics
Thrombophilia evaluation	History of thrombotic event Preoperative thrombophilia panel Institute anticoagulation by risk stratification

thrombophilic traits to receive fixed-rate intravenous heparin postoperatively if their microvascular anastomoses are uncomplicated.[14]

On implementation of the risk-stratified anticoagulation protocol, the authors' group noted lower rates of total (3.0% vs 19.0%, respectively) and partial (10.0% vs 37.0%, respectively) flap loss in the risk-stratified compared with non-stratified controls. In the setting of postoperative thrombosis, successful limb salvage rates remained 0.0%, regardless of protocol. Adequate anticoagulation is necessary to reduce the risk of thrombosis and ultimately limb loss.[14]

Thrombophilia Evaluation

Patients with hereditary or acquired factors for thrombophilia are at significant risk for higher rates of microvascular thrombosis and subsequent flap failures.[14,15] In the authors' practice, all patients are screened by thorough history taking and a standard preoperative thrombophilia panel. Implementation of this preoperative assessment revealed that a majority of patients undergoing FTT for lower extremity salvage had at least 1 thrombophilic trait and more than 30% had 3 or more thrombophilic traits. This evaluation helps inform the postoperative anticoagulation regimen; the authors risk-stratify patients with any historical risk factor or 3 or more

Surgical Planning

The authors' flap selection algorithm is driven by defect characteristics, vascular quality, donor site morbidity, patients' body habitus, and thus flap bulk. The senior authors most commonly utilize the anterolateral thigh (ALT) or vastus lateralis (VL) flap for reconstruction of chronic wounds. The rectus abdominis and latissimus dorsi serve as alternate donor sties when the thigh is unsuitable or in the case of prior flap failure. Donor site morbidity is lowest for ALT and VL, especially when utilizing partial harvest of the VL tailored to the defect as is standard in the authors' practice; thus, flaps from the descending branch of the lateral femoral circumflex artery are preferred.

If a patient has limited subcutaneous tissue, the authors select a fasciocutaneous ALT flap. In obese patients with prohibitive amounts of subcutaneous tissue, the authors favor VL flaps. When patients fall in-between these extremes, the authors prefer a fasciocutaneous ALT flap for plantar defects to avoid a plantar skin graft and a VL flap for nonplantar defects. Otherwise, for defects requiring significant dead space elimination, the authors prefer a VL flap.[16] The superficial circumflex iliac artery perforator (SCIP) flap also may be considered when a fasciocutaneous flap is desired but the bulk of an ALT flap is prohibitive.

Appropriate surgical planning also entails proper understanding of the angiosome theory. There are 6 angiosomes, or 3-dimensional blocks of tissue fed by a source artery, in the foot and ankle. Branches of the posterior tibial artery supply 3 plantar angiosomes: the calcaneal branch feeds the medial and plantar heel, the medial plantar artery feeds the plantar instep, and the lateral plantar artery feeds the lateral midfoot and forefoot. Two anterolateral angiosomes come from the peroneal artery: the anterior perforating branch feeds the anterolateral ankle and the calcaneal branch of the peroneal feeds the hindfoot. The anterior tibial artery and its continuation, the dorsalis pedis, supply the single anterior foot and ankle angiosome. The angiosomes are outlined in **Fig. 2**.

The angiosome principle determines which areas heal appropriately and critically informs optimal incision placement. Incisions in the foot and ankle should be made in between angiosome boundaries to limit perfusion compromise. For example, the authors' group makes incisions at the glabrous junction on the lateral foot and slightly above the glabrous junction on the medial foot. Vascular surgeons can use angiosomal theory to guide revascularization of source arteries contributing to wound formation and propagation.

SURGICAL PROCEDURE

The chronic wound population is challenging, often with limited and compromised vascularity. The authors' group has adopted use of a longitudinal slit arteriotomy end-to-side arterial anastomoses (LS-ETSA) to minimize intimal insult.[17] The flap artery is prepared with a 70° bevel in the direction of the flap to obtain a final 20° resting angle; the final incision length should be 1.3-times the flap artery diameter. The recipient artery is secured with large Acland clamps (S&T, Neuhausen, Switzerland). Incision is made in the area of least calcification, usually evident as the only area with visible pulsatility and confirmed by feel. Vessel calcification often can be visualized and palpated before an incision is made when a vessel is under the microscope. Calcification appears as white, linear marks on a vessel wall. During microsurgery, it may present as crumbling intima or areas where microsurgical needles have difficulty passing through. In recipient vessels with calcification, an inside-to-outside technique tacks plaque against the vessel wall and prevents intimal shearing. When an outside-to-inside approach is used on a calcific vessel, the needle may push the intima out and cause further intimal shearing. When both the recipient and donor vessels are calcified and at risk of intimal shearing, the authors perform a saphenous vein interposition graft. This allows maintaining an inside-to-outside technique on both the flap and the recipient artery. In all cases, the authors utilize a continuous stitch to allow for maximal visualization during anastomosis (**Fig. 3**).

This technique allows FTT success even in patients with highly unfavorable recipient vessels. The authors have not encountered issues with microvascular steal despite routine use of LS-ETSA. Dual venous anastomoses to the deep venous system and/or superficial system when the deep system is unsuitable or additional anastomoses are indicated are performed with GEM Microvascular Anastomotic Coupler (Synovis MCA, Birmingham, Alabama). An implantable Cook-Swartz Doppler Probe (Cook Medical, Bloomington, New Jersey) is used for real-time feedback during inset, because venous congestion may occur in settings of limited soft tissue and efforts to tailor the flap to the defect. Attempts at aggressive flap inset easily can impinge on the low-pressure venous system and result in early flap takeback.

POSTOPERATIVE CARE AND EXPECTED OUTCOME

Postoperative care for the lower extremity FTT patient should be tailored to the individual. The authors' team suggests the following postoperative care protocol for most patients undergoing FTT. Patients are brought to a specialized unit for initial flap monitoring. Flap monitoring should include a combination of clinical examination (color, temperature, capillary refill, and so forth) and Doppler assessment of signals from the arterial and venous system. The interval between flap checks is increased from every 15 minutes to 4 hours by postoperative day 2 to day 3.

In the absence of complications, patients may begin a graduated dangling protocol around postoperative day 5 to day 7. Once the flap shows stability after 45 minutes of continuous gravitational dependence, patients may be discharged safely

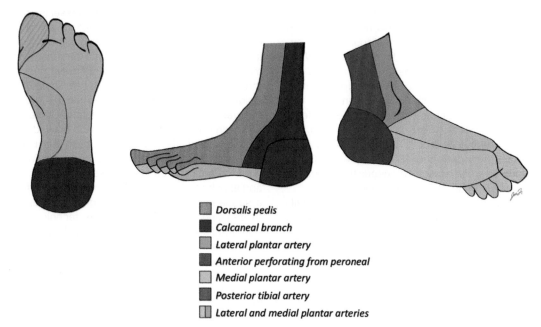

Dorsalis pedis
Calcaneal branch
Lateral plantar artery
Anterior perforating from peroneal
Medial plantar artery
Posterior tibial artery
Lateral and medial plantar arteries

Fig. 2. Angiosomes of the foot and ankle. (*Courtesy of* J. Day, Washington, DC, USA.)

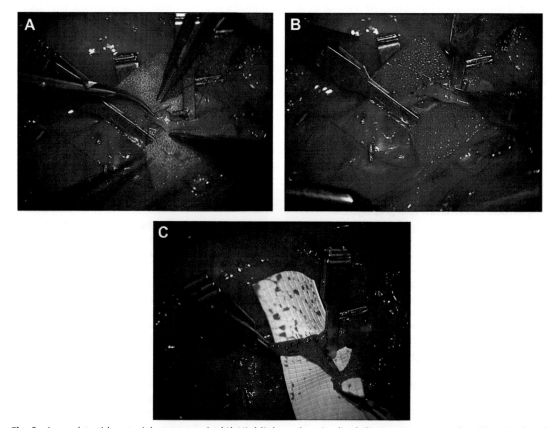

Fig. 3. An end-to-side arterial anastomosis. (*A*) Highlights a longitudinal slit arteriotomy made with a 70° bevel before the anastomosis is complete. (*B*) demonstrates the appearance of the donor and recipient vessels immediately after the anastomosis has been secured (*C*) highlights the final appearance of an end to side anastomosis.

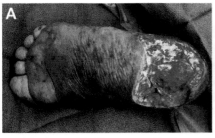
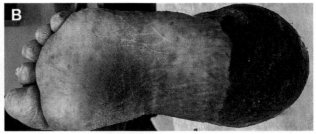

Fig. 4. A plantar hindfoot wound before reconstruction (*A*) and after coverage with a VL flap harvested from the ipsilateral side (*B*).

from the hospital. This typically occurs on postoperative day 7 to day 10. Patients are able to start physical rehabilitation approximately 4 weeks after surgery. Strict non–weight-bearing protocols are in place for the first 4 weeks, but progressive weight bearing can begin 4 weeks to 6 weeks after surgery.

MANAGEMENT OF COMPLICATIONS

As with all FTT procedures, the most morbid complications are caused by microvascular compromise and thrombosis. A well-managed anticoagulation regimen is critical in management of these potential complications, which begins intraoperatively during the FTT procedure.[14] Should postoperative thrombotic complications or microvascular compromise occur, the authors initiate weight-based intravenous heparin at the time of flap takeback.

REVISION OR SUBSEQUENT PROCEDURES

Although the success rate of FTT for lower extremity chronic wounds continues to improve, a cohort of patients inevitably requires revision or subsequent procedures. It is imperative to follow these patients frequently for diabetic foot checks and for managing custom shoe gear to prevent recurrence. The authors have published flap success rate of 93% and a long-term lower limb salvage rate of 79% for recalcitrant diabetic foot ulcers treated with FTT.[18] Despite flap survival, some patients do require additional procedures and infrequently eventual amputation. It is critical to analyze and correct any biomechanical abnormality that exists in the foot and ankle to prevent wound recurrence or transfer lesions. Although FTT is a highly efficacious method of wound coverage, successful limb salvage requires ongoing multidisciplinary management beyond the FTT procedure.

CASE DEMONSTRATION
Case 1

A 54-year-old man presented to the authors' service with a plantar hindfoot wound. The patient's medical history was notably complex—uncontrolled diabetes, kidney transplant after end-stage renal disease, and peripheral vascular disease. The patient underwent several débridements to clean tissue and was reconstructed successfully with a free VL flap from the ipsilateral side of the defect. The patient has progressed to complete healing and has returned to ambulation (**Fig. 4**).

Case 2

A 60-year-old woman presented to the authors' service with a dorsal foot wound and exposed

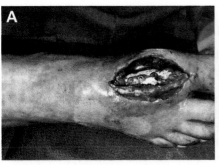
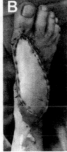
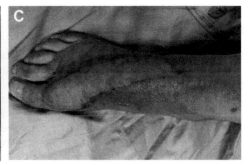

Fig. 5. A dorsal foot wound before reconstruction (*A*), immediately after coverage with a SCIP flap (*B*), and several months after reconstruction (*C*).

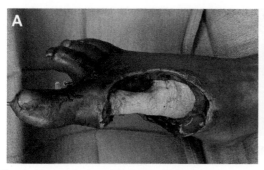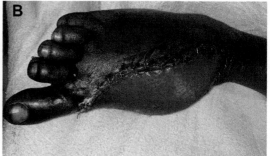

Fig. 6. Traumatic dorsal foot wound before reconstruction (*A*) and after coverage with an ALT flap (*B*).

fusion hardware at the first metatarsophalangeal joint (MPJ). After MPJ fusion with dorsal plating, the surgical site dehisced, a wound developed, and multiple débridements were needed to achieve a clean wound bed. Preoperative angiogram demonstrated 3-vessel runoff to the foot, and venous studies indicated patent deep veins with no evidence of reflux. Hypercoagulability work-up yielded positive antinuclear antibody but did not meet inclusion for high-risk anticoagulation protocols. The patient successfully underwent a SCIP flap from the ipsilateral side of the wound (**Fig. 5**).

Case 3

A 52-year-old man presented to clinic with a wound on the dorsum of the foot secondary to a gunshot wound. He had no past medical history and took no regular medications. After débridement of devitalized tissue, the resultant wound was 10 cm × 12 cm × 5 cm. The ipsilateral ALT flap was harvested. Initially, an end-to-end anastomosis was performed between the perforator and the anterior tibial artery. The anastomosis was kinked and could not be relieved via fat grafting. The anastomosis was redone via an end-to-side method with improved flow. The patient has continued to heal well and is able to ambulate (**Fig. 6**).

DISCUSSION

With improvements in patient work-up, comorbid condition optimization, and surgical technique, outcomes for patients with lower extremity wounds continue to improve. Successful treatment starts with coordinated multidisciplinary care. A multidisciplinary team must be involved in all aspects of treatment—from preoperative patient evaluation and optimization to continued postoperative management of flap compromise or wound recurrence.

The team's primary objectives include vascular assessment and intervention as needed, hypercoagulability work-up, infection eradication, and biomechanical examination. In addition, venous outflow assessment, including the presence of reflux or high venous pressures as well as chronic or acute deep vein thrombosis, is important. When these measures are taken, FTT routinely can achieve long-term wound coverage and limb salvage, even in the highly comorbid tertiary wound center population. Limb salvage with FTT relies on at least a single vessel runoff, highlighting the importance of vascular optimization. The authors' group's systematic approach to vascular assessment and anticoagulation has improved the likelihood of maintaining a successful vascular connection.

Future work should demonstrate functional outcomes and cost utility of limb salvage modalities in the chronic lower extremity wound. Further investigations also need to assure quality of limb salvage care delivery. The current methods for quality assessment are imperfect, and the effects of low-quality limb salvage care are devastating. Mortality rates after development of a chronic wound remain inordinately high, even with limb salvage. These facts highlight the next frontier for chronic wound providers to tackle to ensure high-quality care and life-sparing technique development.

SUMMARY

For patients with chronic lower extremity wounds, the key tenets of the reconstructive approach include aggressive wound preparation and early FTT to achieve definitive coverage, thus avoiding major LEA. Successful treatment relies on coordinated multidisciplinary care to address preoperative patient evaluation and optimization, ensure operative success, and continue postoperative management of flap compromise or wound recurrence. When these measures are taken, FTT routinely can achieve long-term wound coverage and limb salvage in the highly comorbid tertiary wound center population.

CLINICS CARE POINTS

- With definitive coverage by local and free flaps, as many as 80% of LEAs for chronic wounds can be avoided.
- All comorbid conditions must be evaluated and managed by the multidisciplinary team before attempting closure to maximize chance for success. Diabetic patients with an hemoglobin A_{1c} over 6.5% have a 4-times risk of dehiscence, necessitating preoperative glucose management. As many as 27.5% of the authors' patients require vascular intervention before closure.
- Flap selection must take into account defect characteristics, vascular quality, donor site morbidity, patients' body habitus, and flap bulk. Common free tissue donor sites for lower extremity coverage include the ALT or VL.
- Especially in patients with arterial disease, end-to-side anastomosis of donor and recipient vessels preserves distal flow.
- Postoperative care must entail thorough monitoring for flap compromise and prompt return to the operating room if needed.

DISCLOSURE

The authors have no financial disclosures, commercial associations, or any other conditions posing a conflict of interest to report.

REFERENCES

1. Järbrink K, Ni G, Sönnergren H, et al. Prevalence and incidence of chronic wounds and related complications: a protocol for a systematic review. Syst Rev 2016. https://doi.org/10.1186/s13643-016-0329-y.
2. Nussbaum SR, Carter MJ, Fife CE, et al. An economic evaluation of the impact, cost, and medicare policy implications of chronic nonhealing wounds. Value Health 2017;21:27–32.
3. Olsson M, Järbrink K, Divakar U, et al. The humanistic and economic burden of chronic wounds: a systematic review. Wound Repair Regen 2019;27(1):114–25.
4. Robbins JM, Strauss G, Aron D, et al. Mortality rates and diabetic foot ulcers: is it time to communicate mortality risk to patients with diabetic foot ulceration? J Am Podiatr Med Assoc 2008;98(6):489–93.
5. Oh TS, Lee HS, Hong JP. Diabetic foot reconstruction using free flaps increases 5-year-survival rate. J Plast Reconstr Aesthet Surg 2013;66(2):243–50.
6. Driver VR, Fabbi M, Lavery LA, et al. The costs of diabetic foot: the economic case for the limb salvage team. J Vasc Surg 2010;52(3 SUPPL): 17S–22S.
7. Evans KK, Attinger CE, Al-Attar A, et al. The importance of limb preservation in the diabetic population. J Diabet Complications 2011;25(4):227–31.
8. Mathes SJ, Nahai F. Reconstructive Surgery: Principles, Anatomy & Technique. Vol. 2. New York: Churchill Livingstone; 1997. St. Louis: Quality Medical.
9. Economides JM, DeFazio MV, Golshani K, et al. Systematic review and comparative meta-analysis of outcomes following pedicled muscle versus fasciocutaneous flap coverage for complex periprosthetic wounds in patients with total knee arthroplasty. Arch Plast Surg 2017;44(2):124–35.
10. Gottlieb LJ, Krieger LM. From the reconstructive ladder to the reconstructive elevator. Plast Reconstr Surg 1994;93:1503–4.
11. Janhofer DE, Lakhiani C, Kim PJ, et al. The utility of preoperative arteriography for free flap planning in patients with chronic lower extremity wounds. Plast Reconstr Surg 2019;143(2):604–13.
12. Janhofer DE, Lakhiani C, Kim PJ, et al. The utility of preoperative venous testing for lower extremity flap planning in patients with lower extremity wounds. Plast Reconstr Surg 2020;145(1):164e–71e.
13. Fernando M, Crowther R, Lazzarini P, et al. Biomechanical characteristics of peripheral diabetic neuropathy: a systematic review and meta-analysis of findings from the gait cycle, muscle activity and dynamic barefoot plantar pressure. Clin Biomech 2013;28(8):831–45.
14. DeFazio M, Economides J, Anghel E, et al. Lower extremity free tissue transfer in the setting of thrombophilia: analysis of perioperative anticoagulation protocols and predictors of flap failure. J Reconstr Microsurg 2019;35(04):270–86.
15. Wang TY, Serletti JM, Cuker A, et al. Free tissue transfer in the hypercoagulable patient: a review of 58 flaps. Plast Reconstr Surg 2012;129(2):443–53.
16. Black CK, Zolper E, Ormiston L, et al. Free vastus lateralis muscle vs anterolateral thigh flaps for coverage of lower extremity defects in the chronic wound population: a comparison of early and late outcomes. Ann Plast Surg 2020;85:S54–9.
17. Black C, Fan KL, Defazio MV, et al. Limb salvage rates and functional outcomes using a longitudinal slit arteriotomy end to side anastomosis for limb threatening defects in a high-risk patient population. Plast Reconstr Surg 2020;1. https://doi.org/10.1097/prs.0000000000006791.
18. Lu J, Defazio MV, Lakhiani C, et al. Limb salvage and functional outcomes following free tissue transfer for the treatment of recalcitrant diabetic foot ulcers. J Reconstr Microsurg 2019;35:117–23.

Microsurgical Reconstruction of the Lower Extremity in the Elderly

Andreas Gohritz, MD[a,1], Rik Osinga, MD[a,b,1], Alexander Haumer, MD, PhD[a],
Dirk Johannes Schaefer, MD[a,b,*]

KEYWORDS

- lower extremity reconstruction • Orthoplastic surgery • Microsurgery
- Microvascular reconstruction

KEY POINTS

- The steadily growing elderly population implies an increasing need of complex lower extremity reconstruction in patients beyond the seventh decade of life.
- Microsurgery has evolved from a means of last resort to a standardized and safe procedure for leg salvage and prevention of amputation, avoiding potentially life-threatening consequences.
- Multiple comorbidities (eg, diabetes, malnutrition, critical limb perfusion, impaired renal and cardiac function) increase host-related risk factors and require optimization before reconstructive surgery.
- Preoperative multidisciplinary planning, including modern imaging and intraoperative management, is key to reduce complications.
- Microsurgery is not contraindicated because of advanced age per se (biological age supersedes chronologic age) and can often successfully restore ambulation, mobility, and quality of life in the elderly.

 Video content accompanies this article at http://www.plasticsurgery.theclinics.com/.

INTRODUCTION

Individuals of advanced age are the fastest growing subpopulation in many countries, such as Europe and the United States, with an increasing incidence of complex lower extremity wounds of orthopedic, oncologic, vascular, and medical origin. According to epidemiologic data, the number of people aged over 65 years is projected to increase by 135% between 2000 and 2050, and the population aged over 85 years, which is the group most likely to need health and long-term care services, is estimated to increase by 350% within that period.[1] Centenarians may increase from 200,000 in 2020 to 500,000 to 4 million in 2050.

Historically, elderly patients were discouraged from microsurgical reconstructions because of the higher incidence of medical comorbidities and lack of organ system reserve to withstand the lengthy and physically demanding intervention.[2] Today, microsurgical operations have become very reliable because of advances in anesthesia and operative techniques with significantly reduced perioperative morbidity and

[a] Department of Plastic, Reconstructive, Aesthetic and Hand Surgery, University Hospital Basel, Spitalstrasse 21, Basel CH-4031, Switzerland; [b] Centre for Musculoskeletal Infections, University Hospital Basel, Spitalstrasse 21, Basel CH-4031, Switzerland
[1] Contributed equally to this manuscript and are shared first authors.
* Corresponding author. Department of Plastic, Reconstructive, Aesthetic and Hand Surgery, University Hospital Basel, Spitalstrasse 21, Basel, CH-4031, Switzerland,
E-mail address: dirk.schaefer@usb.ch

Clin Plastic Surg 48 (2021) 331–340
https://doi.org/10.1016/j.cps.2021.01.008
0094-1298/21/© 2021 Elsevier Inc. All rights reserved.

mortality.[2,3] Microsurgery is no longer considered to be the last resort when everything else has failed, but rather selected routinely to provide one-stage reconstructions (reconstructive elevator), for example, in orthoplastic surgery.[1,4,5] Salvage of leg function and thus preserving mobility are of essential importance for patients of advanced age who live longer, more active lives and for whom mobility is conditio sine qua non for self-subsistent autonomy. A shift of age limits can even be observed toward the "very old" (>80 years) and occasionally until the age of 100 years (centenarians).[6]

The purpose of this article is to discuss strategies for microsurgical reconstruction of the lower extremity in the elderly population to further reduce perioperative and postoperative risks and complications providing in good functional results.

INDICATIONS

Microsurgical flaps are the procedure of choice for large soft tissue and composite tissue defects throughout the lower extremity, especially in elderly patients who often present with risk factors, such as diabetes, vascular compromise, and osteoporosis. The following indications are given:

- High-energy lower-leg injuries
- Open fractures of the lower extremity: grade III tibial fractures with substantial tissue loss and associated high rates of infection, nonunion, prolonged hospital stay, and sometimes amputation; in these cases, regional musculocutaneous flaps may cause functional and aesthetic deficits and may not achieve sufficient coverage
- Chronic osteomyelitis (eg, owing to trauma or diabetes, with multiple resistant organisms, bone defects, and extensive scarring and fibrosis from previous treatment attempts, which frequently contraindicate the application of local flaps)
- Fracture-related infection and periprosthetic joint infection
- Foot and ankle defects (with exposed bones and tendons or loss of weight-bearing plantar surface, which may preclude local flaps, cause prolonged immobilization and hospitalization, eg, because of multiple surgeries)
- Chronic wounds owing to vascular disease, radiation, diabetes, inflammatory disease, or infection
- Postoncologic resections (eg, owing to soft tissue sarcoma) usually creating complex soft tissue defects[7]

CONTRAINDICATIONS

Microsurgical procedures may not be feasible in cases of/if

- General inoperability (poor general health, bedridden, low life expectancy, high risk for severe morbidity/mortality)
- Bony stabilization impossible
- No adequate donor vessels available/reconstructable (revascularization impossible)
- Multiresistant bacteria/no antibiotic treatment available
- Lack of compliance (eg, drug abuse, psychiatric/mental illnesses)

PREOPERATIVE EVALUATION AND SPECIAL CONSIDERATIONS
Classification: Age Versus Frailty

There is great heterogeneity in the literature defining age and what is considered an "aged" or "elderly" population, with earlier studies including even patients in their 50s. More recently, several different classifications were suggested, such as young-old (>65 years) versus old-old or very old (>80 years) or super seniors (nonagenarians or centenarians).[8–10]

Treatment Objectives

The primary goals of lower extremity reconstruction using microsurgical techniques are similar in the elderly as in their younger counterparts:

- Stable and infection-free soft tissue and bony reconstruction
- Preservation of pain-free function/ambulation and autonomous mobility
- Timely return to previous living status and social condition
- Restoration of body integrity and quality of life
- Minimization of immobilization and confinement to bed
- Maximizing of quality of life in palliative situations

Principles and Strategy

Modern strategies regarding microsurgical reconstruction in elderly patients are based on the following presumptions:

- Age alone does not contradict microsurgery
- Biological age supersedes chronologic age
- Microsurgery is a safe and standardized procedure (low donor-site morbidity and complication rate)
- Interdisciplinary settings produce high success rates

- Thorough preoperative surgical planning and 2-team approach are crucial to reduce operative time

Decision Making

In order to choose the best reconstruction method for the affected elderly individual, the following questions need to be addressed:

- Thorough 3-dimensional analysis of the size and components of the defect
- Exclusion/identification of infecting agents
- Analysis of osseous integrity/stability
- Assessment of the vascular status
- Individual patient's expectations and needs
- Assessment and preoperative improvement of relevant comorbidities
- Contraindications (as above)
- Available treatment options
- Assessment of valid treatment alternatives (eg, locoregional flaps, limb shortening, arthrodesis, amputation)
- Planning of backup strategies (life boats)
- Multidisciplinary problem analysis and treatment plan (radiology, oncology, internal medicine, geriatrics, infectiology, orthopedics, plastic surgery, anesthesiology, physiotherapy, ethical round-table discussion)

Preoperative Patient Evaluation

When microsurgical reconstruction is considered in a patient of advanced age, special attention must be paid to balancing what is technically feasible against what is medically and ethnically reasonable. In order to optimize the patient's status before surgery, preoperative patient evaluation includes the following:

- Comorbidities (above all, cardiovascular, pulmonary, nephrologic, hepatic diseases, immune status)
- Impaired perfusion (arteriosclerosis)
- Restrictions of wound healing (diabetes, autoimmune disease, locoregional flaps critical)
- Prenutrition (proteins, calories)
- Prehabilitation

Perioperative Management

- Bridging of preexisting anticoagulation protocol
- Restrictive volume management and use of vasoactive agents
- Control of cardiovascular and pulmonary function
- Maintain kidney and liver function
- Consultation of geriatrics

Preoperative Planning and Imaging

When planning a free tissue transfer in elderly patients, the vascular situation is of primary interest and should be investigated in advance by clinical examination and modern imaging (computed tomography [CT]/MRI angiography, phlebography, arteriography). In the case of macroangiopathy or microangiopathy, the possibility of vascular intervention, such as bypass, stent, arteriovenous (AV) loop, or vein graft, should always be considered before lower extremity amputations.

SURGICAL PROCEDURE

To minimize medical complications, any factor reducing the intraoperative strain for the elderly patient and speeding up the procedure should be identified and optimized:

- One-stage procedure if possible
- Debridements and biopsies in regional anesthesia
- Vascular procedures to improve inflow (preferred as separate operation)
- Short operative time (ideally <3 hours), for example, by careful preoperative planning (eg, by 3-dimensional imaging or CT angiography), limited incisions in a "longitudinal fashion,"[11] intraoperative utilization of vascular coupler devices, meticulous coagulation
- Scrupulous attention to detail yields great benefit, as elderly individuals tolerate complications poorly
- Regional (spinal) anesthesia and sitting position (beach chair)

The surgical and anesthetic teams should be experienced in dealing with elderly patients and opt for safe and speedy reconstructions:

- Two-team approach (simultaneous flap elevation, preparation of recipient site, donor-site closure)
- Experienced surgical, anesthetic, and nursing staff, no teaching procedure
- Workhorse flaps with long, reliable, and constant pedicles from the lower extremity (gracilis or anterolateral thigh [ALT] flaps) or other donor sites (groin, latissimus dorsi, parascapular, extended lateral arm flaps)
- Primary closure of donor site
- Avoid repositioning
- End-to-side or flow-through anastomosis, venous bypass, or grafting if necessary

- 8-0 or 7-0 sutures with stronger needles in case of arteriosclerotic plaques
- Punch hole for removal of plaques or use of vein grafts
- No clamps on vessel; instead, use of tourniquet or intraluminal occlusion devices as frequently used in cardiac surgery

Special indications include composite defects and reconstruction of osteocutaneous, tendocutaneous, and extensor apparatus defects, exposed prosthesis, and foot reconstruction.[12]

POSTOPERATIVE CARE AND EXPECTED OUTCOME

A scheduled intensive care unit (ICU) stay is frequently necessary to assure postoperative safety and provide timely intervention in cases of postoperative complications. A trend toward increased nondirect surgery-related complications in elderly patients has been observed. Cardiac (heart infarction), pulmonary (pneumonia, embolus), and renal complications are of particular importance and require postoperative control:

- Intensive care or immediate care unit 12 to 48 hours
- Flap monitoring for early detection of perfusion problems
- Restrictive fluid management
- Maintaining body temperature
- blood pressure management (vasoactive agents)
- Nursing and physiotherapy
- Nutrition
- Early mobilization and flap dangling
- Pain control
- Delirium prophylaxis
- Social service
- Rehabilitation

MANAGEMENT OF COMPLICATIONS

Complication rates, mortality, and morbidity can be reduced by respecting the concepts mentioned above. Early detection is important to avoid fast deterioration of the older patient with smaller organ system reserve and complication tolerance. General complications of organ functions and mental status should be addressed in a multidisciplinary approach. Local complications at the donor and recipient site should be treated after thorough causative analysis and with short delay. In case of rare flap loss, a back-up strategy, including nonmicrosurgical concepts, should be considered to avoid repetitive major surgery, and putting the patient in jeopardy.

CASE DEMONSTRATIONS (UP TO 4 CASES)

Case 1

A 72-year-old male patient presented with multiple saw-cutting injuries over the left laterodorsal ankle, including complete cut of the Achilles tendon, peroneal tendons, and distal fibular fracture. Early fracture-related infection was diagnosed after wound breakdown 10 days later. After thorough debridement (**Fig. 1**), a composite soft tissue defect of 7 × 18 cm was reconstructed with a free, extended, neurotized, tendocutaneous lateral arm flap, including triceps tendon, to reconstruct the 4-cm defect of the peroneal tendons (**Fig. 2**) with excellent functional results after 6 months (Video 1) and minimal donor site morbidity in the form of hypesthesia in a small area of the forearm (**Fig. 3**).

Case 2

A 90-year-old male patient presented with a large wound (**Fig. 4**) over a chronically infected composite osteosynthesis of the lower leg and ankle arthroplasty (**Fig. 5**). Debridement was necessary because of acute fracture-related infection, and the multidisciplinary decision was made to avoid amputation and reconstruct the soft tissue defect with a split vastus lateralis ALT flap, establish a chronic fistula medially, and not exchange the osteosynthesis/arthroplasty material. With the established fistula, no acute reinfection has occurred (**Fig. 6**); 6 months later, the patient is playing golf again.

Case 3

A 76-year-old male patient developed a combined soft tissue defect over the right medial ankle and heel after necrotizing fasciitis (**Fig. 7**). The angiological examination revealed a single-vessel runoff fed by the fibular artery. The vascular surgeon provided a recipient artery by using an ipsilateral

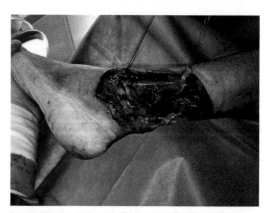

Fig. 1. Lateral intraoperative view of the ankle after debridement. The proximal and distal peroneal tendons are held with sutures posterior to the fibular plate.

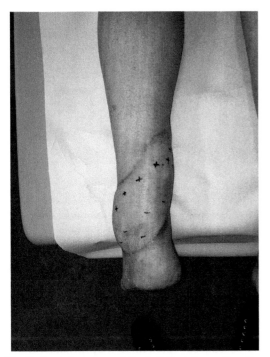

Fig. 2. Posterior view of the left foot 6 months after reconstruction with a neurotized extended composite lateral arm flap. The flap is regaining sensation as indicated by the patient's markings.

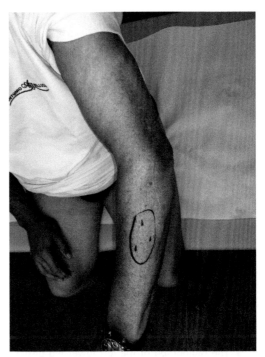

Fig. 3. The left arm shows no functional deficit and minimal loss of sensation distal to the flap harvest site. This is provoked as the inferior lateral cutaneous nerve had been harvested to neurotize the flap (see **Fig. 2**).

saphenous vein graft attached onto the fibular artery in an end-to-side manner (arrow in **Fig. 8**) used for end-to-end anastomosis of a free contralateral gracilis flap covered with a thick split-thickness instep skin graft and good postoperative result 2 months later (**Fig. 9**).

Case 4

An 82-year-old female patient underwent multiple orthopedic operations after periprosthetic joint infection of the ankle, prosthesis removal, nonvascularized osseous reconstruction with an allograft, implant-associated infection, consequent implant removal, debridement, shortening of the leg, and ankle arthrodesis with full-ring external fixation, accompanied by critical soft tissues (**Fig. 10**). The angiological examination showed a single-vessel runoff with the anterior tibial artery intact, and a free ALT flow-through flap was raised on a T-segment (**Fig. 11**) to reconstruct the soft tissue envelope through the ring-fixator, which remained in place. Four months later, the soft tissues are intact (**Fig. 12**), and bony consolidation can be seen radiologically (**Table 1**).

DISCUSSION

Microsurgery has revolutionized lower extremity reconstruction as in concepts of orthoplastic surgery and is increasingly required in elderly patients, a subpopulation that is continuously growing in Europe and the United States. In these patients, however, treatment decisions need careful consideration, as postoperative complications seem to become more relevant after the age of 70 years. Alternative treatment options, for

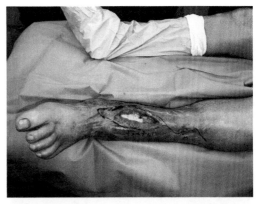

Fig. 4. Intraoperative view right before debridement with the cement of the composite osteosynthesis largely exposed. The marked resection lines indicate an estimated defect of 15 × 7 cm and show the foreseen access to the anterior tibial vessels proximally to the defect.

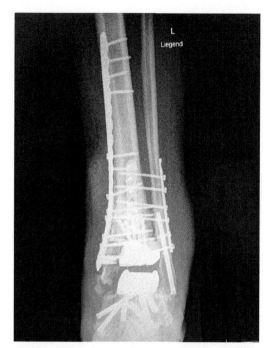

Fig. 5. The radiograph of the left lower leg displays arthrodesis of the subtalar joint, ankle prosthesis, and lower leg composite osteosynthesis with cement over the distal tibia after periprosthetic fracture.

example, amputation, lead to high mortalities and reduced quality of life in this patient cohort. [13] The influence of advanced age has been discussed regarding patient survival, complication rate, and functional outcomes in the literature. An overall number of 5951 cases of free tissue transfer were controlled for comorbidities by Jubbal and colleagues,[14] and age itself was not found to be significantly associated with complications.

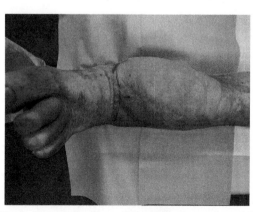

Fig. 6. Six months after soft tissue reconstruction with a split vastus lateralis ALT. No acute infection has occurred with the new fistula fully established (middle distal flap).

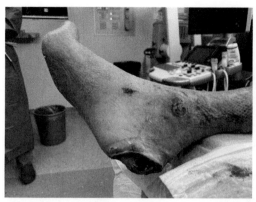

Fig. 7. Preoperative view with a combined small soft tissue defect over the medial ankle and large defect over the right heel. The patient had been bedridden because of necrotizing fasciitis of the contralateral left lower leg and sepsis leading to amputation of the left lower leg.

However, advanced chronologic age was significantly associated with increased mortality. Ustun and colleagues[15] performed a systematic review and meta-analysis of free flaps in patients of advanced age and could not detect any difference in elderly versus young flap success rates or surgical complications; however, they did find significantly more medical complications and mortality in elderly patients. Therefore, the investigators recommend assessment of "physiologic" age instead of chronologic age in patients for free tissue reconstruction. Serletti and colleagues[3] examined 100 patients aged older than 65 years retrospectively and found that chronologic age did not predict flap complications, but higher American Association of Anesthesiology (ASA)

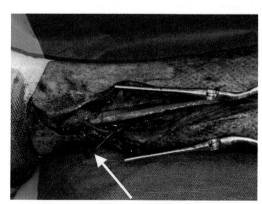

Fig. 8. Intraoperative view showing the venous graft ready for arterial flap anastomosis (*arrow*). It had been harvested from the saphenous vein and anastomosed in an end-to-side manner to the fibular artery (single vessel runoff) by the vascular surgeon.

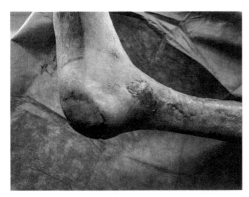

Fig. 9. Two months postoperatively, the gracilis flap, covered with instep split-thickness skin graft for the weight-bearing surface, has completely healed.

scores and length of operative time were significant predictors of postoperative surgical morbidity. This finding emphasizes that compared with the chronologic age, biological age is considered more relevant today, taking into account evaluation measures, such as the ASA classification. In addition to biological age, the term "frailty" describes the consequences of age-associated functional losses that lead to increased

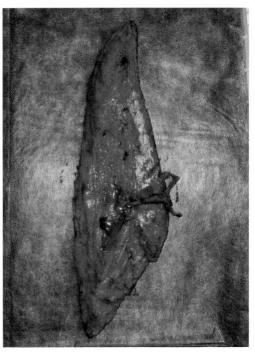

Fig. 11. The undersurface of the single-perforator ALT flap was raised with a vascular T-segment to insert it as a flow-through flap.

vulnerability of the entire organism regarding external and internal stressors and even permanent disability. The "frailty index" according to Rockwood and colleagues[16] summarizes all existing deficits.

In order to reduce postoperative complications in this important patient group, preoperative multidisciplinary planning and intraoperative

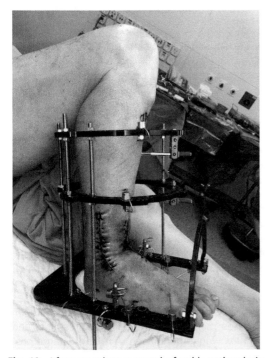

Fig. 10. After complete removal of ankle arthrodesis, allograft, and osteosynthesis material, the soft tissues around the medial and lateral incisions are critical in this single-vessel runoff leg with only the anterior tibial vessels intact.

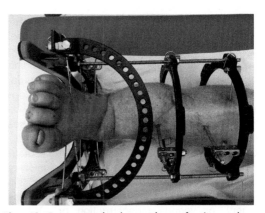

Fig. 12. Four months later, the soft tissues have completely healed with preservation of the perfusion of the foot. The antibiotic therapy to treat the osteomyelitis had been stopped 1 month earlier without recurrence of infection, and the bone is healing.

Table 1
Summary of the consensus statement of the Deutschsprachige Arbeitsgemeinschaft für Mikrochirurgie der Peripheren Nerven und Gefässe (German-speaking Working Group of Microsurgery of the Peripheral Nerves and Vessels)

Indication in patients of advanced age	Patient expectations/wishes, physical strain, quality of life, comorbidities, alternative therapies, salvage options, multidisciplinarity, ethical council
Preoperative preparation	Utilization of workhorse flaps, specific vascular diagnostics, for example, duplex, CT/MRI angiography, conventional/interventional techniques, phlebography, need for AV loop/bypass, patient decree, precautionary power of attorney
Comorbidities and perioperative management	Relevance of cardiologic, nephrologic, pulmonary, and hematologic comorbidities, application of "frailty assessment," possibility of prehabilitation
Particular considerations in postoperative phase	Perfusion monitoring, pain therapy, coagulation management, intensified pressure sore prophylaxis, mobilization, education of medical and nursing staff regarding treatment of elderly patients, prevention, and treatment of delirium

From Ludolph I, Lehnhardt M, Arkudas A, et al. [Plastic reconstructive microsurgery in the elderly patient - Consensus statement of the German Speaking Working Group for Microsurgery of the Peripheral Nerves and Vessels]. *Handchir Mikrochir Plast Chir.* 2018;50(2):118-125; with permission.

management are key. Interestingly, this may be especially important in the very old patient groups, as the high incidence of medical comorbidities increases beyond the age of 80 years. A large retrospective cohort study examined 211 patients 70 years or older at a single institution undergoing free tissue flap surgery and revealed significantly higher rates of medical complications in the octogenarian group when compared with septuagenarians.[17]

Careful patient selection based on medical comorbidities and overall functional status should be taken in a multidisciplinary setting (expert board) and consulted by an expert from internal medicine (infectious disease specialist and geriatric), septic orthopedic surgeon, plastic surgeon,[18] vascular surgeon, and interventional radiologist to individually assess opportunities to improve vascular supply of the leg. In planning complex reconstruction, especially after trauma, magnetic resonance angiography, CT angiography, or conventional angiography should be routinely performed.[19,20] As an alternative in cases with no further risk factors and local reconstruction, duplex ultrasound is safe and highly diagnostic to identify appropriate arterial perfusion of the recipient vessel. In the lower extremity, this may include catheter intervention, stent, bypass surgery, or venous reconstruction or AV-loop intervention.[21–24]

During the microsurgical operation, not only the surgeons but also the anesthetic and nursing teams should be experienced in dealing with elderly patients, as they are more prone to have complications related to the anesthesia and the long duration of the procedure, for example, hypothermia, hyperhydration with imbalanced diuresis, or hypotonic or hypertonic episodes, which require intervention. Intraoperatively, every factor to reduce the strain for the patient and to speed up the operation should be identified and optimized, for example, by using a 2-team approach and allowing simultaneous operating at the donor and recipient sites, keeping the intervention short, successful, and safe.[25] Vascular aging in the lower extremity demonstrates increased structural changes in the arterial system with reduction of arterial elasticity; above all, in posttraumatic damage, diabetes mellitus or peripheral neurovascular pathologic condition increases the difficulty of microsurgical reconstruction of soft tissue and limits the generalization of previous results that have been obtained from breast or head and neck reconstruction. As an example, in a study of 44 microsurgical salvages for posttraumatic leg defects of the lower leg by Xiong and colleagues[19], the preoperative clinical situations of the elderly cohort were characterized by high rates of peripheral neurovascular pathologic condition (diabetes mellitus, peripheral artery disease) and complex wound conditions. A relatively large proportion (36%) of this cohort had only 1 or 2 lower-leg arteries patent, which further increased the difficulty and risk of free flap transfer. Besides, most defects were located in the distal lower leg and accompanied by exposure of bone or hardware.

Such problematic wound situations in geriatric patients require an individually adapted surgical procedure. Safe and speedy reconstructions by workhorse flap techniques with easy vascular access, reliable anatomy and long pedicles and vascular coupler devices should be used.[13]

The authors share the opinion that elderly patients should at least be admitted to an intermediate care unit or to an ICU for closer postoperative monitoring and nursing postoperatively and to enable timely intervention during a minimum of 12 to 24 hours, which is performed in many microsurgical centers even for healthy patients ("flap ICU"). Further postoperative care of these patients, including mobilization, ambulation, and physiotherapy, should be initiated as early as possible.

SUMMARY

Microsurgical reconstruction in the lower extremity can be performed safely with high success rate and manageable complications in elderly patients. The prerequisites include (i) a comprehensive preoperative interdisciplinary assessment of the patient and optimization of risk factors, (ii) meticulous preoperative planning, (iii) intraoperative adaptation of anesthesia and efficient surgical technique, and (iv) specialized postoperative monitoring and early mobilization according to the specific needs of the patient of advanced age (see **Table 1**).

CLINICS CARE POINTS

- A multidisciplinary team approach makes microsurgery a safe and succesful procedure.
- Age-related pathologies (atherosclerosis above all) demand thorough preoperative planning.
- Intraoperative stress can be reduced by regional anaesthesia, a sitting position (beach-chair) and a short operative time through a two-team approach.
- Reliable workhorse flaps provide easy vascular access with limited incisions, reliable anatomy and long vascular pedicles for speedy and safe soft-tissue reconstruction.
- Postoperative intensive / intermediate care helps to detect and manage complications early, provide immediate interventions and avoid fast deterioration due to limited physiological reserve.
- Early flap dangling, mobilization and physiotherapy minimize sequelae of prolonged immobilization and support rapid functional and social reintegration.

DISCLOSURE

The authors have no disclosures to declare.

SUPPLEMENTARY DATA

Supplementary data related to this article can be found online at https://doi.org/10.1016/j.cps.2021.01.008.

REFERENCES

1. Klein HJ, Fuchs N, Mehra T, et al. Extending the limits of reconstructive microsurgery in elderly patients. J Plast Reconstr Aesthet Surg 2016;69(8):1017–23.
2. Goldberg JA, Alpert BS, Lineaweaver WC, et al. Microvascular reconstruction of the lower extremity in the elderly. Clin Plast Surg 1991;18(3):459–65.
3. Serletti JM, Higgins JP, Moran S, et al. Factors affecting outcome in free-tissue transfer in the elderly. Plast Reconstr Surg 2000;106(1):66–70.
4. Azoury SC, Stranix JT, Kovach SJ, et al. Principles of orthoplastic surgery for lower extremity reconstruction: why is this important? J Reconstr Microsurg 2021;37(1):42–50.
5. Coskunfirat OK, Chen HC, Spanio S, et al. The safety of microvascular free tissue transfer in the elderly population. Plast Reconstr Surg 2005;115(3):771–5.
6. Heidekrueger PI, Heine-Geldern A, Ninkovic M, et al. Extending the limits of microsurgical reconstruction in patients with moderate to very severe obesity: single-center 6-year experiences. J Reconstr Microsurg 2017;33(2):124–9.
7. Lin CH. The role of free tissue transfer. In: Pu LLQ, Levine JP, Wei FC, ed. Reconstructive surgery of the lower extremity. New York: Thieme Publishers, 2013. p. 327–44.
8. Forman DE, Berman AD, McCabe CH, et al. PTCA in the elderly: the "young-old" versus the "old-old. J Am Geriatr Soc 1992;40(1):19–22.
9. Katlic MR, Coleman J. Surgery in centenarians. In: Rosenthal RA, Zenilman ME, Katlic MR, editors. Principles and practice of geriatric surgery. Switzerland: Springer Nature; 2020. p. 51–66.
10. Halaschek-Wiener J, Tindale LC, Collins JA, et al. The super-seniors study: phenotypic characterization of a healthy 85+ population. PLoS One 2018; 13(5):e0197578.
11. Osinga R, Fulco I, Schaefer DJ. Soft-tissue reconstruction in exposed total knee arthroplasty. In: Gravvanis A, Kakagia DD, Ramakrishnan V, editors. Clinical scenarios in reconstructive microsurgery. Switzerland: Springer Nature; 2020 (Accepted).
12. Osinga R, Eggimann MM, Lo SJ, et al. Orthoplastics in periprosthetic joint infection of the knee: treatment concept for composite soft-tissue defect with

extensor apparatus deficiency. J Bone Jt Infect 2020;5(3):160–71.

13. Wahmann M, Wahmann M, Henn D, et al. Geriatric patients with free flap reconstruction: a comparative clinical analysis of 256 cases. J Reconstr Microsurg 2020;36(2):127–35.

14. Jubbal KT, Zavlin D, Suliman A. The effect of age on microsurgical free flap outcomes: an analysis of 5,951 cases. Microsurgery 2017;37(8):858–64.

15. Ustun GG, Aksu AE, Uzun H, et al. The systematic review and meta-analysis of free flap safety in the elderly patients. Microsurgery 2017;37(5):442–50.

16. Rockwood K, Song X, MacKnight C, et al. A global clinical measure of fitness and frailty in elderly people. CMAJ 2005;173(5):489–95.

17. Howard MA, Cordeiro PG, Disa J, et al. Free tissue transfer in the elderly: incidence of perioperative complications following microsurgical reconstruction of 197 septuagenarians and octogenarians. Plast Reconstr Surg 2005;116(6):1659–68 [discussion 1669–671].

18. Schmidt VJ, Hirsch T, Osinga R, et al. [The interdisciplinary microsurgeon - results of the consensus workshop of the German Speaking Society for Microsurgery of Peripheral Nerves and Vessels]. Handchir Mikrochir Plast Chir 2019;51(4):295–301.

19. Xiong L, Gazyakan E, Wahmann M, et al. Microsurgical reconstruction for post-traumatic defects of lower leg in the elderly: a comparative study. Injury 2016;47(11):2558–64.

20. Xiong L, Gazyakan E, Kremer T, et al. Free flaps for reconstruction of soft tissue defects in lower extremity: a meta-analysis on microsurgical outcome and safety. Microsurgery 2016;36(6):511–24.

21. Bruner S, Jester A, Sauerbier M, et al. Use of a cross-over arteriovenous fistula for simultaneous microsurgical tissue transfer and restoration of blood flow to the lower extremity. Microsurgery 2004;24(2):114–7.

22. Tukiainen E, Kallio M, Lepantalo M. Advanced leg salvage of the critically ischemic leg with major tissue loss by vascular and plastic surgeon teamwork: long-term outcome. Ann Surg 2006;244(6):949–57 [discussion 957–948].

23. Cavadas PC. Arteriovenous vascular loops in free flap reconstruction of the extremities. Plast Reconstr Surg 2008;121(2):514–20.

24. Momeni A, Lanni MA, Levin LS, et al. Does the use of arteriovenous loops increase complications rates in posttraumatic microsurgical lower extremity reconstruction?-A matched-pair analysis. Microsurgery 2018;38(6):605–10.

25. Herold C, Gohritz A, Meyer-Marcotty M, et al. Is there an association between comorbidities and the outcome of microvascular free tissue transfer? J Reconstr Microsurg 2011;27(2):127–32.

Lower Extremity Reconstruction in the Pediatric Population

Arin K. Greene, MD*, Christopher L. Sudduth, MD, Amir H. Taghinia, MD

KEYWORDS

- Lower extremity • Pediatric • Constriction ring • Lymphedema • Syndactyly • Nevus • Trauma
- Vascular anomalies

KEY POINTS

- Indications for pediatric lower extremity reconstruction often are related to congenital conditions.
- Principles generally follow adult lower limb reconstruction with special considerations for long-term functional and aesthetic outcomes.
- Immobilization of the extremity can help ensure protection of the limb postoperatively.
- Removal of large skin lesions before ambulation can reduce the risk of complications.

INTRODUCTION

The pediatric population is unique because many of the indications for lower extremity reconstruction are congenital conditions. The most common diseases managed by plastic surgeons are syndactyly, macrodactyly, constriction rings, lymphedema, congenital nevi, and vascular anomalies. Defects following extirpation and traumatic injuries are treated similarly to adults. Because of the pediatric age group, aesthetic outcomes are particularly emphasized by patients and families.

INDICATIONS AND CONTRAINDICATIONS

Diagnosis of lower extremity disorders is made by history and physical examination. Indications for operative management are based on the type of congenital condition or defect.

Constriction Ring

Constriction ring is most common in the toes but can affect any area of the leg (**Fig. 1**A). The spectrum ranges from superficial scarring to deep bands. Functional disability, growth disturbance, joint deformity, lymphedema, and congenital

amputation can occur. Operative management is indicated to improve the appearance of a deformity as well as to correct any functional problems. Mild constriction rings not causing significant problems do not require intervention.

Lymphedema

Approximately 95% of patients with lymphedema do not require operative intervention and can be managed successfully with compression strategies (eg, stockings, pneumatic pump).[1] Operative treatment is performed to improve the appearance of the limb if significant psychosocial morbidity is present, to reduce the number of infections, and to enhance the ability to ambulate and wear clothing (**Fig. 1**B).

Syndactyly

Syndactyly most commonly involves the second webspace (**Fig. 1**C). In Apert syndrome, syndactyly affects all 4 webspaces and bone coalition is rare distally. Syndactyly of the foot usually does not cause major functional problems. Most children are able to run and participate in sports. Treatment is usually requested by parents in early

Department of Plastic and Oral Surgery, Boston Children's Hospital, Harvard Medical School, 300 Longwood Avenue, Boston, MA 02115, USA
* Corresponding author.
E-mail address: arin.greene@childrens.harvard.edu

Clin Plastic Surg 48 (2021) 341–347
https://doi.org/10.1016/j.cps.2020.12.010
0094-1298/21/© 2020 Elsevier Inc. All rights reserved.

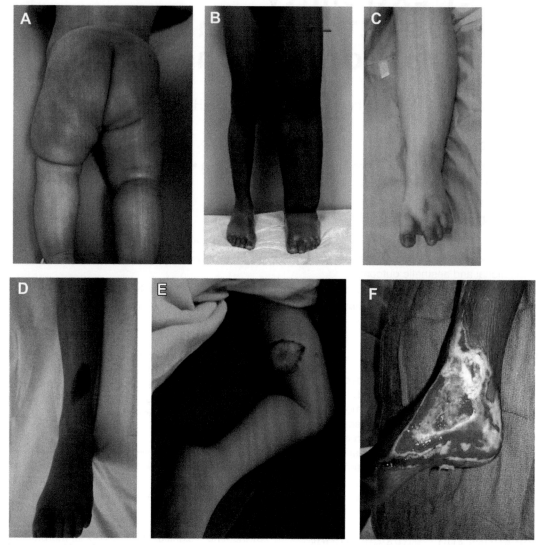

Fig. 1. Examples of pediatric conditions requiring lower extremity reconstruction. (*A*) Constriction ring. (*B*) Primary lymphedema. (*C*) Syndactyly. (*D*) Congenital pigmented nevus. (*E*) Involuted infantile hemangioma. (*F*) Traumatic injury.

infancy or by patients during teenage years to improve the appearance.

Reconstruction Following Lesion Removal/Trauma

Giant nevi are at risk for developing melanoma and are excised if possible. Small, medium, and large nevi are removed if they appear atypical or are causing a significant deformity (**Fig. 1**D). Vascular anomalies typically are removed if they are symptomatic during infancy (eg, bleeding, infection, pain) or in childhood if they are causing a deformity (**Fig. 1**E). Defects resulting from lesion extirpation or trauma are managed similarly to adults (**Fig. 1**F). Usually adequate local tissue is available

to cover bone or hardware proximal to the knee. Large areas of exposed bone or hardware involving the knee and mid-tibia may be covered using regional gastrocnemius or soleus flaps. Significant tissue loss involving the lower one-third of the leg can require free tissue transfer.

PREOPERATIVE EVALUATION AND SPECIAL CONSIDERATIONS

Congenital anomalies do not require operative intervention unless they are causing a functional or "cosmetic" problem. The lower extremity is an unfavorable location to remove large lesions of the integument because skin redundancy is minimal and gravity favors swelling, which increases stress on the incision line. Placement of a cast or a removable knee brace after lesion excision should be considered to ensure better healing and avoid dehiscence. It is best to perform elective procedures after 6 months of age because the infant's physiology approximates that of an adult, which reduces the risk of anesthesia. Because most infants begin ambulating at approximately 12 months of age, it is preferable to remove lesions before this time to reduce the risk of suture line dehiscence. If patients present after 12 months of age with lesions causing a deformity only (eg, infantile hemangioma, benign pigmented nevus), then removing the lesion before 4 years of age will eliminate the deformity before the child's long-term memory and self-esteem begins to form. Some parents will prefer to wait until a child is old enough to participate in the decision to extirpate a lesion, which can occur in late childhood or early adolescence.

Constriction Ring

Operative treatment of a constriction ring should address the functional and aesthetic issues of the limb. Collaboration with an orthopedic surgeon is required in cases of joint involvement. For bands involving the legs or thighs, excision and flap advancement is performed. It is most favorable to treat before ambulation to take advantage of the extra soft tissue of an infant and easier immobilization.

Lymphedema

Patients are asked about risk factors for lymphedema (eg, family history, travel to areas endemic for filariasis, removal of or radiation to inguinal lymph nodes). Physical examination shows pitting edema and inability to pinch the dorsal skin of the foot (positive Stemmer sign). Definitive diagnosis of lymphedema is obtained with lymphoscintigraphy; the test is 96% sensitive and 100% specific for the disease.[1] Individuals who are operative candidates (eg, repeated infections, large limb affecting activities of daily living) undergo MRI to determine if they have excess subcutaneous adipose hypertrophy that would benefit from suction-assisted lipectomy.

Syndactyly

Syndactyly most commonly affects the second webspace. Syndactyly usually does not result in lost function and patients are able to excel in physical activities. Operative intervention most often is performed to improve the deformity. Correction in infancy is advantageous before ambulation to reduce the risk of complications. Another common

time to correct the syndactyly is during adolescence when patients become more self-conscious about their appearance. Before surgical correction, radiography is performed to determine if osseous fusion is present.

Reconstruction Following Lesion Removal/ Trauma

Congenital nevi are evaluated by a dermatologist to determine if the lesion is concerning for malignancy. Patients with giant nevi larger than 2% total body surface area undergo MRI of the brain and spinal cord to rule out melanosis of the central nervous system. Most vascular malformations are evaluated by MRI to determine the extent of the lesion. Plain radiography is used to rule out fractures and foreign bodies following major traumatic injuries.

Almost all skin lesions can be removed by lenticular excision and linear closure; large areas may be managed by serial excision. Occasionally, large circumferential lesions require skin grafting or tissue expansion. Reconstruction of traumatic defects is based on the size, location, and depth of the wound. Superficial areas can be allowed to heal secondarily (with or without vacuum-assisted wound closure). Larger defects may be closed with delayed primary closure. Skin grafts are necessary if the wound cannot be closed linearly by advancing skin flaps. In the pediatric population, skin grafts should be avoided if possible because they cause a worse deformity than a linear scar and patients often will request that the graft be removed. Localized areas of exposed bone or tendon can be managed with vacuum-assisted wound closure to decrease the area of the wound and generate granulation tissue amenable to skin grafting. Large areas of exposed bone, tendon, or hardware in the lower leg require regional muscle flap closure or free tissue transfer.

SURGICAL PROCEDURES
Constriction Ring

We favor the technique described by Upton and Tan.[2] Bands that are deep and narrow are favorable because they provide extra soft tissue to restore contour. The ring is marked and the skin is excised. Separate adipofascial and skin flaps are raised. The adipofascial flaps are mobilized and closed and then the skin flaps are approximated ideally away from the line of closure of the adipofascial flaps. Z-plasties are advocated extensively in the literature but are rarely needed. If the ring is deep or if there are multiple closely spaced rings, then a staged approach is considered (**Fig. 2**).

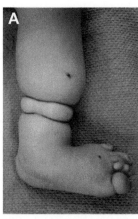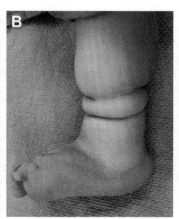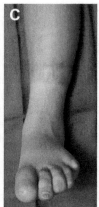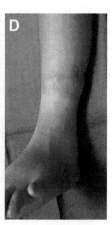

Fig. 2. Constriction ring of the lower extremity. (*A, B*) Preoperative appearance. (*C, D*) After circumferential excision, advancement of cephalad and caudad fasciocutaneous flaps, and skin closure. (*From* Greene AK, Taghinia. Lower Extremity. In: Greene AK (ed). *Pediatric Plastic and Reconstructive Surgery*. New York, NY: Thieme; 2018; with permission.)

Lymphedema

Suction-assisted lipectomy is our preferred operative technique for extremity lymphedema because it gives consistently favorable results with minimal morbidity.[3] The technique removes the abnormally hypertrophied subcutaneous adipose tissue and reduces excess extremity volume (**Fig. 3**). Liposuction improves lymphatic flow and function but does not cure the disease, and thus patients must continue their compression regimen. The procedure is performed using tumescent technique without a tourniquet. Fifteen to 20 1-cm incisions are made from the ankle to the hip and the adipose is removed with a 5-mm Becker cannula and/or a 5-mm power-assisted cannula. Patients are admitted overnight and allowed to ambulate immediately. Six weeks after their skin has contracted, they are fitted for new compression garments.

Reconstruction Following Lesion Removal/Trauma

Small defects or areas on the foot that would necessitate complicated reconstruction can be allowed to heal secondarily. Almost all skin lesions can be removed by lenticular excision and linear closure; large areas are managed by serial excision (**Fig. 4**).[4,5] Occasionally, large circumferential lesions require skin grafting or tissue expansion because serial excision can be performed only if

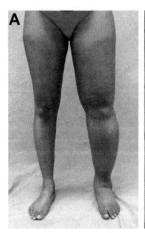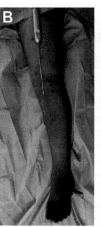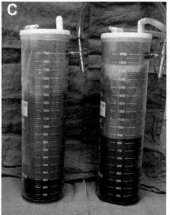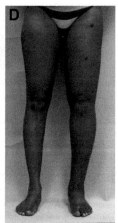

Fig. 3. Adolescent-onset primary lymphedema of the left lower extremity. (*A*) Preoperative appearance. (*B*) Intraoperative view of subcutaneous adipose removal using suction-assisted lipectomy. (*C*) Lipoaspirate. (*D*) Postoperative result. (*From* Greene AK, Taghinia. Lower Extremity. In: Greene AK (ed). *Pediatric Plastic and Reconstructive Surgery*. New York, NY: Thieme; 2018; with permission.)

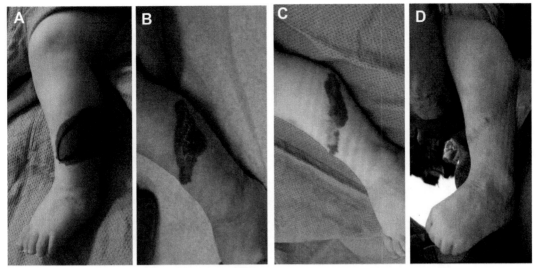

Fig. 4. Removal of a large congenital nevus. (*A*) Preoperative appearance. Outline illustrates the initial area to be resected. (*B*) After first-stage resection. (*C*) Following second-stage serial excision. (*D*) Final appearance after third stage removal. (*From* Greene AK, Taghinia. Lower Extremity. In: Greene AK (ed). *Pediatric Plastic and Reconstructive Surgery.* New York, NY: Thieme; 2018; with permission.)

normal skin is present on either side of the lesion. Wounds with exposed bone can be allowed to heal secondarily (if the area is small), or closed with approximation of adjacent tissues. Localized areas of exposed bone or tendon can be managed with vacuum-assisted wound closure. Large areas of exposed bone, tendon, or hardware require regional muscle flap closure (eg, gastrocnemius, soleus) or free tissue transfer (**Fig. 5**).[4]

Syndactyly

Using a tourniquet, dorsal and plantar triangular flaps are designed for commissure reconstruction (**Fig. 6**).[6] Plantar zig-zag incisions, similar to those used for release of hand syndactyly are not required. Straight-line releases are used that rarely cause contractures. The resulting defects are covered with full-thickness skin grafts from the lower

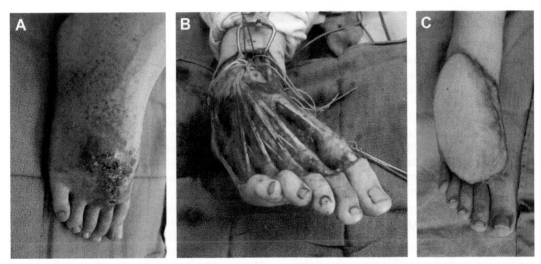

Fig. 5. An arteriovenous malformation of the foot was managed with complete extirpation and reconstruction with a free tissue transfer. (*A*) Preoperative appearance. (*B*) Following resection. (*C*) Inset of anterolateral thigh free flap. (*From* Greene AK, Taghinia. Lower Extremity. In: Greene AK (ed). *Pediatric Plastic and Reconstructive Surgery.* New York, NY: Thieme; 2018; with permission.)

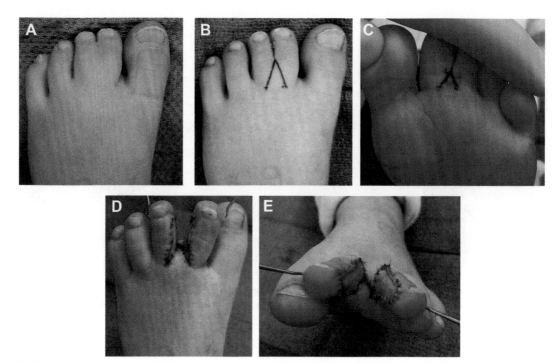

Fig. 6. Toe syndactyly treated with dorsal and plantar triangular flaps. (*A*) Preoperative appearance. (*B, C*) Markings of the flaps that are raised sharply in the subdermal plane. Once the syndactyly has been released, the flaps are transposed into the commissure. (*D, E*) Full-thickness skin grafts from the lower abdomen are used to resurface the skin defects on each side of the web. (*From* Greene AK, Taghinia. Lower Extremity. In: Greene AK (ed). *Pediatric Plastic and Reconstructive Surgery.* New York, NY: Thieme; 2018; with permission.)

abdomen. Three weeks of cast immobilization and non–weight bearing is used to maximize graft take. The ideal time to perform the operation is in infancy just before the patient begins to ambulate.

POSTOPERATIVE CARE AND EXPECTED OUTCOME

We have a low threshold to immobilize the lower extremity following operative intervention. The leg is an unfavorable area for suture line healing because of limited skin laxity to close incisions and the negative effects of gravity on edema. Placing the patient in a cast or knee immobilizer reduces the risk of complications. An exception to immobilization is after suction-assisted lipectomy for lymphedema. These patients do not have suture lines and they are encouraged to ambulate to reduce their risk of deep vein thrombosis.

MANAGEMENT OF COMPLICATIONS

The most common complication following a procedure on the lower extremity is suture line dehiscence. The larger and more distal the skin defect, the greater the risk of wound breakdown. Suture line dehiscence can be minimized by leaving

sutures in place for a longer period and placing the patient in a case or knee immobilizer for 2 to 3 weeks to limit stress on the incision line. A knee immobilizer may be removed when the patient is sleeping.

REVISION OR SUBSEQUENT PROCEDURES

Constriction ring reconstruction typically is satisfactory after 1 procedure. If a residual depression remains after an initial procedure, fat grafting or dermal-grafts could be used to augment the tissue in the area. Following liposuction for lymphedema, the underlying lymphatic function can be improved and recurrent adipose deposition is rare. Repeat liposuction could be performed if subcutaneous adipose deposition occurs. When we perform staged excision of skin lesions (eg, congenital nevus, vascular anomalies), we wait at least 3 months in-between stages to allow the skin adjacent to the nevus to regenerate.[5] Occasionally after correction of syndactyly, the webspace can experience recurrent webbing. After waiting 1 year to allow for maximal scar maturation, additional skin grafting and local flaps can be performed to further deepen the webspace.

DISCUSSION

Lower extremity reconstructive problems in children are different from adults. Several congenital disorders exist that are not managed in the adult population. Principles of extirpation of lesions and reconstruction can be similar to adults. Advantages of performing lower extremity reconstruction in children is that they typically do not have adult comorbidities that can complicate operations (eg, smoking history, diabetes, peripheral vascular disease). Because the pediatric population does not have arterial or venous disease, they can best tolerate wide skin undermining and closure of wounds linearly.

A disadvantage of surgery in the pediatric population is that patients are less likely to follow postoperative instructions. Consequently, immobilization of the extremity should be performed after an operation. Children and their parents are less tolerant of scars and the aesthetic outcome is more of a focus compared with adults. For example, patients often return requesting scar revisions and excision of skin grafts because they are concerned with their appearance, particularly during adolescence. Children's legs are often exposed during school or sports and their peers can comment on their deformity. Consequently, the pediatric population can require more revisions to achieve the best aesthetic result compared with adult patients.

In general, children should be managed as low on the reconstructive ladder as possible. Most constriction rings can be corrected by advancement of proximal and distal fasciocutaneous flaps and closure without Z-plasties. Most patients with lymphedema do well as long as they maintain an active life-style and body mass index. Suction-assisted lipectomy effectively reduces the size of a lymphedematous extremity in patients who are having significant morbidity. Large skin lesions (eg, congenital pigmented nevi, vascular anomalies) can be removed with serial excision; skin grafts and tissue expansion should be avoided when possible. Large traumatic defects are managed similarly to adults. Exposed neurovascular structures and bone may require regional muscle flap coverage or free tissue transfer. Syndactyly rarely causes functional problems and is most often corrected during infancy before ambulation, or during adolescence when patients become more concerned about the appearance of the deformity.

SUMMARY

Lower extremity reconstruction in the pediatric population has advantages and disadvantages compared with adults. Children typically are healthier and have a lower risk of complications from flap transfer or wide skin undermining than adults with diabetes, peripheral vascular disease, or smoking history. However, children are less likely to follow postoperative instructions and thus immobilization of the leg is important to minimize complications. Indications for lower extremity reconstruction in pediatrics can be unique and often involves congenital deformities. Consequently, patients are best managed by pediatric plastic surgeons familiar with these conditions (eg, vascular anomalies, lymphedema, syndactyly, giant nevi, constriction bands).

CLINICS CARE POINTS

- Problematic constriction rings are best treated with excision prior to ambulation when extra soft tissue is present; orthopedic consultation is required for all cases of joint involvement.
- Lymphedema rarely requires operative intervention but when indicated suction-assisted lipectomy is the preferred technique and may result in improved lymphatic function.
- Reconstruction following trauma or lesion removal is based on the size, location and depth of the resulting defect.
- Syndactyly can be managed with dorsal and plantar triangular flaps using straight-line releases and is ideally performed in infancy before the patient begins to ambulate.

DISCLOSURE

The authors have no conflicts of interest to declare.

REFERENCES

1. Maclellan RA, Greene AK. Lymphedema. Semin Pediatr Surg 2014;23(4):191–7.
2. Upton J, Tan C. Correction of constriction rings. J Hand Surg Am 1991;16(5):947–53.
3. Greene AK, Voss SD, Maclellan RA. Liposuction for swelling in patients with lymphedema. N Engl J Med 2017;377(18):1788–9.
4. Greene AK, Taghinia AH. Lower extremity. In: Greene AK, editor. Pediatric plastic and reconstructive surgery. New York (NY): Thieme; 2018.
5. Hassanein AH, Rogers GF, Greene AK. Management of challenging congenital melanocytic nevi: outcomes study of serial excision. J Pediatr Surg 2015;50(4):613–6.
6. Marsh DJ, Floyd D. Toe syndactyly revisited. J Plast Reconstr Aesthet Surg 2011;64(4):535–40.

Lower extremity reconstruction for limb salvage and functional restoration - The Combat experience

Ian McCulloch, MD, MRes[a], Ian Valerio, MD, MS, MBA[b,c],*

KEYWORDS

- Limb salvage • Limb restoration • Functional extremity reconstruction • Lower extremity injury
- Residual limb • Microsurgery • Peripheral nerve • Combat casualty care

KEY POINTS

- Lessons learned in extremity restoration and residual limb care secondary to combat trauma rapidly transfer among military and civilian centers as well as vice versa.
- Experience of surgical and medical teams treating extremity injuries has a direct impact on decision making and algorithm adoption, which have a positive impact on treatment measures and outcomes.
- Microsurgical techniques and advancements in orthoplastic surgery, including perforator and chimeric flaps; peripheral nerve surgery, including repair strategies and nerve transfer applications; and bone as well as soft tissue regeneration techniques and regenerative medicine increasingly have been applied to restoration of war-related traumatic lower extremity injuries.
- Functional limb restoration and residual limb patients require rehabilitation and potential ongoing surgical care measures that can span their lifetimes after initial traumatic injury recovery.
- An integrative, collaborative multidisciplinary team approach to extremity injury treatment and ongoing care needs is a desired state and ultimate goal.

BACKGROUND

Plastic surgery has a long history of innovation when faced with wartime challenges.[1-3] Most surgeons attribute the birthplace of modern plastic surgery to the European trenches of World War I. The protection of vital structures and relative exposure of the face saw the return of many soldiers with devastating facial injury. These challenges allowed Morestin, Valadier, and later Gilles to establish new techniques to reconstruct the maxillofacial injuries.[4] In World War II, the advent of militarized aviation led to a greater proportion of shrapnel injuries and fuel tank explosions. Sir Archibald McIndoe pioneered modern burn care and used many of the techniques described by Gilles to reconstruct his badly disfigured patients. These men who were willing to undergo cutting edge procedures for a chance at

a The Massachusetts General Hospital and Harvard Medical School, 55 Fruit Street, WACC 435, Boston, MA 02114, USA; b The Uniformed Services University of the Health Sciences, Bethesda, MD 20814, USA; c Medical Corps, U.S. Navy Active Reserve Component, Division of Plastic and Reconstructive Surgery, Massachusetts General Hospital and Harvard Medical School, 55 Fruit Street, WACC 435, Boston, MA 02114, USA
* Corresponding author. Medical Corps, U.S. Navy Active Reserve Component, Division of Plastic and Reconstructive Surgery, Massachusetts General Hospital and Harvard Medical School, 55 Fruit Street, WACC 435, Boston, MA 02114.
E-mail address: ivalerio@mgh.harvard.edu

Clin Plastic Surg 48 (2021) 349–361
https://doi.org/10.1016/j.cps.2021.01.005
0094-1298/21/Published by Elsevier Inc.

rehabilitation self-named themselves, "The Guinea Pig Club."[5] During the same period, Dr Sterling Bunnell's contributions, as a consultant to the US Army,[6] directly increased the understanding and treatment of hand injuries in which time he personally treated more than 20,000 combat-related hand injuries. His efforts led to the definitive textbook and background for all hand surgery training programs for decades and beyond.[7]

Modern conflict presents extremity reconstructive surgeons with a new set of challenges when treating combat casualties returning from the war theater. The recent conflicts in Iraq and Afghanistan now represent the longest sustained engagement in American military history. Analysis of the injuries incurred by American combat casualties reveal a marked increase in the proportion of complex extremity injury compared with injuries of the same type sustained in previous wars.[8,9] This observation within the US military medical care setting was paralleled by a comparative British study, which also reported approximately half of all injuries to trauma patients were to the extremity, with the largest proportion affecting the knee and/or lower leg.[10] This shift in injury patterns can be attributed to several factors. First, modern warfare has brought about the widespread use of individual protective body armor and Kevlar (DuPont, Wilmington, DE) helmets. These protective measures have greatly reduced life-threatening thoracic and head injury, yet, in turn, created an increase in extremity injury following combat-related trauma.[11] Additionally, the higher rates of indirect ambush attacks and utilization of improvised explosive devices (IEDs) by enemy combative forces and terrorists have increased the proportion of ballistic injuries incurred to the lower extremities. These weapons and associated high-energy blasts often result in composite tissue defects consisting of open fracture(s) with variable comminution patterns, severe soft tissue losses, and potential concomitant thermal injury as well as high rates of contamination with various particulates and foreign debris (**Fig. 1**).[12] Given the threat of exsanguination from extremity injuries suffered during combat, algorithms have been implemented for the improved use of tourniquet application, leading to a tremendous reduction in hemorrhagic deaths while further increasing the number of combat casualties requiring extremity reconstruction and restoration measures.[13,14]

Reconstructive surgeons have advanced beyond the more simplistic concept of "limb salvage" to that of "functional limb restoration" (**Figs. 2** and **3**). The goal of limb salvage is to

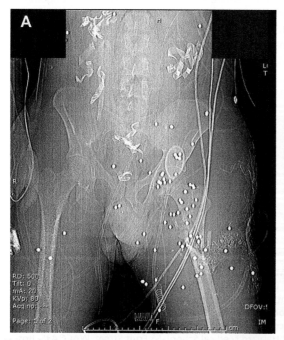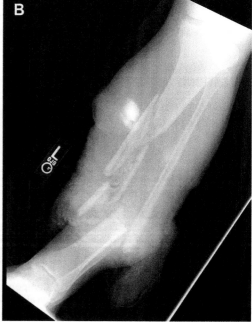

Fig. 1. (*A*) Radiographic images of patient illustrating the widespread injuries from IED blast exposure after transfer to in-theater military treatment facility from the initial battlefield injury setting. Various contaminated foreign bodies embedded within soft tissue injuries consisting of abdominal and small bowel perforations, perineal region injuries, and left open femur as well as open (*B*) grade 3B tibia/fibula fractures.

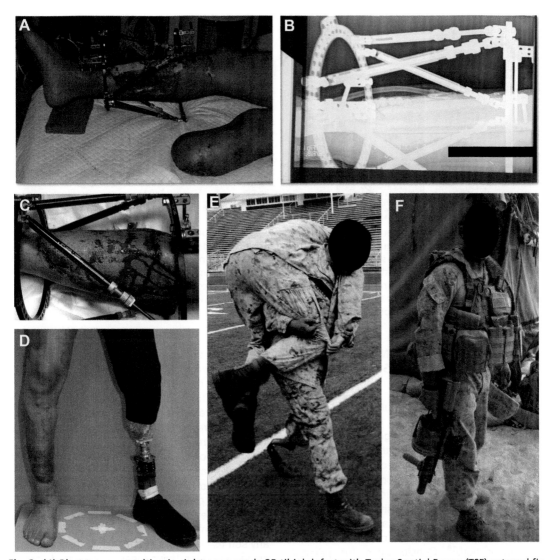

Fig. 2. (*A*) Blast trauma resulting in right open grade 3B tibial defect with Taylor Spatial Frame (TSF) external fixator in place. (*B*) Corresponding plain film showing fracture. The left lower extremity is status post–below-knee amputation following blast. Patient also suffered left ulna open grade 3B defect. (*C*) Right lower extremity following a latissimus free flap reconstruction for soft tissue coverage and skin grafting. Place back in TSF for stabilization and (*D*) out of fixator and able to bear weight. (*E, F*) The patient also underwent free anterolateral thigh flap and skin grafting to left upper extremity wounds. Now status post–successful upper and lower extremity salvages, including left residual limb optimization. (*E*) Able to showcase his abilities to perform and (*F*) returned to active duty and redeployed after complete rehabilitation from combat injuries.

recover the form and function of the lower extremity to the greatest extent possible. A salvaged limb that has ongoing neuropathic pain and/or significant functional deficits, however, is not nor should no longer be considered a success. Therefore, the primary idealized goal of extremity reconstruction is to restore the function and stability of the injured lower extremity while minimizing neuropathic pain and related disabilities—that is, functional limb restoration. This article highlights the lessons learned; outlines various principles, concepts, and best-known practices; and reflects on techniques that aid in functional limb restoration from lower extremity injuries suffered by wounded warriors. How an integrated, collaborative care model **(Fig. 4)** for ongoing lifelong care either for limb restoration or residual limb patients is the desired state to optimize the care of those patients suffering from severe lower extremity injury(-ies) also is presented.

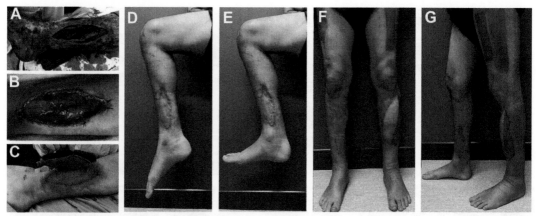

Fig. 3. Patient with bilateral open grade 3B tibial injuries following blast injury. (*A*) Wound following initial injury. (*B*) Following serial débridement, Integra dermal matrix is applied to the wound in preparation for further reconstruction. (*C*) Split-thickness skin graft placed with application of negative pressure wound therapy. (*D–G*) The bilateral tibial injuries reconstructed as follows: right lower extremity defect reconstructed with pedicled medial hemisoleus flap and skin grafting; left lower extremity defect reconstructed with free anterolateral thigh flap respectively. This series shows the patient 1-year post–reconstruction procedures. He is able to ambulate and continue duties after traumatic combat injuries.

INITIAL CONSIDERATIONS AND TRIAGING LOWER EXTREMITY INJURIES ON THE BATTLEFIELD

Regardless of whether an injury occurs on the battlefield or in civilian life, severe extremity trauma first should be managed by life-saving measures, including stopping the bleed or rapid tourniquet application, followed by assessment and establishment of supportive airway and breathing measures (circulation, airway, and breathing).[15] A primary survey should be conducted expeditiously to identify any active hemorrhage that can be controlled by direct pressure or tourniquet application.[16] Consideration for primary

amputation should be made only in instances where there are no options for limb preservation that would convey some return to function or form of the affected limb. Reports have shown that there are few indications for primary amputation if limb preservation is not a threat to a patient's life. Limb preservation at index operations may allow time for emotional acceptance of eventual amputation and has been shown to be cost effective in at least 1 study.[17]

Once the patient is stabilized, a thorough secondary survey, including comprehensive physical lower extremity examination, should document any soft tissue losses, identify any non–life-threatening vascular injury(-ies), associated nerve

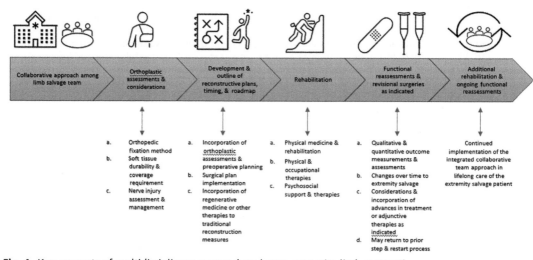

Fig. 4. Key concepts of multidisciplinary approach to lower extremity limb restoration.

injury(-ies), muscle-tendon deficits, and concomitant bony injury(-ies). Initial radiographs to determine the extent of bony injury using a portable radiograph once in the military trauma bay because orthopedic injury should heighten the suspicion for neurovascular injury. These studies should not interfere, however, with a more diagnostic computed tomography (CT) with or without angiography scan when indicated. These studies can provide more robust examination of soft tissue defects and vascular integrity when combined with a lower extremity angiogram.[18]

DAMAGE CONTROL AND MANAGEMENT OF LOWER EXTREMITY WOUNDS

Once life-threatening injuries are stabilized, the orthoplastic surgical management of a mangled or severely injured lower extremity can be broken down into the treatment of the associated bone, neurovascular, and soft tissue injuries. Consideration of the orthopedic fixation method, nerve injury assessment and management, and soft tissue coverage for durability and tolerance of potential revisional surgeries to be collectively employed should be outlined and mapped among the integrated team. Unstable fractures and joints should be stabilized initially with in-line traction, Kirschner wires, external fixators, or plaster splints prior to eventual definitive fixation[12] (see **Fig. 2**). Soft tissue injuries must undergo early, aggressive, and serial débridement as well as irrigation of all nonviable skin, muscle, and other soft tissues of the lower extremity, typically every 2 days to 3 days.[19–21] These measures rid the wound of nonviable tissues, which are a nidus for infection, while subsequently diluting any contaminants to the wound bed of the extremity. Most ballistic and high-energy trauma patients should be treated initially with broad-spectrum antibiotic therapy. In general, a short course using broad-spectrum antibiotics is recommended in any open fracture trauma,[22] but coverage should be tailored to the nature of the injury and the microbiome of the environment in which the injury occurred.[23] There have been reports of reduced risk of infection of traumatic lower extremity wounds when using antibiotic-impregnated polymethyl methacrylate beads to deliver a concentrated source of antibiosis at the site of injury, while various orthoplastic surgeons have utilized absorbable antibiotic beads to aid in local infection reduction control measures.[24] Several publications support the use of negative-pressure wound therapy with or without incorporation of irrigation solutions (eg, instillation of saline or topical irrigant solutions), such as Dakin solution (sodium hypochlorite) or Vashe solution (hypochlorous acid), when awaiting time to definitive orthoplastic reconstruction and soft tissue coverage.[25–28]

LOWER EXTREMITY VASCULAR INJURY

The initial assessment for vascular injury should include examination of hard signs, including active hemorrhage; large, expanding, or pulsatile hematoma; bruit or thrill over the wound; absent distal pulses; and any distal ischemic manifestations, such as pallor, paresthesia, or poikilothermia.[29] Kelly and colleagues[30] suggested that physical examination alone has sensitivity to rule out ischemic injury. Once vascular injury is suspected, prompt CT angiography is paramount for diagnosing the level of injury and allows for more precise surgical planning prior to the operating room. If perfusion must be restored but definite vascular repair either is not advisable due to patient condition or infrastructure capabilities, the use of temporary shunting has been championed.[31,32] Rasmussen and colleagues used data analysis of combat casualties suffering extremity injuries with vascular compromise in Iraq to conclude that the use of shunts was an effective stopgap to temporize perfusion during immediate evacuation rather than attempt reconstruction in remote locations.[33] These findings have been extrapolated to civilian trauma centers where temporary shunting has been employed for certain extremity trauma.

In scenarios where shunting is not feasible, the redundant nature of the lower leg circulation allows for ligation of 1 of the 3 dominant vessels (anterior tibial, posterior tibial, and peroneal) without compromising the perfusion to the foot. Burkhardt and colleagues[34] suggested that revascularization can be deferred if 1 tibial vessel remains patent if the foot is warm and well appearing on clinical examination. If both anterior and posterior tibial arteries are injured, distal bypass often is required. Perfusion via only the peroneal artery typically is inadequate for foot salvage.[34] Outside of distal bypass procedures, the authors' group also has utilized flow-through flap options for concurrent soft tissue coverage and reconstitution of arterial and venous outflow in severe combat-related dysvascular lower extremity injuries. Ligation of larger and more proximal vessels at the level of the thigh can be more perilous. Arterial ligation at this level is more likely to lead to distal ischemia and should be monitored closely postoperatively. Venous ligation often leads to acute hypertension due to inadequate outflow. Ideally, vascular repair should occur within 6 hours from injury because there is evidence that ischemia time longer than 6 hours portends increased risk of amputation.[35] The most common flaps employed as flow-through flaps consisted of the anterolateral thigh flap with and without inclusion of the vastus lateralis muscle utilizing the descending branch of the lateral circumflex vessels, the omentum and its gastroepiploic vessels; the rectus abdominis and perforator flap variants (muscle-sparing free transverse or vertical rectus abdominis and/or the deep inferior epigastric perforator flaps) based on the deep inferior epigastric vessels, the subscapular based vessels supplying the latissimus, thoracodorsal artery perforator; scapular and parascapular flaps, as well as the osseous-, osteocutaneous, and osteomyocutaneous flaps utilizing the fibula and its parent peroneal vessel system.

Postoperative monitoring of vascular repair should include baseline graft duplex studies or ankle-brachial index values to assess efficacy of revascularization.[36] Routine duplex study often is regarded as the best noninvasive method for surveillance of repair patency.[37] Careful clinical monitoring via physical examination of distal perfusion may be as effective as intensive.[38] The intermediate postoperative period (3–18 months) often is the time where a significant number of repairs fail.[36] Failure in this time period most often is a result of myointimal hyperplasia with vein grafts. Late failure often is a result of naturally progressive atherosclerosis.[39]

LOWER EXTREMITY NERVE INJURY

Peripheral nerve injuries that are incurred following a combat injury represent a complex surgical problem. The mechanism of injury from penetrative or ballistic force often results in severe orthoplastic injury that can cause transection, stretch, or shear injuries on nearby peripheral nerves. Although damage to upper extremity nerves can have more deleterious effects on function given their relationship to the hand, major peripheral nerves in the lower extremity were also associated with poor outcome, historically.[40,41] A thorough clinical examination along with electrodiagnostic testing accompanied by magnetic resonance imaging (MRI) can inform the surgeon regarding the extent of the peripheral nerve injury. There also is utility in high-definition ultrasound as a diagnostic tool, particularly when metal fragments are retained or anatomy is grossly distorted, thus limiting the reliability of MRI or electromyographic studies.[42]

Once peripheral nerve injuries are identified and documented, established and newly founded indications for repair increasingly have been pursued in combat casualty extremity trauma in an effort to reduce functional deficits and neuropathic pain development. Cleanly transected nerves, although less common in war-related extremity trauma, can be repaired primarily with end-to-end suture techniques if the resultant repair does not result in unfavorable tension after neurolysis and preparation of the nerve. One of the key principles employed is sharp débridement of the peripheral nerve to healthy fascicles when possible to permit better nerve regeneration and repair. If a tension-free coaptation cannot be achieved after debridement and preparation of the nerve, reconstructive surgeons can employ several adjunctive techniques to aid in peripheral nerve repair. Specifically, small gaps less than 1 cm can be repaired with nerve conduit to aid in achieving a tension-free repair.[43] Larger gaps exceeding 1 cm in length often require either nerve autograft or processed cadaveric nerve allograft for reconstruction of the nerve. In general, selection of appropriate donor nerves for autograft or allograft should consider the size of segmental gap encountered, the proximity to recipient nerve motor end plates or distal target end organ for reinnervation, redundancy of donor nerves, synergism of donor muscles to target muscles, and size matching for effective nerve repair and regeneration.[44]

In combat casualties suffering complex injury patterns, a subacute repair can at times be advantageous. In these situations, the extent of nerve injury often does not present itself until edema resolution and resulting scar formation occur. In these cases, nerve ends often are marked during initial exploration with spanning Prolene (Ethicon, Cincinnati, OH) or nylon sutures for delayed repair procedures. Definitive reconstruction ideally is performed within 3 weeks to 6 weeks of the initial injury. This delay also may have the added benefit of allowing for adequate débridement, treatment of concomitant injury, declaration of soft tissues, and control of infection in the affected extremity. Delay should not exceed 3 months following injury because Jonsson and colleagues[45] reported that this may represent a critical time point after which repair strategies have significantly worse outcomes, and delay in repair can lead to less optimal outcomes, especially regarding critical motor end plate reinnervation.

Residual paralysis from nerve injury that does not achieve meaningful functional recovery via nerve repair can be treated with tendon transfers, nerve transfers, and/or neurotized flap reconstruction in certain cases. In the lower extremity, the most effective reconstructive method to preserve stability and prevent foot deformity in peroneal nerve palsy continues to be tibial tendon transfer (tibialis posterior to tibialis anterior) or the Ninkovic procedure (lateral gastrocnemius muscle and tendon transfer with neurotization via transfer of the peroneal nerve to the lateral sural nerve to the lateral gastrocnemius muscle).[44,46–48]

Apart from motor nerve injury, damage to sensory nerves can result in neuropathic pain that mirrors phantom limb pain (PLP) or the perception of discomfort in a limb that is no longer present as seen in residual limb patients. This poorly understood phenomenon can occur in up to 85% of patients with traumatic loss of limb and can be experienced in patients suffering major peripheral nerve injury to their salvaged limb.[49] In addition, the formation of symptomatic neuroma at peripheral nerve blind endings can result in neuropathic pain further irritated by pressure, light touch, and even temperature variation.[50] Knowing this, targeted muscle reinnervation (TMR) or regenerative peripheral nerve interface (RPNI) often are employed as measures to mitigate the formation of neuroma and prevent neuropathic pain in not only residual limb patients but also patients undergoing functional limb restoration in cases where nerve reconstruction cannot be had (eg, large segmental nerve injuries where autografting or allografting is not likely to contribute to complete functional nerve recovery) (**Figs. 5–8**). Using these techniques, peripheral nerve endings without end-organ targets are transferred to recipient motor nerves and freshly denervated motor end plates of residual muscle or to free muscle grafts to allow for more organized neurite outgrowth and reinnervation of the target muscle and muscle grafts. Armed with the promise of these initial results,

reconstructive surgeons often now apply these techniques in a prophylactic manner for lower extremity patients with traumatic nerve injuries, which in turn has shown to have a significant effect in the prevention of neuroma and PLP[51] (see **Figs. 7** and **8**). This preemptive approach to treating PLP and symptomatic neuroma has been shown to decrease pain severity in patients following traumatic amputation and in limb restoration patients.[51–53]

SOFT TISSUE COVERAGE

As discussed previously, the mechanism for injury within the conflict in the Middle East is associated with high volume of lower extremity wounds, multiple extremity trauma, and at times massive loss of soft tissue and amputation.[54] The ultimate goal of reconstruction is return to function. Reconstructive considerations begin with primary closure or local tissue advancement if excess tissue is available. More often, in the lower extremity, a pedicled flap or free autologous tissue flap is used for definitive wound coverage.[55,56] Fasciocutaneous, various perforator, osseous, and muscle-based flaps all have been use with excellent rates of success in lower extremity reconstruction.[57,58] Throughout the course of the recent conflicts, a transition to higher applications of fasciocutaneous and perforator-based flaps has been evident especially in delayed reconstruction and restoration procedures (**Fig. 9**). The benefits of these flaps are many, including relative ease in re-elevation for subsequent procedures (such as delayed nerve grafting,

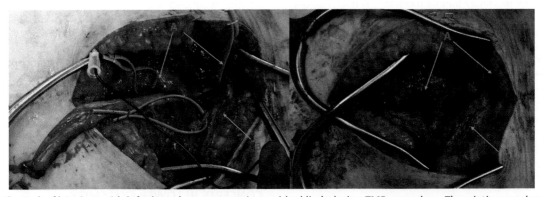

Fig. 5. (*Left*) Patient with left above-knee amputation residual limb during TMR procedure. The sciatic nerve has been dissected and the recipient motor nerves identified and labeled prior to TMR nerve transfers. The 2 superior vessel loops mark motor nerve branches of the biceps femoris muscle, the inferior vessel loop marks a motor nerve branch to semitendinosus muscle. Each nerve branch is stimulated to confirm the muscle target. (*Right*) Same left residual above-knee amputation limb. The sciatic nerve has been divided into 3 components (peroneal nerve and tibial nerve split into 2) and transferred to recipient motor nerves and motor end plates. One tibial nerve segment and the peroneal nerve transferred to separate motor nerve branches of the biceps femoris muscle. The second tibial nerve branch was transferred to the motor nerve branch of the semitendinosus muscle. Successful transfers confirmed with proximal nerve stimulation firing distant target muscles.

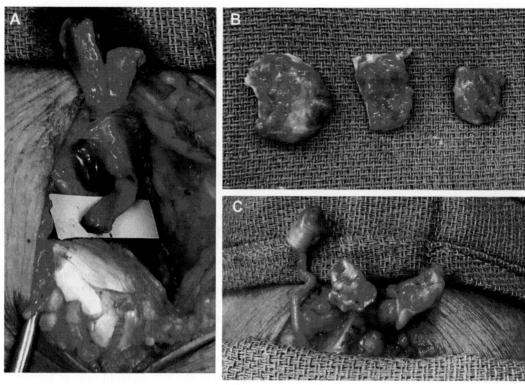

Fig. 6. (*A*) Above-knee amputation residual limb during RPNI procedure. The sciatic nerve is dissected into 3 components (sciatic nerve split into its peroneal nerve segment and 2 separate tibial nerve segments). (*B*) Free muscle grafts harvested. (*C*) Free nerve endings following placement as 3 RPNIs for prevention of painful neuroma.

tendon repair, and/or tenolysis) and sparing of core muscles needed for rehabilitation and recovery.[59] In contrast, muscle flaps have been shown—via laboratory study—to more effectively reduce infectious colonization and promote healing of fractures in lower extremity trauma models.[60] A useful adjunctive technique to perforator-based flaps, however, is the incorporation of small portion of muscle to place over an underlying fracture when of interest. This technique does not add significant time to the procedure, can spare the function of the muscle because only a small portion is included, and can provide a chimeric flap with multiple orientation pattern options for complex soft tissue coverage. Flap choice, ultimately, should take into consideration the extent of the soft tissue defect, timing, and surgical resources, including the skill set of the surgeon.[61]

OPTIONS FOR FLAP RECONSTRUCTION

Tintle and colleagues[62] developed algorithms for both upper and lower extremity combat wound reconstruction. Pedicled tensor fascia latae, rectus femoris, and rectus abdominus flaps were used in reconstruction of the proximal leg. Injuries to the middle third were reconstructed with

pedicled gastrocnemius/soleus flaps or free flaps. The distal leg reconstructions employed free flaps for pedicled sural artery or dorsalis pedis flaps. The authors have previously reported their own outcome data for 359 flap procedures conducted on US wounded warriors injured in Iraq and Afghanistan between 2003 and 2012, 60% of which were performed for lower extremity reconstruction.[59] For this cohort, a variety of soft tissue flap options were used, including fasciocutaneous flaps, muscle flaps, and perforator flaps as well as chimeric flaps with distinct muscle, bone, and fasciocutaneous components. This retrospective review highlighted the importance of tailoring the limb restoration algorithm to each injury pattern encountered.[59]

REGENERATIVE MEDICINE AND FUTURE CONCEPTS IN LOWER EXTREMITY RECONSTRUCTION

Wartime injuries—in particular, ballistic injuries— often result in massive tissue losses and concomitant bony defects, leaving behind a lack of tissue donor sites for reconstruction. Recently, military surgeon teams have begun to study the utility of incorporating regenerative medicine techniques into their

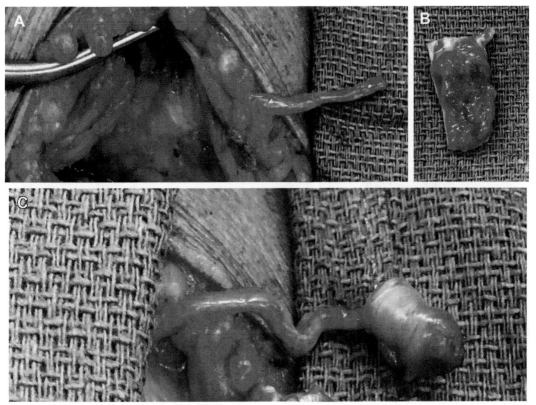

Fig. 7. Example of RPNI for neuroma and pain control of noncritical sensory nerve of the lower extremity. (*A*) Noncritical sensory nerve (saphenous nerve) with gap that is too large to be amenable to reconstruction with either an autograft or allograft. (*B*) Free muscle graft for RPNI. (*C*) RPNI of saphenous nerve where free muscle graft is wrapped over stump of peripheral nerve.

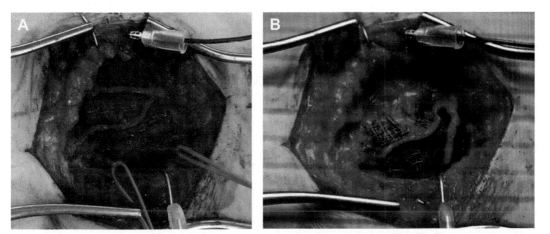

Fig. 8. Example of TMR for neuroma and pain control of noncritical sensory nerve of the lower extremity. (*A*) Noncritical sensory nerve (lateral femoral cutaneous nerve [LFCN] of the thigh) with ongoing neuroma and neuropathic pain in extremity salvage patient. (*B*) TMR with formal nerve transfer of the LFCN to 2 separate motor branches and accompanying motor end plates of the vastus lateralis muscle.

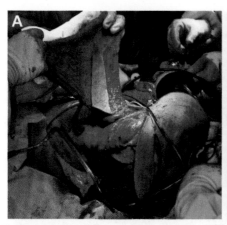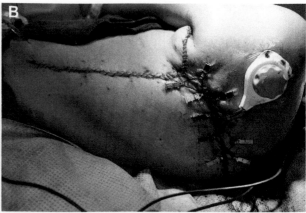

Fig. 9. Example of utilizing multiple flaps and/or creation of chimeric flaps from the subscapular system. (*A*) Intra-operative photo after completed harvest of a scapular osteocutaneous flap for left ulnar reconstruction, a myocutaneous latissimus flap for right lower extremity open grade 3B tibial coverage, and a serratus flap used for right dorsal hand coverage reconstruction, respectively. These 3 free flaps were transferred to cover, reconstruct, and salvage 3 separate limbs, including wounds of the bilateral upper extremities and lower extremity. (*B*) Complex closure and external tissue expander placement to chimeric subscapular system flap donor site.

armamentarium to augment traditional reconstructive algorithms used for these complex extremity injuries. For instance, large segmental bone losses have been treated successfully with allograft mesenchymal stem cells (MSCs) in combination with cadaveric bone grafts as well as vascularized bone grafts in isolation or via the Capanna technique.[63] In theory and application, these pluripotent MSCs can serve as an osteoconductive scaffold and contain osteogenic cells capable of forming bony structures de novo.[64] Early results of these MSC-based allograft and vascularized autograft reconstructions are promising.

Regenerative medicine also may supplement the current management of soft tissue defects. Dermal regenerative matrices, extracellular matrices, such as human-derived, bovine-derived, and porcine-derived materials, have been shown to assist in coverage of devitalized vital structures, including exposed bone, resulting in tissue regenerates suitable for definitive skin grafting[63] (see **Fig. 3**). These regenerative extracellular matrix materials have beneficial properties that help to establish granulating tissue, including the stimulation of neoangiogenesis, and blood vessel development and to support the chemotaxis of progenitor cells that favor regeneration of more native tissues over scar formation.[61,62,65]

CLOSING

During periods of high-intensity conflicts and military engagement, advancements and evolutions in extremity care have been evident, given the significant injuries many combat casualties present. The high volume of cases and lower extremity injuries that result from armed conflict often present challenges for reconstructive surgeons and teams treating war-related injuries. The armed conflicts of yesterday and today, as well as future engagements, while spanning different times or eras, have presented and will present similar challenges and calls for innovation and further advancements. The recent modern war theater operations in Iraq and Afghanistan have presented an opportunity to move beyond the concept of limb salvage and instead strive for an idealized goal of functional limb restoration. Building on the basic concepts pioneered by giants of the reconstructive field and incorporating modern techniques, the goal is to strive to restore function and stability of injured lower extremities while preventing neuropathic pain and related disability to improve the care and outcomes for those suffering from extremity injuries.

CLINICS CARE POINTS

- Evolution and adoption of perforator flaps for lower extremity reconstruction have occurred throughout recent conflicts and mirrored those seen in civilian centers.
- Limb restoration is desired goal as recovery of pain-free form, function, and stability over the remaining lifetime for a patient who has experienced a devastating lower extremity injury.
- An integrated, collaborative care model for extremity injured patients requiring limb restoration as well as those undergoing limb loss requires ongoing and lifelong care and is a model for centers to exemplify when possible.

- Advances in cell-based therapies and regenerative medicine adjuncts to optimize limb restoration have been fostered and implemented for extremity injuries seen during recent conflicts.
- Microsurgical innovation for the reconstruction of composite tissue and severe combat-related extremity injuries has been achieved in restoring bone and soft tissue defects as well as addressing peripheral nerve injuries to reduce pain and recover function.

DISCLOSURE

Dr I. McCulloch has no commercial or financial conflicts of interest to declare. Dr I. Valerio is an advisor and/or consultant to Axogen Inc, Integra Lifesciences Inc, and Stryker Corporation, none of which is relevant to the work presented in this article, and no financial proceeds from commercial interests were obtained in writing or assistance with publication of this article.

REFERENCES

1. Howard JT, Kotwal RS, Stern CA, et al. Use of combat casualty care data to assess the US military trauma system during the Afghanistan and Iraq conflicts, 2001-2017. JAMA Surg 2019. https://doi.org/10.1001/jamasurg.2019.0151.
2. Sabino JM, Slater J, Valerio IL. Plastic surgery challenges in War Wounded I: flap-based extremity reconstruction. Adv Wound Care 2016. https://doi.org/10.1089/wound.2015.0656.
3. Casey K, Sabino J, Jessie E, et al. Flap coverage outcomes following vascular injury and repair. Plast Reconstr Surg 2015. https://doi.org/10.1097/prs.0000000000000769.
4. Mazzola R, Mazzola I. History of reconstructive and aesthetic surgery 'in' P. Neligan *Plastic Surgery*. Elsevier; 2013. p. 21.
5. Macnamara AF, Metcalfe NH. Sir Archibald Hector McIndoe (1900-1960) and the Guinea Pig Club: the development of reconstructive surgery and rehabilitation in the second World war (1939-1945). J Med Biogr 2014. https://doi.org/10.1177/0967772013480691.
6. Brown T. Hand surgery in World war II. J Bone Jt Surg 1956. https://doi.org/10.2106/00004623-195638040-00040. Edited by S. Bunnell, M.D. Washington, Office the Surgeon General, Department of the Army, 1955. $3.75.
7. Green SA. Giants in orthopaedic surgery: sterling bunnell MD. Clin Orthop Relat Res 2013. https://doi.org/10.1007/s11999-013-3303-1.
8. Owens BD, Kragh JF, Macaitis J, et al. Characterization of extremity wounds in operation Iraqi freedom and operation enduring freedom. J Orthop Trauma 2007. https://doi.org/10.1097/BOT.0b013e31802f78fb.
9. Belmont PJ, Schoenfeld AJ, Goodman G. Epidemiology of combat wounds in operation Iraqi freedom and operation enduring freedom: orthopaedic burden of disease. J Surg Orthop Adv 2010; 19(1):2–7.
10. Chandler H, MacLeod K, Penn-Barwell JG, et al. Extremity injuries sustained by the UK military in the Iraq and Afghanistan conflicts: 2003–2014. Injury 2017. https://doi.org/10.1016/j.injury.2017.05.022.
11. Belmont PJ, McCriskin BJ, Hsiao MS, et al. The nature and incidence of musculoskeletal combat wounds in Iraq and Afghanistan (2005-2009). J Orthop Trauma 2013. https://doi.org/10.1097/BOT.0b013e3182703188.
12. Shin EH, Sabino JM, Nanos GP, et al. Ballistic trauma: lessons learned from Iraq and Afghanistan. Semin Plast Surg 2015. https://doi.org/10.1055/s-0035-1544173.
13. Kragh JF, Dubick MA, Aden JK, et al. U.S. military use of tourniquets from 2001 to 2010. Prehosp Emerg Care 2015. https://doi.org/10.3109/10903127.2014.964892.
14. Kragh JF, Nam JJ, Berry KA, et al. Transfusion for shock in US military war casualties with and without tourniquet use. Ann Emerg Med 2015. https://doi.org/10.1016/j.annemergmed.2014.10.021.
15. Stop the Bleed. Available at: https://www.facs.org/Publications/Newsletters/COT-News/Summer2017/bcon.
16. Scalea TM, DuBose J, Moore EE, et al. Western trauma association critical decisions in trauma: management of the mangled extremity. J Trauma Acute Care Surg 2012. https://doi.org/10.1097/TA.0b013e318241ed70.
17. Chung KC, Saddawi-Konefka D, Haase SC, et al. A cost-utility analysis of amputation versus salvage for gustilo type IIIB and IIIC open tibial fractures. Plast Reconstr Surg 2009. https://doi.org/10.1097/PRS.0b013e3181bcf156.
18. Ritter J, O'Brien S, Rivet D, et al. Radiology: imaging trauma patients in a deployed setting. Mil Med 2018. https://doi.org/10.1093/milmed/usy063.
19. Bowyer G. Débridement of extremity war wounds. J Am Acad Orthop Surg 2006. https://doi.org/10.5435/00124635-200600001-00012.
20. Yaremchuk MJ, Brumback RJ, Manson PN, et al. Acute and definitive management of traumatic osteocutaneous defects of the lower extremity. Plast Reconstr Surg 1987. https://doi.org/10.1097/00006534-198707000-00002.
21. Anglen JO. Wound irrigation in musculoskeletal injury. J Am Acad Orthop Surg 2001. https://doi.org/10.5435/00124635-200107000-00001.

22. Lane JC, Mabvuure NT, Hindocha S, et al. Current concepts of prophylactic antibiotics in trauma: a review. Open Orthop J 2012. https://doi.org/10.2174/1874325001206010511.

23. Hospenthal DR, Murray CK, Andersen RC, et al. Guidelines for the prevention of infections associated with combat-related injuries: 2011 update endorsed by the infectious diseases society of America and the surgical infection society. J Trauma Inj Infect Crit Care 2011. https://doi.org/10.1097/TA.0b013e318227ac4b.

24. Burtt KE, Badash I, Leland HA, et al. The efficacy of negative pressure wound therapy and antibiotic beads in lower extremity salvage. J Surg Res 2020. https://doi.org/10.1016/j.jss.2019.09.055.

25. Fang R, Dorlac WC, Flaherty SF, et al. Feasibility of negative pressure wound therapy during intercontinental aeromedical evacuation of combat casualties. J Trauma Inj Infect Crit Care 2010. https://doi.org/10.1097/TA.0b013e3181e452a2.

26. Couch KS, Stojadinovic A. Negative-pressure wound therapy in the military: lessons learned. Plast Reconstr Surg 2011. https://doi.org/10.1097/PRS.0b013e3181fd344e.

27. Hehr JD, Hodson TS, West JM, et al. Instillation negative pressure wound therapy: an effective approach for hardware salvage. Int Wound J 2020. https://doi.org/10.1111/iwj.13283.

28. West J, Wetherhold J, Schulz S, et al. A novel use of next-generation closed incision negative pressure wound therapy after major limb amputation and amputation revision. Cureus 2020. https://doi.org/10.7759/cureus.10393.

29. Pasquale MD, Frykberg ER, Tinkoff GH. Management of complex extremity trauma. Bull Am Coll Surg 2006.

30. Kelly SP, Rambau G, Tennent DJ, et al. The role of CT angiography in evaluating lower extremity trauma: 157 patient case series at a military treatment facility. Mil Med 2019. https://doi.org/10.1093/milmed/usz028.

31. Eger M, Golcman L, Goldstein A, et al. The use of a temporary shunt in the management of arterial vascular injuries. Surg Gynecol Obstet 1971;132(1):67–70.

32. Fox CJ, Patel B, Clouse WD. Update on wartime vascular injury. Perspect Vasc Surg Endovasc Ther 2011. https://doi.org/10.1177/1531003511400625.

33. Rasmussen TE, Clouse WD, Jenkins DH, et al. The use of temporary vascular shunts as a damage control adjunct in the management of wartime vascular injury. J Trauma Inj Infect Crit Care 2006. https://doi.org/10.1097/01.ta.0000220668.84405.17.

34. Burkhardt GE, Cox M, Clouse WD, et al. Outcomes of selective tibial artery repair following combat-related extremity injury. J Vasc Surg 2010. https://doi.org/10.1016/j.jvs.2010.02.017.

35. Perkins ZB, Yet B, Glasgow S, et al. Meta-analysis of prognostic factors for amputation following surgical repair of lower extremity vascular trauma. Br J Surg 2015. https://doi.org/10.1002/bjs.9689.

36. Mills JL, Fujitani RM, Taylor SM. The characteristics and anatomic distribution of lesions that cause reversed vein graft failure: a five-year prospective study. J Vasc Surg 1993. https://doi.org/10.1016/0741-5214(93)90023-F.

37. Lundell A, Lindblad B, Bergqvist D, et al. Femoropopliteal-crural graft patency is improved by an intensive surveillance program: a prospective randomized study. J Vasc Surg 1995. https://doi.org/10.1016/S0741-5214(95)70241-5.

38. Mills JL, Bandyk DF, Gahtan V, et al. The origin of infrainguinal vein graft stenosis: a prospective study based on duplex surveillance. J Vasc Surg 1995. https://doi.org/10.1016/S0741-5214(95)70240-7.

39. Bandyk DF. Surveillance after lower extremity arterial bypass. Perspect Vasc Surg Endovasc Ther 2007. https://doi.org/10.1177/1531003507310460.

40. Roganović Z, Pavlićević G, Petković S. Missile-induced complete lesions of the tibial nerve and tibial division of the sciatic nerve: results of 119 repairs. J Neurosurg 2005. https://doi.org/10.3171/jns.2005.103.4.0622.

41. Roganovic Z. Missile-caused complete lesions of the peroneal nerve and peroneal division of the sciatic nerve: results of 157 repairs. Neurosurgery 2005. https://doi.org/10.1227/01.NEU.0000186034.58798.

42. Smith JK, Miller ME, Carroll CG, et al. High-resolution ultrasound in combat-related peripheral nerve injuries. Muscle Nerve 2016. https://doi.org/10.1002/mus.25216.

43. Pfister BJ, Gordon T, Loverde JR, et al. Biomedical engineering strategies for peripheral nerve repair: surgical applications, state of the art, and future challenges. Crit Rev Biomed Eng 2011. https://doi.org/10.1615/CritRevBiomedEng.v39.i2.20.

44. Ray WZ, Mackinnon SE. Nerve problems in the lower extremity. Foot Ankle Clin 2011. https://doi.org/10.1016/j.fcl.2011.01.009.

45. Jonsson S, Wiberg R, McGrath AM, et al. Effect of delayed peripheral nerve repair on nerve regeneration, Schwann cell function and target muscle recovery. PLoS One 2013. https://doi.org/10.1371/journal.pone.0056484.

46. Wiesseman GJ. Tendon transfers for peripheral nerve injuries of the lower extremity. Orthop Clin North Am 1981;12(2):459–67.

47. Leclère FM, Badur N, Mathys L, et al. Nerve transfers for persistent traumatic peroneal nerve palsy: the Inselspital bern experience. Neurosurgery 2015. https://doi.org/10.1227/NEU.0000000000000897.

48. Giuffre JL, Bishop AT, Spinner RJ, et al. Partial tibial nerve transfer to the tibialis anterior motor branch to treat peroneal nerve injury after knee trauma. Clin

Orthop Relat Res 2012. https://doi.org/10.1007/s11999-011-1924-9.

49. Ehde DM, Czerniecki JM, Smith DG, et al. Chronic phantom sensations, phantom pain, residual limb pain, and other regional pain after lower limb amputation. Arch Phys Med Rehabil 2000. https://doi.org/10.1053/apmr.2000.7583.

50. Buchheit T, Van De Ven T, Hsia HLJ, et al. Pain phenotypes and associated clinical risk factors following traumatic amputation: results from veterans integrated pain evaluation research (VIPER). Pain Med 2016. https://doi.org/10.1111/pme.12848.

51. Valerio IL, Dumanian GA, Jordan SW, et al. Preemptive treatment of phantom and residual limb pain with targeted muscle reinnervation at the time of major limb amputation. J Am Coll Surg 2019. https://doi.org/10.1016/j.jamcollsurg.2018.12.015.

52. Souza JM, Cheesborough JE, Ko JH, et al. Targeted muscle reinnervation: a novel approach to postamputation neuroma pain. Clin Orthop Relat Res 2014. https://doi.org/10.1007/s11999-014-3528-7.

53. Dumanian GA, Potter BK, Mioton LM, et al. Targeted muscle reinnervation treats neuroma and phantom pain in major limb Amputees: a randomized clinical trial. Ann Surg 2019. https://doi.org/10.1097/SLA.0000000000003088.

54. Tintle SM, Forsberg JA, Keeling JJ, et al. Lower extremity combat-related amputations. Spring 2010; 19(1):35–43.

55. Casey K, Sabino J, Jessie E, et al. Flap coverage outcomes following vascular injury and repair: Chronicling a decade of severe war-related extremity trauma. Plast Reconstr Surg 2015. https://doi.org/10.1097/PRS.0000000000000769.

56. Connolly M, Ibrahim ZR, Johnson ON. Changing paradigms in lower extremity reconstruction in war-related injuries. Mil Med Res 2016. https://doi.org/10.1186/S40779-016-0080-7.

57. Yazar S, Lin CH, Wei FC. One-stage reconstruction of composite bone and soft-tissue defects in traumatic lower extremities. Plast Reconstr Surg 2004. https://doi.org/10.1097/01.PRS.0000138811.88807.65.

58. Yildirim S, Gideroğlu K, Aköz T. Anterolateral thigh flap: Ideal free flap choice for lower extremity soft-tissue reconstruction. J Reconstr Microsurg 2003. https://doi.org/10.1055/s-2003-40578.

59. Sabino J, Polfer E, Tintle S, et al. A decade of conflict: flap coverage options and outcomes in traumatic war-related extremity reconstruction. Plast Reconstr Surg 2015. https://doi.org/10.1097/PRS.0000000000001025.

60. Harry LE, Sandison A, Pearse MF, et al. Comparison of the vascularity of fasciocutaneous tissue and muscle for coverage of open tibial fractures. Plast Reconstr Surg 2009. https://doi.org/10.1097/PRS.0b013e3181b5a308.

61. Bremner LF, Mazurek M. Reconstructive challenges of complex battlefield injury. J Surg Orthop Adv 2010;19(1):77–84.

62. Tintle SM, Gwinn DE, Andersen RC, et al. Soft tissue coverage of combat wounds. J Surg Orthop Adv 2010;19(1):29–34.

63. Fleming ME, Bharmal H, Valerio I. Regenerative medicine applications in combat casualty care. Regen Med 2014. https://doi.org/10.2217/rme.13.96.

64. Rush SM. Trinity evolution: mesenchymal stem cell allografting in foot and ankle surgery. Foot Ankle Spec 2010. https://doi.org/10.1177/1938640010369638.

65. Mitchell KB, Gallagher JJ. Porcine bladder extracellular matrix for closure of a large defect in a burn contracture release. J Wound Care 2012. https://doi.org/10.12968/jowc.2012.21.9.454.

Moving?

Make sure your subscription moves with you!

To notify us of your new address, find your **Clinics Account Number** (located on your mailing label above your name), and contact customer service at:

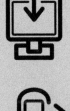

Email: journalscustomerservice-usa@elsevier.com

800-654-2452 (subscribers in the U.S. & Canada)
314-447-8871 (subscribers outside of the U.S. & Canada)

Fax number: 314-447-8029

Elsevier Health Sciences Division
Subscription Customer Service
3251 Riverport Lane
Maryland Heights, MO 63043

*To ensure uninterrupted delivery of your subscription, please notify us at least 4 weeks in advance of move.

Printed and bound by CPI Group (UK) Ltd, Croydon, CR0 4YY

08/05/2025

01864697-0011